Visual Electrodiagnosis in Systemic Diseases

Documenta Ophthalmologica Proceeding Series volume 23

Editor H. E. Henkes

Springer-Science+Business Media, B.V. 1980

Visual Electrodiagnosis in Systemic Diseases

Proceedings of the
17th I.S.C.E.V. Symposium
Erfurt, June 5–10, 1979

Edited by

E. Schmöger and J. H. Kelsey

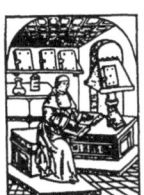

Springer-Science+Business Media, B.V. 1980

Distributors:

for the United States and Canada

Kluwer Boston, Inc.
190 Old Derby Street
Hingham, MA 02043
USA

for all other countries

Kluwer Academic Publishers Group
Distribution Center
P.O. Box 322
3300 AH Dordrecht
The Netherlands

Library of Congress Cataloging in Publication Data   CIP

    International Society for Clinical Electroretinography
      Vision
      Visual electrodiagnosis in systemic diseases.

      (Documenta ophthalmologica : Proceedings series ;
  v.23)
      1. Electroretinography--Congresses. 2. Ocular
manifestations of general diseases--Congresses.
I. Schmöger, Elisabeth. II. Kelsey, J.H. III. Title. IV. Series. (DNLM: 1. Eye manifestations--
Congresses. 2. Electroretinography--Congresses.
3. Electrooculography--Congresses. W3 D0637 v. 23
1979 / WW475 1605v 1979)
RE79.E4158 1980   616.07'547   80-20630
ISBN 978-94-009-9182-8   ISBN 978-94-009-9180-4 (eBook)
DOI 10.1007/ 978-94-009-9180-4

Cover design: Max Velthuijs

© Springer Science+Business Media Dordrecht 1980
Originally published by Dr W. Junk bv Publishers in 1980
Softcover reprint of the hardcover 1st edition 1980

PREFACE

The research workers at the Eye Clinic of the Medical Academy of Erfurt are proud of having been entrusted, for the second time, with the organization of the yearly ISCEV symposium. Twelve years ago the 6th Symposium was held in Erfurt. This time we turned to Reinhardsbrunn, an old castle situated in the vicinity of Erfurt on the fringes of the wonderful mountainscape of the Thuringian Forest. Reinhardsbrunn castle serves today as a holiday hotel and convention place. It seemed to us to be the right place for carrying on the discussions in a comfortable and informal way after the actual sessions were over.

Comparing the scientific reports read at the 6th and 17th Symposium, both organized in Erfurt, one readily becomes aware of the impressive advances in our rapidly developing field of interest. The technical and, more specifically, the electronic advancements have been enormous, especially in the field of recording and processing the visually evoked cortical potentials. Actually, the addition of this special field of study to our realm, led to the renaming of the Society some years ago. Moreover, it became more and more obvious that interdisciplinary cooperation between ophthalmologists, physiologists, physicists, technologists and mathematicians is essential. This is also reflected in the composition of our membership.

As far as the themes of this symposium are concerned, we selected two main topics. The first being: "Visual electrodiagnosis in systemic diseases" which topic serves also as the title of the Proceedings. The second topic is "Visual electrophysiology and localized stimulation."

Though in the course of time, scientific knowledge has extended and has differentiated more and more, there is still much left to be discovered before we will be able to grasp and interpret correctly the electrical events which play a role in normal and abnormal visual function. We are convinced that the 17th Symposium has brought important contributions in this respect.

We wish to express our gratitude to all who have contributed to the preparatory work and thus to the success of this symposium. We too extend our sincere thanks to the Board of the ISCEV who entrusted us with the arrangements. Especially we thank Professor Henkes, President of the ISCEV, who was always prepared to give us friendly advice in the preparations. We are also greatly indebted to the GDR Ministry of Health and the local authorities who made this meeting possible. We are indebted too, to the coworkers of the Eye Clinic of Erfurt who did their utmost before and during the congress, allowing smooth functioning of the organization.

We must not fail to acknowledge the services rendered by the scientific translator and lecturer, Mr. H. W. Kleifield at Erfurt, who revised the English text of the papers from the socialist countries. We extend our sincere thanks too to Mr. J. H. Kelsey at London, who did a great deal of editing. Last but not least we are grateful to all participants for their contributions and their share in the discussions.

We want to recall the memory of our Board member Dr. J. T. Pearlman, who intended to participate in this meeting. He looked forward very much to this occasion, offering his linguistic assistance during the preparations of the symposium. Shortly before the beginning of this symposium, we were informed of his untimely death. We will remember him as a wise, friendly and highly esteemed colleague.

Those attending the 17th ISCEV Symposium will certainly agree that this meeting underlines once more the necessity for further close cooperation in the special fields discussed, viz. visual electrodiagnosis and local stimulation in visual electrophysiology.

ELISABETH SCHMÖGER
Chairman of the 17th ISCEV Symposium

CONTENTS

Part Two: Visual electrophysiology and localized stimulation

ERG

PART ONE

VISUAL ELECTRODIAGNOSIS
IN SYSTEMIC DISEASES

ERG AND EOG IN SYSTEMIC DISEASES
(MAIN REPORT)

E. SCHMÖGER
(*Erfurt, G.D.R.*)

ABSTRACT

This report is an introduction to the contributions concerning visual electrodiagnosis in systemic diseases. The ERG and EOG in all the diseases in which the retina is involved cannot be described in full detail here. This report is restricted to some typical diagnoses of diseases classed in chapters such as systemic infections, vascular changes, diabetes, endocrine and metabolic disorders, diseases of liver and kidney, syndromes, and finally retrolental fibroplasia.

It is my intention to give a survey of ERG and EOG investigations in systemic diseases as an introduction to the following papers. There are, indeed, a great many diseases in which the retina in one way or another is involved. On the other hand, in a great number of cases we are unable to differentiate the disturbed electric answer of the retina with our latest knowledge and technical supports. There are interesting interrelations between systemic disorders and the retina; some of them, however, being of seldom occurrence. For this reason it will be impossible for one laboratory to perceive these conditions on the whole. So my report mainly refers to the latest publications on the topic and I trust that this introduction will be useful.

Let me start with the *systemic infections* and only mention two examples of virus infections:

Pigmentary retinopathy due to maternal *rubeola* during the first trimester of pregnancy is well known. It is one of the three ocular main symptoms in connatal rubella (apart from cataract and glaucoma), and does not begin before some months after birth. The active virus is to be found in the tissues up to the second year of life. This retinopathy generally leaves the retina functionally intact and the ERG normal. Several authors have seen such children years later and have confirmed the stationary character of the disease. The insignificant disturbance of the retina by a virus infection during the first trimester can be explained by the state of retinal development beginning to differentiate not before the fourth month of pregnancy. In more severe post-natal acquired cases of rubeola retinopathy there is no assurance that the condition will not be progressive (Franceschetti *et al.* 1958, Krill 1967, Scheie *et al.* 1972).

In the case of *measles* there may occur an acute blindness with neuroretinitis, retinal edema, retinal hermorrhages and stallate macula lesion, usually within a period from 4 to 11 days after the appearance of exanthema, ERG is severely disturbed or extinguished, the EOG ratio might be depressed. During the course of months and years there will be the appearance and progression of pigmentary retinopathy. A satisfactory vision and some ERG response may return, but often ERG remains extinguished and the visual field restricted. Therefore extremely guarded long-term prognosis should be given. (D'Epinay and Martenet 1972; Franceschetti, Dieterle and Schwarz 1958; Hentsch and Külz 1969; Scheie and Morse 1972). The differential diagnosis between the pigmentary retinopathy including an extinguished ERG due to this postnatal infection and that of a primary heredity can be derived from the sudden loss of vision in the case mentioned in the first instance.

VASCULAR DISEASES

In systemic arterial hypertension and arteriosclerosis the ERG can be subnormal in spite of normal ophthalmoscopic findings, but usually the ERG disturbance is in agreement with the arteriosclerotic state. In cases of central retinal vascular occlusions the clinical and electrodiagnostic findings may vary within wide limits. This is summarized in Table 1. (Algvere 1968; Asayama *et al.*

Table 1. Retinal vascular affections.*

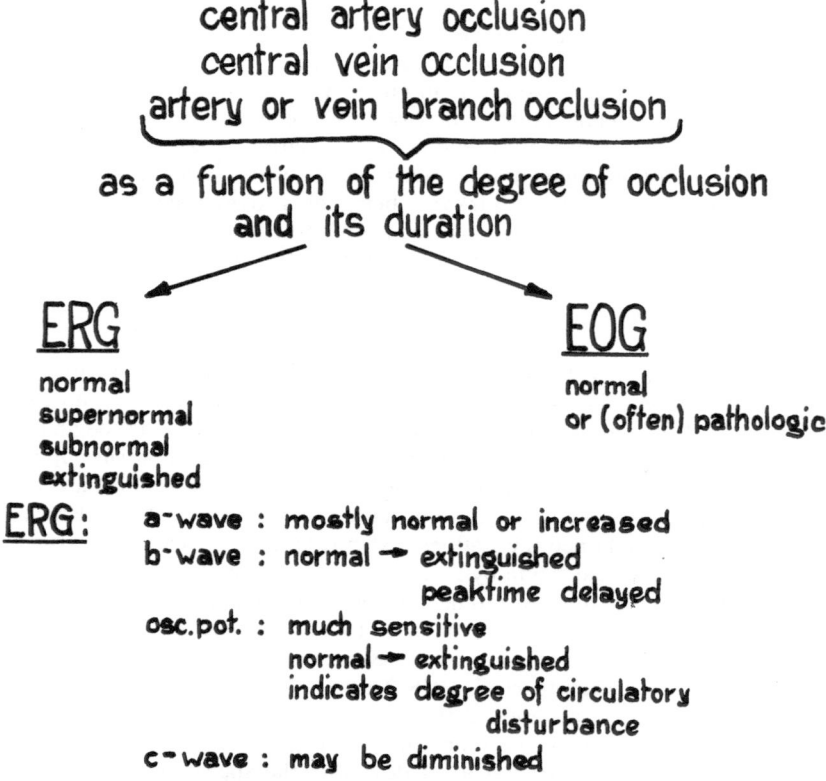

* References: see text.

1965; Babel et al. 1977; Burian 1963; François, De Rouck and Cambie 1973; Gliem 1968; Heilemann and Bastian 1968; Henkes and van der Kam 1954; Karpe and Germanis 1961; Kojima et al. 1965; Krill et al. 1962; Kurachi et al. 1965; McLeod 1973; Müller and Haase 1968; Ponte 1966, Ponte and Lodato 1977; Svěrák and Peregrin 1968; Textorius 1978; Textorius et al. 1978; Usami 1965; Wulfing 1963; Yonemura 1965; Younessian 1962). It is of interest that EOG and c-wave are diminished in retinal vascular occlusions, since the pigment epithelium is said to be the main source of both, and they should therefore be unimpaired. Additional disturbed choroidal circulation may take place or there is some contribution to these potentials from the inner retinal parts (Gliem 1968, Textorius 1978). Nilsson (1971) reported on an obvious correlation between a markedly reduced b-wave amplitude, as a sign of severe functional damage in cases of arterial or vein obstructions and greatly prolonged retinal circulation time, measured by retinal angiography. In consideration of these two items he takes them as a basis for selecting patients with reversible damage for fibrinolytic therapy.

Arteritis temporalis and *pulseless disease* are further indications for making electrophysiologic investigations. If there are affected the posterior ciliary arteries only, as it is usual in arteritis temporalis, ERG and EOG are normal. A subnormal or abolished b-wave in the ERG indicates additional circulatory disturbances in the retina (Burian 1963, McLeod 1973, Younessian 1962). In *pulseless disease* the oscillatory potentials are said to be the most sensitive ones in the early beginning of this disease, where fundus oculi ophthalmoscopically may appear normal (Asayama 1965; Krill et al. 1962; Kurachi et al. 1965; Wulfing 1963; Yonemura 1965).

DIABETES

From the beginning of the clinical electroretinography there has been an interest in diagnosis of early retinal changes in diabetics by means of an ERG. Classical ERG investigation, however, did not show any marked changes in ERG or EOG before the advanced retinopathy had taken place (many authors, e.g. François and De Rouck 1954; Gliem et al. 1971; Henkes et al. 1966; Karpe, Kornerup and Wulfing 1958).

The latest knowledge about the origin of diabetic retinopathy has been summarized best by Gjötterberg (1974) shown in Table 2. It is the vicious circle that constitutes the basis of the electrodiagnostic findings.

It was in the *first ISCERG Symposium*, held in Stockholm 1961, that *Yonemura* and co-workers demonstrated that oscillatory potentials disappear or greatly diminish in cases with slight retinopathy or even before changes could be seen ophthalmoscopically in the retina of diabetics. This was in contrast to retinal arteriosclerosis, where oscillatory potentials even in advanced stages were existing. Since that time the interest in these potentials has much increased and many investigators have confirmed *Yonemura's* findings. The oscillatory potentials whose origin in the inner nuclear layers is assumed but not confirmed, are most sensitive to impairment of retinal circulation and according to Simonsen (1966) probably insulin-sensitive, too. The a-wave has a low and the b-wave an intermediate sensitivity in relation to that of the

5

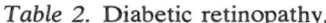

Table 2. Diabetic retinopathy.

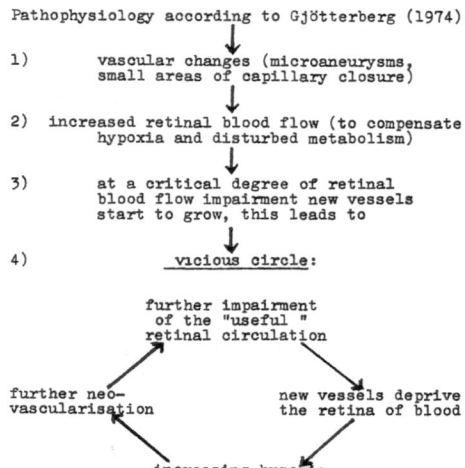

Pathophysiology according to Gjötterberg (1974):

↓

1) vascular changes (microaneurysms, small areas of capillary closure)

↓

2) increased retinal blood flow (to compensate hypoxia and disturbed metabolism)

↓

3) at a critical degree of retinal blood flow impairment new vessels start to grow, this leads to

↓

4) vicious circle:

further impairment of the "useful " retinal circulation

further neo-vascularisation

new vessels deprive the retina of blood

increasing hypoxia

oscillatory potentials as far as diabetic retinopathy is concerned. Hypernormal b-wave may be an expression of early ischemic damage, but there is no marked reduction occurring prior to the seriously deteriorated retinal circulation.

Follow-up studies by Simonsen (1974) in more than 100 young diabetics have confirmed the considerable value of the oscillatory potentials in the prognostic evaluation of diabetic retinopathy, especially with a view to the possibility of proliferative development.

The diagnostic conclusions can be drawn as follows: Oscillatory potentials in the ERG on the one hand, and fluorescein angiography of the fundus oculi on

Table 3. ERG and the Endocrines.

Endocrine gland	Type of dysfunction	Type of ERG (b-wave)	Author(s)
Thyroid	Hyperthyroidism	Supernormal	TORRENTS *et al.* PEARLMAN-BURIAN WIRTH-STIRPE
	Hypothyroidism	[o] Nor.-Supernor. Subnormal	WIRTH TORRENTS *et al.* PEARLMAN-BURIAN
	Induced Hypethyr.	[oo] Normal [ooo] Supernormal	WIRTH PEARLMAN-BURIAN
Adrenal medulla	Phaeochromocitoma	Normal	WIRTH
	After adrenaline injection	Normal	WIRTH *et al.*
Adrenal cortex	Cushing disease	Supernormal	WIRTH
	Addison disease	? ?	—

[o] Including so-called 'transition stages'.
[oo] T_3 Glaxo, 20 μg 6 times, total dose 1440 μg.
[ooo] Cytomel (L-triiodothyronine), total dose 2200 μg.

(A. Wirth, 1966)

the other hand are supplementary methods in diagnostics of diabetic retino-phaty. The former provide measurable values of the *overall* retina, the latter a picture of the vessles, which discloses perfusion disturbances of the *posterior* retinal parts.

Other endrocrine disorders with relation to hormonal influence on ERG were mainly studied by Wirth and coworkers (1955, 1966, 1967). This will be best demonstrated by a table given by Wirth in the Gent Symposium 1966 (Table 3). The different hormones let the b-amplitude significantly increase or de-crease. I feel obliged to remind of Pearlman and Burian (1964), who in a case of severe thyreotoxicosis found the highest ERG amplitudes they ever have registred (1964). EOG obviously would not be affected considerably by hormones.

RENAL DISEASES

Concerning the diseases of kidney I do not want to refer to hypertensive retinopathy, but direct your attention to chronic uremia, in the state the b-wave usually is diminished. The interest in the bioelectric changes increases with the number of dialyse cases and of renal transplantations, since renal retinopathy has changed its appearance. Perossini and Tota (1977) as well as

Table 4. Renal diseases.

ERG and EOG affected in:	ERG	EOG	remarks
(1) *Alport syndrome* autosom. dominant inherit. progress. nephropathy	normal subnormal or extinguished	normal or flat	as a function of the severity of retinal dystrophy
(2) *Nephronophthise* autosom. recess. inherit. progress. nephropathy			
children:	extremely decreased or extinguished		if greatly impaired vision (cong. retinal dystrophy)
juvenile cases:	subnormal		milder retinal dystrophy
heterozygotes:	scotopic decreased		
(3) *Nephropathic cystinosis* autosom. recess. inherit.	normal or subnormal		tapetoret. degeneration?

References: Abraham *et al.* 1974; François *et al.* 1972; Hochgesand *et al*; 1974, Huck *et al.* 1976; Puech *et al.* 1976; Read *et al.* 1973; Severin 1975.

Zimmerman *et al.* (1973) could not perfectly clear up the conditions. They found the b-wave usually more reduced in the course of periodic haemodialysis than before, but in the individual case no significant difference before and after dialysis. They think that haemodialytic treatment interferes with the electrolytic equilibrium.

The conditions in some hereditary progressive nephropathies affected with tapetoretinal degeneration will be represented in Table 4.

LIVER DISEASES

Liver diseases play a role in vitamin A deficiency and lead to some reduction in scotopic ERG and in EOG, a significant relation to the severity of liver cirrhosis could not be found but vitamin A therapy led to some improvement in the dark adaptation curve and ERG. (Straub 1965; B. Schmidt 1966, 1969; Dehon *et al.* 1977). Hypovitaminosis A, due to undernourishment or malabsorption, leads to more extensive hemeralopia with marked scotopic and photopic ERG and EOG reductions. The first who clearly demonstrated these electrodiagnostic facts was Bornschein (and co-worker) 1973. It is of interest that both conditions can be improved by a vitamin A therapy. However, long-term cases of vitamin A deficiency eventually end in irreversible retinal pigmentary degeneration (Bors and Fells 1971; Duke-Elder 1967; Genest 1966; Thaler *et al.* 1976).

SYNDROMES

Numerous syndromes involve the retina in form of tapetoretinal degeneration of the macular or peripherical type. In spite of being seldom they are of practical and theoretical importance. By advancing the knowledge about the metabolic deficiencies, retinal degeneration and other symptoms might be prevented thanks to a therapeutic support. A cytological or biochemical diagnosis before birth or in heterocygotes can be made in some instances.

To deal with all the ERG and EOG changes in the numerous syndromes would be beyond my capability. I will try to direct your attention only to some interesting points in the following tables. There are:

Syndromes without known metabolic disorder (Table 5). *In Usher's syndrome* the partial hearing defect is stationary, whereas vision and ERG impairment always are progressive. Vestibular involvement uses to be combined only with those cases of congenital deafness which are joined with pigmentary retinopathy. (Abrahan *et al.* 1977; De Haas *et al.* 1970; Holland *et al.* 1972). In *Cockane's syndrome* the hearing defect is progressive. Since retinal degeneration is well known in this disease, a pathologic ERG and EOG would be expected, but I did not find any relevant report. – *Laurence–Moon–Bardet–Biedl's syndrome* also belongs to this group, and ERG may help for an early diagnosis (Ehrenfeld *et al.* 1970, Prosperi *et al.* 1977).

Lipidoses

(Table 6). The different forms of the so-called *amaurotic family idiocy* are hereditary metabolic disorders and belong to the lipidoses. The most important

Table 5. Progressive retinal pigmentary degeneration in syndromes (metabolic disorders unknown).*

	additional symptoms	ERG	EOG
Usher's syndrome autosomal recessive inheritance	congenital (partial) deafness (stationary) often combined with vestibulary involvement	↓↓↓ or ∅	flat?
carriers may show:	gyrate retinal atrophy or atypical fundus anomalies and some disorders in retinal function (dark adaptation)	normal <u>abnormal</u> only in cases with gyrate atrophy	=
Cockayne's syndrome recessive inheritance	progressive infantile deafness mental retardation, skeletal and neurological abnormalities photosensibility of skin	↓↓↓ ? or ∅	flat?
Laurence-Moon-Bardet-Biedl's syndrome mostly recess. inherit.	hypogenitalism, adipositas, mental retardation, polydactyly and other abnormalities (variable manifestations)	↓↓↓ or ∅	flat?

↓ = reduced
∅ = extinguished

* References: see text.

9

Table 6. Retinal pigmentary degeneration in hereditary metabolic disorders (Lipidoses).

clinical classification	metabolic disorder	type of retinal degeneration	onset	course of life	ERG	EOG	systemic symptoms
infantile: <u>Tay-Sachs</u> (amaurotic family idiocy)	gangliosidosis	macular	1st to 2nd year	2 years	normal	?	severe psycho-motoric deterioration
<u>Niemann-Pick</u>	phospholipidosis	macular (60% of cases)	1st year	a few years	?	?	similar to Tay-Sachs
late infantile: <u>Bielschowski</u> (amaurotic family idiocy)	neuronal ceroid lipofuscinosis	macular (peripheral)	2nd to 4th year	years	↓↓ or ∅	?	mental retard., neurological disorders (progressive)
juvenile: <u>Batten-Mayou</u> <u>Spielmeyer-Vogt</u> (amaurotic family idiocy)	"	macular peripheral	5th to 10th year	years	=	L/D ratio↓ or flat	psycho-motoric disorders

| ↓ = reduced   ∅ = extinguished |

References: Beckerman and Rapin 1975; Bolmers *et al.* 1974; Copenhaver and Goodman 1960; Göttinger und Minauf 1971; Harden *et al.* 1973; Honda and Sudo 1976; Pilz *et al.* 1968; Pinckers et Bolmers 1974; Raitta and Santavuori 1974; Stanescu *et al.* 1973; Thiel und Behnke 1971; Thranberend und Adachi-Usami 1973.

points that can be borne in mind easily may be summarized as follows:

The earlier the onset	— the severer the mental retardation,
the later the onset	— the more peripheral the retinal degeneration,
the more peripheral the retinal degeneration	— the more diminished the ERG and EOG.

In most cases the cytological or biochemical diagnosis will be feasible before birth or in heterozygotes.

Mucopolysaccharidoses (MPS)

In those hereditary metabolic disorders the following points are of interest (Table 7): All but one are autosomal recessive inherited, only Hunter's disease is of sex linked recessive inheritance. From an electrodiagnostic point of view it is more important that in MPS IV (Morquio) retinal involvement is unknown, ERG and EOG normal. The same is the rule in MPS VI (Marateaux-Lamy), whereas all the other very often involve the retina and show subnormal or extinguished ERG and EOG.

The last group of these disorders (Table 8) includes two syndromes (*Batten-Kornzweig's* and *Menke's kinky hair syndrome*) in which all symptoms may be reversible by an early parenteral vitamin A therapy or copper therapy, respectively. Recovery is to be estimated also in ERG recordings provided that the therapy begins early. Of course, these will be only the first steps for solving the problems involved.

The study of the above-mentioned syndromes has to take into account their changed *classification* within the last years in relation to the advanced knowledge about metabolic disorders (Cogan 1978).

In consideration of all the above-mentioned syndromes *we summarizing can state that atypic cases of retinitis pigmentosa are suspected of being of hereditary metabolic disorders.*

Myotonic dystrophy

On the contrary to the above-mentioned metabolic disorders the myotonic dystrophy Steinert–Batten is not seldom, because it is of autosomal dominant inheritance, as well as the myotonia congenita Thomson. They have to be differentiated since the former involves the retina and shows ERG and EOG changes, whereas the latter has no eye symptoms, ERG and EOG, therefore, are normal. However, the retinopathy in myotonic dystrophy seems to be a mild form and of stationary character. Most of these cases have a reduced ERG (ERP, b-wave, oscillat. potentials) and L/D ratio of EOG is often abnormal. (Babel and Tsacopoulos 1970, Burian and Burns 1966, Mausolf *et al.* 1972, Remky 1972, Stanescu and Michiels 1975, 1976, Stewart and Rubin 1972, Tamai and Holland 1975).

Some further syndromes which are of electrodiagnostic interest will be the *uveo-meningeal syndromes* of *Vogt-Koyanagi-Harada* and of *Behçet*, where ERG and EOG change in parallel with the clinical course (Godel *et al.* 1978, Hatt and Niemeyer 1976, Nagaya 1972). Some *skin diseases* involve the

Table 7. Retinal pigmentary degeneration in hereditary metabolic disorders (Mucopolysaccharidoses).

clinical classification	type of metabolic disorder	inheritance	retinal degenerat.	corneal clouding	systemic symptoms skeletal	systemic symptoms mental	ERG	EOG
Hurler	MPS I H	autosomal recessive	+ (not in all cases)	+++	+++	+++	(normal) subnormal → Ø	subnormal
Scheie	MPS I S (formerly V)	=	=	+++ (progress)	similar but milder than MPS I H		normal abnormal or Ø	?
Hunter severe mild	MPS II	sex linked recessive	=	- +	+++ ++	+++ -	=	abnormal? normal
Sanfilippo	MPS III	autosomal recessive	=	-	+ -	+++ (deafness)	subnormal or Ø	?
Morquio	MPS IV	=	-	++	+++	+	normal	normal
Maroteaux-Lamy	MPS VI	=	- (+)	++	+++	-	normal (abnormal?)	normal (abnorm.?)

References: Abraham et al. 1974; Cogan 1978; Di Ferrante et al. 1974; François 1974; Kennyon et al. 1972.

12

Table 8. Retinal pigmentary degeneration in hereditary metabolic disorders (different disorders).

clinical classification	metabolic disorder	inheritance	(systemic) symtoms	ERG	EOG	onset	
Refsum's syndrome (heredopathia atactica poly-neuritiformis)	phytane acid (chlorophyll metabolism)	autosomal recessive	atypic progressive retinopathy, neurologic disorders	↓↓ ?	flat?		
Batten-Kornzweig's syndrome	acanthocytosis (hypo-)α-beta-lipoproteinemia	autosomal recessive (seldom dominant)	progressive spino-cerebellar degeneration, low or absent levels of serum vitamin A atyp. progr. retinopathy	↓↓ ø	flat?	infancy	all symptoms reversable by early vitamin A therapy (parenteral)
Menke's kinky-hair syndrome	copper absorption disorder	sex linked	progr. neurodegener. disorders, seizures, psycho-motor. retard. structure of hair = kinky	normal ↓↓ (progr. decrease)	?	first months of life	symptoms may be reversable by early copper therapy (parenteral)
Atypic cases of retinitis pigmentosa are suspected of being of hereditary metabolic disorders							

References: François 1975; Friedmann et al. 1978; Levy et al. 1974; Sperling et al. 1972; Yee et al. 1976.

13

retina: It is of interest that L/D ratio in *human albinos* is normal and does not depend on the amount of melanotic pigments. EOG at the same time showed a low base value, a delayed light rise and an earlier dark trough, as found by Gahlot and Hansen (1974). In cases of angioid streaks in *Grönblad–Strandberg syndrome* an abnormal EOG can be presumed to be the conclusion of only a few investigations (Babel *et al.* 1977).

Finally let me refer to the value of the electrodiagnostics in premature infants: It is necessary to follow up the cases of *retinopathia praematurorum* (retrolental fibroplasia) over a long period since we have learned about the possible progression of retinal deterioration for months and years after birth. Bohár and Veli (1977) were able to demonstrate that development of ERG in premature children shows regression with the first signs of retrolental fibroplasia – and may normalize by improving the retinal condition.

In many of the above mentioned diagnoses, VECP may also be taken into consideration, but this was not to deal with in my report. Anyway, it must be said that there is still a great deal to do in this province of research and nothing in here, as in all the other spheres of science can *a priori* be taken for granted.

REFERENCES

Abraham, F.A., D. Cohen & H. Somer. Usher's syndrome: Electrophysiological tests of the visual and auditory systems. *Doc. Ophthalm.* 44: 435–444 (1977).

Abraham, F.A., L. Yanko, A. Licht & R.J. Viskoper. Electrophysiologic study of the visual system in familial juvenile nephronophthisis and tapetoretinal dystrophy. *Amer. J. Ophthal.* 78: 591–597 (1974).

Abraham, F.A., S. Yatziv, A. Russell & E. Auerbach. Electrophysiological and psychophysical findings in Hunter syndrome. *Arch. Ophthal.* (Chic.) 91: 181–186 (1974).

Abraham, F.A., S. Yatziv, A. Russell & E. Auerbach. A family with two siblings affected by Morquio syndrome (MPS IV). *Arch. Ophthal.* (Chic.) 91: 265–269 (1974).

Asayama, Nagata & K. Adachi. The effects of reduced blood flow through the main branches of the aortic arch on the ERG and VER in rabbits. pp. 88–98 in Nakajima, A. (ed.), Retinal degenerations, ERG and optic pathways. Proc. 4th ISCERG Symp. 1965. *Jap. J. Ophthal.* 10: Suppl., Tokyo, 1966.

Babel, J., N. Stangos, S. Korol & M. Spiritus. Ocular Electrophysiology. Thieme, Stuttgart, 1977.

Babel, J. & M. Tsacopoulos. Les lésions rétiniennes de la dystrophie myotonique. *Ann. d'Oculist.* 203: 1049 (1970).

Beckerman, R.L. & I. Rapin. Ceroid lipofuscinosis. *Amer. J. Ophthal.* 80: 73–77 (1975).

Bohár, A. & M. Veli. Frühe ERG-Zeichen der retrolentalen Fibroplasie. *Klin. Mbl. Augenheilk.* 170: 746–749 (1977).

Bolmers, D.J.M., F.J.M. Gabreels, E.M.G. Joosten, A. Gabreels-Festen & A.J.G. Pinckers. Some patients with cerebro-macular degeneration in the cadre of Batten's disease. *Ophthalmologica* (Basel) 169: 241–254 (1974).

Bors, F. & P. Fells. Reversal of the complications of self-induced vitamin A deficiency. *Brit. J. Ophthal.* 55: 210 (1971).

Cogan, D.G. The rise and fall of eponyms. *Arch. Ophthal.* (Chic) 96: 2202 (1978).

Dehon, P. & G. Lavergne. Adapto-électrorétinographie en lumiere blanche et cirrhose de Laennec. *Ann. d'Oculist.* 210: 141–146 (1977).

Duke-Elder, St. Diseases of the retina. p. 496 in: System of Ophthalmology. Vol. 10. Kimpton, London, 1967.

Ehrenfeld, E.N., H. Rowe & E. Auerbach. Laurence–Moon–Bardet–Biedl syndrome in Israel. *Amer. J. Ophthal.* 70: *524–532* (1970).

D'Epinay, S.L. & A.C. Martenet. Zum klinischen Bild und Verlauf der Retinopathie bei Masern. *Ophthalmologica* (Basel) 165: *332–342* (1972).

Di Ferrante, N., B.H. Hyman, W. Klish *et al.* Mucopolysaccharidosis VI (Maroteaux Lamy disease). Clinical and biochemical study of a mild variant case. *Johns Hopkins Med. J.* 135: *42* (1974).

François, J. Ocular manifestations of the mucopolysaccharidoses. *Ophthalmologica* (Basal) 169: *345* (1974).

François, J. Prévention des manifestations oculaires dans les erreurs innées du metabolisme. *Ann. d'Oculist.* 208: *825* (1975).

François, J., M. Hanssens, R. Coppieters & L. Evens. Cystinosis. A clinical and histopathologic study. *Amer. J. Ophthal.* 73: *643–650* (1972).

François, J., A. De Rouck & E. Cambie. Electrophysiological aspects in retinal venous thrombosis. pp. 43–56 in J.T. Pearlman (ed.) Xth ISCERG Symposium 1972. *Doc. Ophthal. Proc. Ser. II.* (1973).

Friedman, E., A. Harden, M. Doivikko & G. Pampiglione. Menkes' disease: new physiological aspects. *J. Neurol. Neurosurg. Psychiat.* 41: *505–510* (1978).

Gahlot, D.K. & E. Hansen. Electro-Oculography in Albinos. *Acta Ophthal.* (Kbh.) 52: *220–224* (1974).

Gjötterberg, M. Studies on the diabetic retinopathy. The value of electroretinography, fluorescein angiography, and adaptometric measurements in clinical examination of diabetics. Stockholm, 1974.

Gliem, H., D.E. Möller & G. Kietzmann. Die bioelektrische Aktivität bei der diabetischen Retinopathie. *Acta Ophthal.* (Kbh.) 49: *353–363* (1971).

Godel, V., M. Blumenthal & L. Regenbogen. Functional evaluation in Harada's disease. *Acta Ophthal.* (Kbh.) 56: *314–321* (1978).

Göttinger, W. & M. Minauf. Netzhautveränderungen bei juveniler amaurotischer Idiotie. *Klin. Mbl. Augenheilk.* 159: *532–538* (1971).

De Haas, E.B.A., G.H.M. van Lith, J. Rijnders, A.L.M. Rümke & Ch. Volmer. Usher's syndrome. *Doc. Ophthal.* 28: *166* (1970).

Harden, A., G. Pampiglione & N. Picton-Robinson. J. Neurol. Neurosurg. *Psychiat.* 36: *61–67* (1973).

Hatt, M. & G. Niemeyer. Elektroretinographie bei Morbus Behçet. *Graefes Arch. Ophthal.* 198: *113–120* (1976).

Hentsch, R. & J. Külz. Beitrag zur sekundären Pigmentdegeneration der Netzhaut bei Masern. *Klin. Mbl. Augenheilk.* 154: *706–712* (1969).

Hochgesand, P., P.D. Steinbach & E. Straub. Augenveränderungen bei Alport-Syndrom. *Klin. Mbl. Augenheilk.* 165: *447–452* (1974).

Holland, M. G., E. Cambie & W. Kloepfer. An evaluation of genetic carriers of Usher's syndrome. *Amer. J. Ophthal.* 74: *940–947* (1972).

Honda, Y. & M. Sudo. Electroretinogram and visually evoked cortical potential in Tay-Sachs disease. *J. pediat. Ophthal.* 13: *226–229* (1976).

Huck, D., H. Meythaler & R. Rix. Alport-Syndrom mit Hornhautbeteiligung und Veränderungen des ERG. *Klin. Mbl. Augenheilk.* 168: *553–556* (1976).

Kenyon, K.R., H.A. Quigley, I.E. Hussels, R.G. Wyllie & M.F. Goldberg. The systemic mucopolysaccharidoses. *Amer. J. Ophthal.* 73: *811–833* (1972).

Kojima, K. *et al.* ERG in diabetes. pp. 120–127 in A. Nakajima (ed.) Retinal Degenerations, ERG and optic pathways. Proc. 4th ISCERG Symp. 1965. *Jap. J. Ophthal.* Vol. 10, Suppl., Tokyo, 1966.

Krill, A.E. The retinal disease of rubella. *Arch. Ophthal.* (Chic.) 77: *445* (1967).

Levy, N.S., W.W. Dawson, B.J. Rhodes & A. Garnica. Ocular abnormalities in Menkes' kinky-hair syndrome. *Amer. J. Ophthal.* 77: *319–325* (1974).

15

Mausolf, F.A., C.A. Burns & H.M. Burian. Morphologic and functional retinal changes in myotonic dystrophy unrelated to quinine therapy. *Amer. J. Ophthal.* 74: *1141–1143* (1972).

Mc.Leod, D. Electroretinal responses in ocular vascular occlusions due to temporal arteritis. *Brit. J. Ophthal.* 57: *921–934* (1973).

Nagaya, T. Use of the electro-oculogram for diagnosing and following the development of Harada's disease. *Amer. J. Ophthal.* 74: *99–109* (1972).

Nilsson, S.E. Human retinal vascular obstructions. *Acta Ophthal.* (Kbh.) 49: *111–133* (1971).

Perossini, M. & G. Tota. Electroretinographic findings in chronic uraemics treated with periodic haemodialysis. pp. 257–263 in: J. François & A. De Rouck, Electrodiagnosis, Toxic Agents and Vision. 15th ISCEV Symp. 1977. Doc. Ophthal. Proc. Ser. Vol. 15, Junk, The Hague, 1978.

Pilz, H., D. Müller, K. Sandhoff & V. ter Meulen. Tay-Sachs'sche Krankheit mit Hexosamidase-Defekt. *Dtsch. med. Wschr.* 93: *1833* (1968).

Pinckers, A. & D. Bolmers. Neuronal ceroid lipofuscinosis (ERG et EOG). *Ann. d'Oculist.* 207: *523–529* (1974).

Ponte, F. & G. Lodato. Electro-oculographic investigations in central retinal vessel occlusions. pp. 155–157 in: J. François & A. De Rouck, Electrodiagnosis, Toxic Agents and Vision. 15th ISCEV Symp. 1977. Doc. Ophthal. Proc. Ser. Vol. 15, Junk, The Hague, 1978.

Prosperi, L., M. Cordella & S. Bernasconi. Electroretinography and diagnosis of the Laurence–Moon–Bardet–Biedl syndrome in childhood. *J. pediat. Ophthal.* 14: *305–308* (1977).

Puech, J.-F., G. Renard, J.-L. Dufier, M.-F. Blanck & L. Polliot. L'eléctrorétinogramme dans la néphronophtise. *Arch. Ophtal.* (Paris) 36: *313–320* (1976).

Raitta, C. & P. Santavuori. Ophthalmological findings in infantile type of neuronal ceroid lipofuscinosis. *Acta Genet.* med. 23: *123–195* (1974).

Read, J., M.F. Goldberg, G. Fishman & I. Rosenthal. Nephropathic cystinosis. *Amer. J. Ophthal.* 76: *791–796* (1973).

Remky, H. Retinopathia myotonica. *Klin. Mbl. Augenheilk.* 161: *372–387* (1972).

Scheie, H.G. & P.H. Morse. Rubeola retinopathy. *Arch. Ophthal.* (Chic.) 88: *341–344* (1972).

Schmidt, B. Electroretinographic investigations in vitamin A substitution of patients suffering from liver-cirrhosis. pp. 374–384 in: D. Başar & Ü. Bengisu, Symposium on Electroretinography, Proc. 7th ISCERG Symp. 1969, Istanbul, 1971.

Severin, M. Augenveränderungen bei familiärer Nephronophthise. *Klin. Mbl. Augenheilk.* 166: *674–686* (1975).

Simonsen, S.E. Prognostic value of ERG (oscillatory potential) in juvenile diabetics. *Acta Ophthal.* (Kbh.) Supl. 123: *223–224* (1974).

Sperling, M.A., D.A. Hiles & J.S. Kennerdel. Electroretinographic responses following vitamin A therapy in A. beta-lipoproteinemia. *Amer. J. Ophthal.* 73: *342–351* (1972).

Stanescu, B. & J. Michiels. Temporal aspects of electroretinography in patients with myotonic dystrophy. *Amer. J. Ophthal.* 80: *224* (1975).

Stanescu, B. & J. Michiels. Retinal degenerations, electroretinographic aspects in patients with myotonic dystrophy. pp. 257–262 in: T. Lawwill (ed.), ERG, VER and Psychophysics. Proc. 14th ISCERG Symp. 1976, Doc. Ophthal. Proc. Ser. 13, Junk, The Hague, 1977.

Stanescu, B., M. Spiritus & J. Michiels. La rétinopathie dans la maladie de Batten–Mayou–Spielmeyer–Vogt. *Arch. Ophtal.* (Paris) 33: *827–834* (1973).

Stewart, H.L. & M.L. Rubin. Visual electrophysiology in myotonia congenita. pp. 5–16 in: Pearlman, T. (ed.), Proc. Xth ISCERG Symp. 1972, Doc. Ophthal. Proc. Ser. II, Junk, The Hague, 1973.

Tamai, A. & M.G. Holland. Ophthalmological studies on myotonic dystrophy. *Folia ophthal. jap.* 26: *194* (1975).

Textorius, O. The c-wave of the human electroretinogram in central retinal artery occlusion. *Acta Ophthal.* (Kbh.) 56: *827–836* (1978).

Thaler, A., P. Heilig & G. Zehetbauer. Der Einfluss von Vitamin A – Mangel auf das Elektrookulogramm. *Graefes Arch. Ophthal.* 199: *187–190* (1976).

Thiel, H.-J. & H. Behnke. Beitrag zur Klinik und Differentialdiagnose der juvenilen amaurotischen Idiotie. *Klin. Mbl. Augenheilk.* 158: *670–677* (1971).

Thranberend, Chr. & E. Adachi-Usami. Elektrophysiologische Untersuchungen bei spätinfantiler und juveniler familiärer amaurotischer Idiotie. *Klin. Mbl. Augenheilk.* 162: *224–233* (1973).

Yee, R.D., P.N. Herbert & D.R. Bergsma. Atypical retinitis pigmentosa in familial hypobetalipoproteinemia. *Amer. J. Ophthal.* 82: *64–71* (1976).

Yonemura *cf.* Kojima 1966 (discussion), 1965.

Younessian, S. L'ERG dans l'artérite temporale. *Ophthalmologica* (Basel) 143: *288* (1962).

Zimmerman, T.J., W.W. Dawson & J.R. Cade. Electroretinographic changes; pre- and postrenal dialysis. *Ann. Ophthal.* 5: *769–772* (1973).

other authors *cf.* E. Schmöger 1972. Klinische Elektroretinographie. pp. 573–712 in: K. Velhagen (ed.), Der Augenarzt, 2nd ed. Vol. II, Thieme, Leipzig.

Author's address:
Prof. Dr. sc. med. Elisabeth Schmöger
Augenklinik der Medizinischen Akademie
Nordhäuser Str. 74
DDR-506 Erfurt
German Democratic Republic

ELECTROPHYSIOLOGICAL STUDIES IN GROENBLAD-STRANDBERG SYNDROME

J. FRANÇOIS AND A. DE ROUCK

(Ghent, Belgium)

ABSTRACT

Fifteen cases (30 eyes) of Groenblad-Strandberg pseudoxanthoma elasticum were examined on the electrophysiological point of view. In only more or less 50% of the cases the results were subnormal. The diamox-test, which may be a functional test of the pigment epithelium, was also abnormal in 50% of the cases. Its significance is still not clear.

MATERIAL AND METHODS

Functional and electrophysiological tests were performed in 15 cases (30 eyes) of Groenblad-Strandberg syndrome (pseudo-xanthoma elasticum). In all patients the diagnosis was confirmed by a histological skin examination. Functional tests included: visual acuity, visual field (Goldmann perimeter), global light sense (Weekers-Goldmann adaptometer: 5' preadaptation at 2000 asb). The electrophysiological tests included:

(1) The ERG was performed in both light (300 lux) and dark adapted states, with white Xenon flashes of various intensities, blue and red filters. The registration was made by means of a Mingograf Elema (time constant 0,6 and 1,2 sec).

(2) The EOG was performed to study the light induced responses as well as the drug induced responses of the standing potential (SP).

(a) Light/dark ratio. The classical EOG was performed according to the technique we have previously described (François et al., 1966).

(b) Diamox-response. The technique of Yonemura et al. (1978) was used: 500 mgr. Diamox were injected intravenously within 60 seconds after the standing potential (SP) was stabilized at a steady level. The SP decreases within 1 to 2 min. and shows a new plateau level 5 to 8 min. after the injection.

All cases were classified in several groups and subgroups, according to the fluoro-angiographic aspect of the fundus lesions. (François and De Laey, 1978).

A. *First group*: eyes showing only a degeneration of the Bruch's membrane either (1) with no other changes than the typical angioid streaks: 4 eyes, or (2) with a dehiscence of the Bruch's membrane from the choriocapillaris, producing a "peau d'orange" appearance (Federman et al., 1976): 3 eyes.

B. *Second group*: one eye, showing subretinal haemorrhages following trauma.

Table 1. Results of the functional tests in 30 eyes with angioid streaks. Visual acuity: F.C. = fingers counting. Classification of the visual field: (A) normal or slight enlargement of the blind spot, (B) relative central scotoma with normal peripheral isopters, (C) absolute central scotoma with normal peripheral isopters; the number following the letter C indicates the extent in degrees of the absolute scotoma. The level of the dark adaptation curve is given at the 15th min. ERG.-Photopic b-wave: maximal amplitude of the absolute scotoma. The state. R.L. = amplitude of the cone b-wave in red light (dark adapted), B.L. = amplitude of the rod b-wave in blue light (dark adapted state), a_m = amplitude of the maximal a-wave in dark adapted state and b_m = amplitude of the maximal b-wave in cone adapted state.

Name	Age	Group	Visual acuity	Visual Field	Dark adaptation	Photopic b-wave	ERG R.L.	ERG B.L.	ERG a_m	ERG b_m	L/D ratio	Diamox test
1 Verv. J.	19	A1	1,0	A	$\bar{5},6$	205	185	270	490	580	210	66
		B	F.C.	C-15	$\bar{5},6$	195	190	275	480	600	216	68
2 De W. J.	50	A1	1,0	A	$\bar{4},3$	210	140	260	480	480	190	
		A1	1,0	A	$\bar{4},3$	200	170	250	470	510	220	
3 Vandenh. M.	34	A2	1,0	A	$\bar{5},8$	180	180	310	450	480	183	65
		A2	1,0	A	$\bar{5},8$	190	190	320	460	510	185	70
4 Fatz. N.	51	A1	1,0	A	$\bar{5},6$	200	280	260	400	440	178	77
		D3	F.C.	C-15	$\bar{5},7$	205	260	280	410	460	177	83
5 De C. H.	17	A2	1,0	A	$\bar{4},0$	200	250	320	400	510	215	78
		D3	F.C.	C	$\bar{4},0$	190	235	310	420	525	186	75
6 De Sch.	51	D2	0,1	C-10	$\bar{4},0$	125	105	190	300	370	145	71
		C	0,9	B	$\bar{4},0$	180	185	290	400	450	171	68

Name		D										
7 Mour. J.	51	D1-C	1,0	A	$\overline{5,3}$	180	160	190	340	340	214	69
		D2	0,6	B	$\overline{5,3}$	180	180	180	320	340	224	79
8 Lip. L.	50	D2	0,2	C-10	$\overline{5,7}$	200	180	220	520	450	205	64
		D2	0,3	C-10	$\overline{5,7}$	200	180	300	520	510	213	62
9 Mor. K.	42	D2	0,1	C-10	$\overline{5,8}$	195	190	260	500	520	218	64
		D3	F.C.	C-20	$\overline{5,8}$	200	175	270	495	505	211	70
10 Lox. P.		D3	0,05	C-15	$\overline{4,2}$	120	110	200	240	340	158	73
		D2	0,4	B	$\overline{4,2}$	160	180	260	300	460	161	73
11 Iem. Y.	52	D3	F.C.	C-45	$\overline{4,2}$	200	240	260	480	520	198	71
		D3	F.C.	C-45	$\overline{4,4}$	190	210	260	460	510	191	75
12 Yer. S.	47	D3	F.C.	C-50	$\overline{4,2}$	100	80	100	260	230	105	80
		D3	F.C.	C-60	$\overline{4,0}$	110	90	120	250	235	110	77
13 De Sch. T.	54	D3	F.C.	C-45	$\overline{4,0}$	130	110	180	320	350	156	73
		D3	F.C.	C-40	$\overline{4,0}$	160	180	280	420	500	180	75
14 Ver. E.	55	D3	F.C.	C-20	$\overline{4,2}$	210	240	300	440	520	217	77
		D3	F.C.	C-25	$\overline{4,1}$	200	230	280	430	500	223	72
15 Tor. M.		D3	F.C.	C-15	$\overline{4,4}$	210	220	220	360	300	127	73
		D3	F.C.	C-15	$\overline{4,2}$	180	280	220	400	430	112	71
Normal values	mean value				$\overline{5,0}$	223	268	330	485	570	180	61
	mean value + 2σ				$\overline{5,7}$	140	180	260	340	440		71
	deviation											

Table 2. Peak-time of cone *b*-wave and diamox response.

| | Peak-time (msec.) cone *b*-wave | | Diamox test | |
	Normal	Pseudo-xanthoma elasticum	Normal	Pseudo-xanthoma elasticum
Number of cases	40,0	30,0	32,0	28,0
mean	32,0	34,6	61,0	72,0
σ^2	3,61	2,26	24,25	25,6
σ	1,9	1,5	4,9	5,05
Difference between means	$34,6 - 32,0 = 2,6$		$72 - 61 = 11$	
Standard error of difference	$S = \sqrt{\dfrac{3,61}{40} + \dfrac{2,26}{30}} = 0,40$		$S = \sqrt{\dfrac{24,25}{32} + \dfrac{25,6}{28}} = 1,3$	

C. *Third group*: one eye with large dystrophic changes of the choriocapillaris and of the pigment epithelium, mainly in the posterior pole.

D. *Fourth group*: eyes with disciform macular degeneration.

(1) *Stage I* of the degeneration, characterized by macular oedema, but without choroidal neo-vascularisation: 1 eye.

(2) *Stage II* of the degeneration, characterized by choroidal neo-vascularisation, detected by fluoro-angiography. New vessels penetrate the ruptured Bruch's membrane and produce subretinal as well as retinal haemorrhages: 6 eyes.

(3) *Stage III* of the degeneration, characterized by the development of fibrous tissue and the formation of a macular scar: 14 eyes.

RESULTS

The results are summarised in Table 1.

(A) The *global light sense* was slightly subnormal in 18 eyes, the thresholds after 15' of dark adaptation being never more than $\overline{4},4$ (60% of cases). No correlation with the fundus changes could be found. The dark adaptation curve

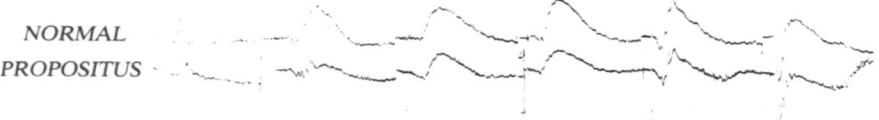

NORMAL
PROPOSITUS

LIGHT adapt. DARK adapt.
WHITE stim.   RED stim.   BLUE stim. WHITE stim. WHITE stim. WHITE stim.
1100 μV   int. I   int. II   int. III
⊢ 20 msec

Fig. 1.

22

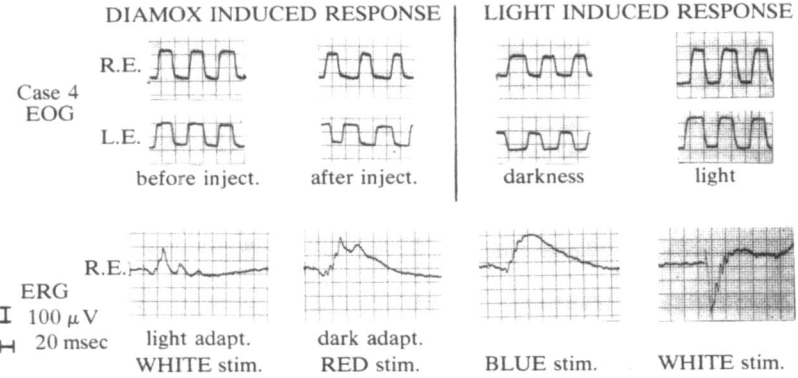

Fig. 2.

of both eyes was higher in the same way, even when the fundus changes were not symmetric.

(B) *ERG*. 1. *Amplitude* Subnormal responses were detected in 14 eyes (46% of cases): in 2 cases only the cone-system was involved, in 4 cases only the rod-system and in 8 cases both systems, mostly in eyes with advanced disciform macular degeneration. Normal ERG records could, however, be obtained even in cases with terminal macular degeneration.

2. *Temporal characteristics*. These characteristics were not obviously modified. The mean peak-time of the cone *b*-waves in photopic conditions, however, was 34,6 msec, while in normal people it is 32,0 msec. The difference is statistically significant (Table 2). The peak-times of the rod *b*-waves showed no statistically significant increase as compared to normal results. The oscillatory potentials were present in all cases (Fig. 1).

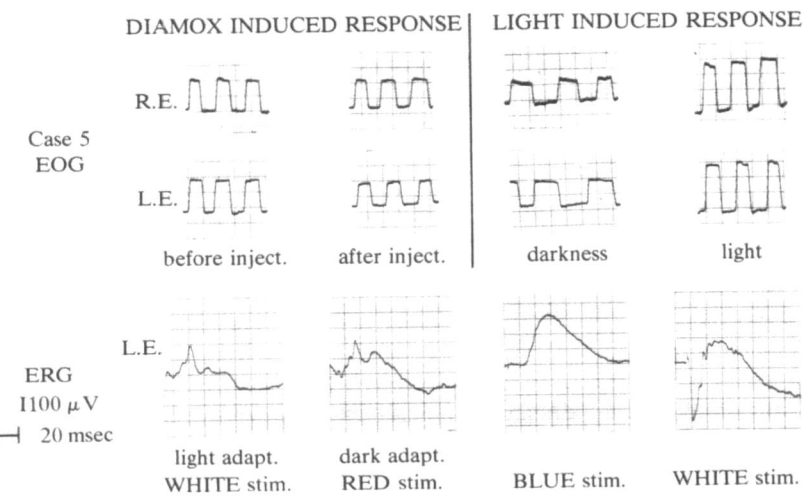

Fig. 3.

DIAMOX INDUCED RESPONSE | LIGHT INDUCED RESPONSE

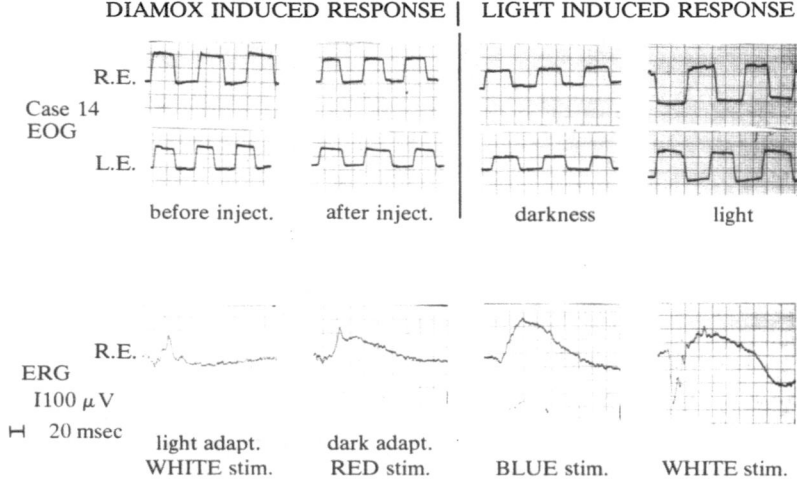

Fig. 4.

(C) *EOC.* 1. *Light-dark ratio.* This ratio was pathological in 8 eyes (26% of cases): between 165 and 130% in 4 cases and below 130% in other 4 cases. In 3 eyes the L/D ratio was more than 165%, but less than 180%. Pathological EOG's were only recorded when also the ERG was subnormal. Normal EOG's could be recorded even in cases with advanced macular degeneration.

2. *Diamox-response.* The reduction in amplitude of the EOG is expressed by the ratio $100 \times A_2/A_1$, A_2 representing the minimal amplitude of the EOG 5 to 8 min after Diamox injection, and A_1 the steady amplitude before the administration of the drug. In normal people this ratio has a mean value of 61, with $\pm 2\sigma$ deviations of 10. In 15 of our patients, the Diamox ratio remained above the 2σ deviation (50% of cases). The Diamox response was abnormal even in eyes without macular or functional changes (Table 2 and Figs. 2 to 4).

DISCUSSION

The Diamox response was first described and investigated by Yonemura *et al.* (1978). They demonstrated experimentally that the drug-effect was preserved in the in-vitro eye cup maintained in an artificial incubating solution. Therefore, cornea, lens, ciliary body, possible changes in intraocular pressure and blood circulation do not contribute essentially to the Diamox-response and one may assume that this Diamox-response represents a test for the pigment epithelium, although the clinical significance still remains obscure. There is, for instance, no concordance with other drug induced standing potential responses, such as the hyperosmolarity response. On the other hand, the Diamox-response remains normal in patients with pigmentary retinopathy (Yonemura *et al.*, 1978) and with longstanding retinal detachment (personal observations). The fact remains, nevertheless, that a significant change of the Diamox-response can be recorded in patients with degenerative changes of the Bruch's

24

membrane and the choroidal vessels. For all these reasons it may be concluded that further investigations are needed.

Electroretinographic and electro-oculographic changes exist in Groenblad-Strandberg syndrome, but only in more or less 50% of cases, so that the electrophysiological tests have only a minor diagnostic value.

REFERENCES

Federman S.L., Shields J.A. & T.L. Tomer. Angioid streaks II fluorescein angiographic features. *Arch. Ophthal.* (Chicago), 93: *951–962* (1972).

François J. & J.J. De Laey. Pseudo-xanthoma elasticum (Syndroom van Groenblad-Strandberg). Tijdschr. Geneesk., 5: *297–302* (1978).

François J., De Rouck A., Verriest, G. & M. Szmigielski. An extended clinical test of the ocular standing potential and its results in some cases of retinal degeneration. Proceedings 4th ISCERG Symp., *Jap. J. Ophthal.*, 10: *267–268* (1966).

Yonemura D., Kawasaki K., Tanabe J. & S. Yamamoto. Susceptibility of the standing potential of the eye to Acetazolamide and its clinical application. *Folio Ophthal. Jap.* 29: *408–415* (1978).

Author's address:
Opthalmological Clinic
University of Ghent
Ghent
Belgium

Docum. Ophthal. Proc. Series, Vol. 23

ERG AND EOG IN SCLERODERMA

ALICJA MOSZCZYŃSKA-KOWALSKA, EWA DRÓBECKA-BRYDAK
AND TADEUSZ KĘCIK

(*Warsaw, Poland*)

ABSTRACT

Twenty patients were examined, in whom various types of sclerodermia were clinically diagnosed. Visual acuity, visual field, dark adaptation, and colour vision were assessed in all the patients. The anterior segment and the fundus were evaluated too. ERG and EOG examinations were performed on all subjects. Fluorescein angiography of the retinal vessels was also made on several patients of this group. In the results it is worth noting that the threshold of dark adaptation was always elevated. Most of the patients showed pathology in the ERG results, expressed by a reduction of amplitude of the b-waves. The LP/DT-ratio in the EOG was also slightly lower. No correspondence was observed between the ERG results and the LP/DT-ratio in the EOG.

INTRODUCTION

Scleroderma is a multisystemic disease with a various clinical symptomatology and is included in connective tissue disease. Ocular changes appearing in scleroderma involve most often the protective apparatus of the eye (Kirkham, 1969), but they also include the anterior (Woodruff, 1977) and posterior segment (Manschot, 1965), Berndt and Hoffman (1977) of the eye and they express the generalized character of the disease (Cernea *et al.* 1975). Circumscribed scleroderma, known as a dermatologoic disease is in a matter of fact, a more benign form of the same process. The aetiology of scleroderma is not known and the pathogenesis is not yet certain. There is evidence of an important role of the nervous, especially vegetative, system in the developing mechanism of all forms of scleroderma (Jabłońska, 1963).

The main features of scleroderma are: induration of collagen, the presence of vascular changes and the atrophic symptoms in later periods. The vascular changes are usually of the type of arteritis with a secondary hypertrophy of endothelium followed by the partial or total occlusion of the arteries (Jabłońska, 1963). The obliteration of the small vessels is characteristic, the bigger vessels remain intact.

Fluorescein angiography (Grennan and Forrester, 1977) and histopathologic evaluation (Farkas *et al.* 1972) show the same type of pathology in the eye. The changes are situated mainly in the choriocapillaries. It may be expected that the changes appearing in choroid may influence the function of the retina impairing its electrical response.

The purpose of our report is to assess ocular function paying special attention on ERG and EOG in the patients presenting different forms of scleroderma.

27

Table 1

Type of scleroderma	Age of patients (years)			
	15–30	31–40	41–50	51–60
Acrosclerosis	1	4	5	7
Sclerosis generalisata		1		2
Sclerosis fasciitis				1
Hemiatrophia faciei secundaria post sclerodermiam	2		1	
Morphea generalisata			1	

MATERIAL AND METHODS

Twenty-five patients (6 M, 19 F) aged 15 to 60 years were examined. Table 1 presents the patients divided into groups depending on their age and diagnosis. The duration of the disease was 1 to 5 years in twelve patients, 6 to 10 years in six patients, 11 to 15 years in four patients and over 20 years in three patients.

All the patients had a general ophthalmic examination including: visual acuity, visual field, anterior and posterior segment, colour vision, dark adaptation (Goldmann-Weekers adaptometer). ERG and EOG were performed using a Retinographor Alvar. Six patients underwent in addition fluorescein angiography. The results of the EOG examination were divided into 3 groups (according to the value of Arden's coefficient)

1. 200–243%

2. 185–199%

3. 130–184%

The patients pupils were dilated with 1% Mydriacyl (Alcon) before ERG and the retina was adapted to darkness for 5 minutes. A xenon lamp was used to elicite the ERG, the duration time of the single flash was 150 μs and its energy was 0.03 and 0.3 J. A Kodak-Wratten 26 filter was used to obtain the red light. The recording was performed using Henkes-Worst contact lens electrode, connected with the pen-writing apparatus. The amplification was 100 μV/cm in combination with a time constant of 0.3 sec. and paper speed 6 cm/sec. The retinal response to single red and white flashes in dark and light adaptation and CFF were estimated.

RESULTS

From the group of 25 patients only one, a 51 year old male, suffering from acrosclerosis for 15 years, was the visual acuity impaired, because of advanced cataract. The rest of the patients had normal vision. All the evaluated patients had a normal visual field. Colour vision estimated by Farnsworth test 100 Hue was normal in most of the patients, only four of them showed uncharacteristic defects. All the patients presented abnormal scotopic adaptation curves, the final threshold was increased one log unit above the mean value. The ocular fundus was normal in 6 patients. In 18 patients the generalized constriction of arteries, especially of the small arteries, was observed. Apart from thinning of

Table 2

Type of scleroderma	EOG (40 eyes)		
	200–243%	185–199%	130–184%
Acrosclerosis	8	7	15
Sclerosis generalisata			2
Hemiatrophia faciei secundaria post sclerodermiam	2		4
Morphea generalisata	2		

the retina, dispersion of pigment at the periphery and depigmentation of the macular area were noticeable. Ophthalmoscopy was impossible to perform on one patient, because of cataract.

All the patients were normotensive and their renal function was normal.

Capillaroscopy performed on the patients with circumscribed scleroderma was within normal limits. All the others had R (Raynaud) and/or S (Scleroderma) type loops in the different phases.

Fluorescein angiography. In 6 patients staining of retinal vessels walls and uneven thinning of epithelium was observed. Those changes involved mainly the periphery and optic disk area. One patient (a 41 year old female suffering from circumscribed scleroderma for 7 years) presented scattered lesions of pigment epithelium with markedly increased spotted fluorescence of the whole retina appearing in the early arterial phase.

In all the examined patients the choroidal vessels could be observed through the retina (this maybe associated with obliteration of the choriocapillaries). Obliteration of the retinal vessels was not observed.

The EOG results obtained from 20 patients (40 eyes) are presented in Table 2 and the ERG results from 25 patients are shown in Table 3. Table number 4 shows the dependence between both EOG and ERG results.

Table 3

Type of scleroderma	Type of ERG (50 eyes)				
				Subnormal	
	Normal	Supernormal	Negative +	wave b 100–170 μV	wave b 50–100 μV
Acrosclerosis	7	2	1	17	7
Sclerosis generalisata				6	
Sclerosis fasciitis					2
Hemiatrophia faciei secundaria post sclerodermiam	2	1	1	2	
Morphea generalisata		1	1		

Table 4

EOG%	Type of ERG				
	Normal	Super normal	Negative +	Subnormal I	II
200–243	2	1	2	6	1
185–199	2	1	—	3	1
130–184	3	2	1	11	4

DISCUSSION

Analysis of the ERG and EOG results demonstrates the frequent decrease of the retinal electric response in patients suffering from scleroderma.

Within the group of 25 patients (50 eyes) only 9 eyes presented normal ERG responses. The responses from the 34 eyes (68%) were subnormal, of those 9 eyes had scotopic b wave below 100 μV. It is noticeable that the pathological responses did not depend on types of the disease and appeared in the both forms, circumscribed and generalized.

The EOG coefficient was decreased below 185% in 21 eyes (52.5%). This concerned also the patients with the circumscribed type of scleroderma. No relationship between ERG and EOG responses was observed during our studies. It should be pointed out that the lowered results of electrophysiological tests were not accompanied by the impaired visual acuity or changes in the visual field, but the ophthalmological changes were slight or none.

Ophthalmoscopic evaluation showed, similar to Dobżanskij (1969), angiopathy and depigmentation in the macular area and periphery in 18 patients. From this group 6 patients had normal or higher b waves and 5 patients had normal EOG coefficient.

From the group of 6 patients with no ophthalmoscopic changes 4 had lowered b waves down to 50 μV and EOG coefficients to 143%. This lack of relationship between ERG, EOG and ophthalmoscopy results is difficult to explain especially because all the evaluated patients had impaired dark adaptation.

The observed differences do not seem to be related to the duration of the disease or to patients' age.

It seems certain that the observed pathology is the result of primary choroid circulation impairment. Fluorescein angiography performed in 6 of our patients showed deterioration of the choriocapillaries in all cases. The most distinct changes occurred in the eyes of the woman with a circumscribed form of the disease. It confirms the previous observations of other authors, that fluorescein angiography allows visualisation of the choriocapillar pathology even before the appearance of retinal changes (Grennan and Forrester, 1977). It also confirms the idea that generalized deterioration of the microcirculation is the basic causative factor in the pathogenesis of both systemic and circumscribed types of scleroderma (Berndt and Hoffman, 1977).

Concluding we would like to stress that we could not find any reports evaluating ERG and EOG results in the patients suffering from scleroderma. It seems that these tests can be used as an additional method to estimate in an indirect way the microcirculation of the eye.

REFERENCES

Berndt, K. & A. Hoffman. Zentralarterinverschlub der Retina bei progressiver Sklerodermic. *Klin. Mbl. Augenheilk.* 171: *597–600*, (1977).

Cernea, P. & G. Dobrescu. Manifestations oculaire dans la sclerodermie. *Ann. Oculist.* 208: *409–505*, (1975).

Dobżanskij, S.J., Gonczarow, B.J. & T.P. Pismak. Porażenije głaz pri skrerodermi. Vest. Oftal. 1: *76–77*, (1969).

Farkas, T., Sylvester, V. & D. Archer. The choroidopathy of progressive systemic sclerosis (scleroderma). *Am. J. Ophth.* 74: *875–886*, (1972).

Grennan, D. & J. Forrester. Involvement of the eye in SLE and Scleroderma. *Ann. of the Rheumatic Diseases* 36: *152–156*, (1977).

Jabłońska, S. Scleroderma and scleroderma-like conditions. PZWL, Warszawa, (1963).

Kirkham, T.H. Scleroderma and Sjögren's syndrome. *Brit. J. Ophthal.* 53: *131–133*. (1969).

Manschot, W.A. Generalized scleroderma with Ocular Symptoms. Ophthalmologica 149: *131–137*, (1965).

Volpi, U., Borgioli M., Colatto, A. & P.L. Amerio. Fluorescein retinographic study in scleroderma/progressive systemic sclerosis. In: *Excerpta Medica* 31: *3*, (1977).

Woodronff, M.E. Diseases of the Uvea – 1976. Review. Am. J. Opt. Physiol. Optics. 54: *338–343*, (1977).

Author's address:
Eye Clinic of the Medical Academy
Lindley'a 4
02-005 Warsaw
Poland

Docum. Ophthal. Proc. Series, Vol. 23

ELECTROPHYSIOLOGICAL EXAMINATION AND CINE-ANGIOFLUOROGRAPHIC STUDY OF VASCULOPATHIES IN MAN

PIERRE SOLÉ, RINALDO ALFIERI
AND FRANCK BACIN

(*Clermont-Ferrand, France*)

ABSTRACT

The purpose of this work is to study the relationship between electrophysiological and circulatory parameters during retinal vascular obstructions in man.

Before and after treatment by urokinase, the following tests were performed: electroretinography using white light (ERG), visual evoked potentials using red monochromatic light (VEP), visual acuity, fluorescein angiography, cine-fluorescein angiography with transit times and vessels lumen width measurement.

The results enable us:

1. On the diagnosis level, to confirm parallelism between ERG (variations of the b_1-wave amplitude and of the ratio b_1/a) and retinal hemodynamic data.

2. On the prognosis level, to show VEP importance. A recanalization, demonstrated by an electroretinographic improvement, does not imply macular functional recovery unless the VEP is equally improved. These facts will then be confirmed by the angiographic appearance of the posterior pole.

INTRODUCTION

Many authors have studied the pathology of retinal circulation in man either principally from an electrophysiological point of view (Henkes, 1953, 1976; Jayle, Boyer and Saracco, 1965; François *et al.*, 1973, 1974; Letrone, 1977; Henkes and van Mierlobensteijn, 1978), or by comparing electrophysiologic and angiographic data (Flower, Speros and Kenyon, 1977; Coscas and Dhermy, 1978). Personally, we wanted to support this last point of view by attempting to establish a quantitative study, on the one hand of the electrophysiologic data by measuring the ratio b_1/a of the values of ERG photopic waves, and on the other hand of the hemodynamic data by measuring angiographic transit times and retinal vessels lumen width (cine-fluorescein angiography).

SUBJECTS AND METHODS

Subjects

Our seven patients were men. Two (55 and 62-year-old) presented a central retinal artery obstruction; two others (43 and 73-year-old) suffered from a central retinal vein obstruction, one with ischemic retinopathy, the other with edematous retinopathy; two others (61 and 66-year-old) had a branch retinal vein obstruction, one with ischemic retinopathy, the other with edematous retinopathy; the last (63-year-old) associated a branch retinal artery obstruction with a branch retinal vein obstruction of the ischemic type.

All these patients were treated by urokinase perfusion (2,000 I.U./kg) during 24 hours, a few of them received a complementary therapy with subcutaneous injections of calcium heparinate (0.12 ml/24 h) during 3 weeks.

Methods

Before and after treatment by urokinase, the following tests were performed in the seven patients: electroretinography, visual evoked potentials, visual acuity, angiography, angiographic transit times and retinal vessels lumen width measurement.

Electroretinography
The stimulation is performed using white light. Therefore the electroretinogram presents essentialy photopic waves: a is a negative deflection, b_1 is a positive one. Schematically (Solé *et al.* 1979; Alfieri and Solé, 1979) the a-wave arises from the photoreceptor level (receptoral component of ERG) while the b-wave demonstrates the activity of bipolar cells (postreceptoral component of ERG). Thus, an ischemia extended only to the internal layers of the retina should only affect the b-wave; accordingly, we determined the ratio b_1/a, before treatment (*i.e.*, r) and after treatment (*i.e.* r'); we also calculate its relative variation $R\% = \frac{r'-r}{r} \times 100$.

Visual evoked potentials
The stimulation is performed using a monochromatic red light (658 nm centered interference filter with 16 nm band pass). For each eye, visual evoked potentials are recorded from homolateral and contralateral occipital scalp. Its presence demonstrates the functional integrity of the macula and of the macular ganglion cells fibers.

Visual acuity
Far vision is measured using Monoyer scale (from 1/20 to 10/10 for the increasing acuity) and close vision is measured using Parinaud scale (from P 14 to P 1.5 for the increasing acuity).

Angiography
Classical angiography was performed. The photographic field being limited to 30° for one picture, we sometimes make a picture assembly in order to evaluate better the extent of retinal circulatory lesions.

Angiographic transit times measurement
This measurement was performed on cine-fluorescein angiography (Vilaire, 1973) using an original system consisting of:
1. *An automatic injector* allowing, on the one hand, a constant duration of the

dye injection (always given at the same place), and on the other hand, a simultaneous triggering of the camera.

2. *A Beaulieu 16 mm camera*, with a 15° angle. It is fitted with a quartz driven engine allowing reduction of the starting inertia and to fix carefully to 25 the rate of frames per second.

3. *A Carl Zeiss retinal chamber* (PT3), fitted with the camera. The light source is a xenon tube (Osram XB0 150W) working on high tension and permanently.

4. *A Elmo 16 AR projector* with frame counter, reverse, and single frame projection. It allows to interpret the film and to measure the index defined by Brunel (1975):

   (a) T1: appearance time of fluorescein at the disc. This, represents theoretically, the measure of arm-retina transit time. Practically, it includes also retinal arterial transit because the filling of the retinal arterial tree is almost concommittant.

   (b) T_2: arrival time of the venous laminar stream at the disc margin; T2 − T1 is therefore a rough estimate of capillary transit time.

   (c) T3: arrival time of complete venous filling at the disc margin; T3 − T2 is therefore an estimate of venous transit time.

In central vessel obstructions times were measured in all the retinal quadrants. For the obstruction of branch retinal vessels, we were able to measure times in comparing pathological and sound areas.

Vessels lumen width measurement
This measure (Brunel, 1975) is performed, by projecting cine-fluorescein angiography frames on a screening table used in the study of pictures obtained in a bubble chamber in corpuscular physics. As it is the fluorescent content that is visualized on the film, we measure, therefore, the vessel lumen width and not the anatomical width. We used arbitrary units for this measure performed before (*i.e.* w) and after treatment (*i.e.* w′); we are only interested in the relative variation $W\% = \dfrac{w' - w}{w} \times 100$.

RESULTS

We shall only detail 3 observations, each one being demonstrative of one type of vascular obstruction.

Case 1

A 62-year-old man with a central retinal artery obstruction in his left eye, was treated with anatomical success three hours after the occurrence of the disease.
ERG (Fig. 1: I)
It shows, in the left eye, a disappearance of b_1-wave that reappears with a good amplitude after treatment, hence R reaches +∞%. This demonstrates a recanalization of the bipolar cell layer of the retina.
VEP (Fig. 2: II)
On the contrary, non recordable before treatment it remains unchanged. This

I. ELECTRORETINOGRAM

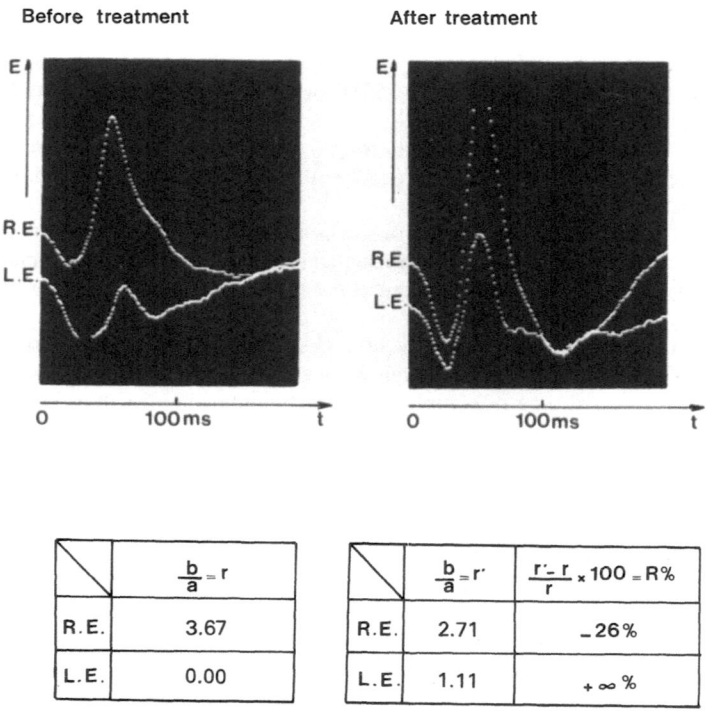

Before treatment

After treatment

	$\dfrac{b}{a} = r$
R.E.	3.67
L.E.	0.00

	$\dfrac{b}{a} = r'$	$\dfrac{r'-r}{r} \times 100 = R\%$
R.E.	2.71	-26%
L.E.	1.11	$+\infty\%$

Fig. 1. Central retinal artery obstruction: electroretinogram. E: potential; t: time; R.E.: right eye; L.E.: left eye.

demonstrates a persisting lesion either of the macula, of the macular fiber bundle, or of both.

Visual acuity (Fig. 2: III)

After treatment there is only light perception in the left eye, corroborating the VEP results.

Angiography (Fig. 3: IV)

Before treatment, angiography of the left eye demonstrates total non perfusion of the posterior pole. After treatment it shows a complete recovery of vascular perfusion, corroborating the ERG results.

Angiographic transit times measurement (Fig. 4: V)

Before treatment the capillary transit time $T2 - T1$ is over 60 s; after treatment it definitely improves but still reaches 15 s. This shortening is in good accordance with ERG and angiography results.

Vessels lumen width measurement (Fig. 4: VI)

After treatment, only the relative variation of the vein is coherent, W reaching $+120\%$, demonstrating arterial recanalization.

II . VISUAL EVOKED POTENTIALS

Before treatment   After treatment

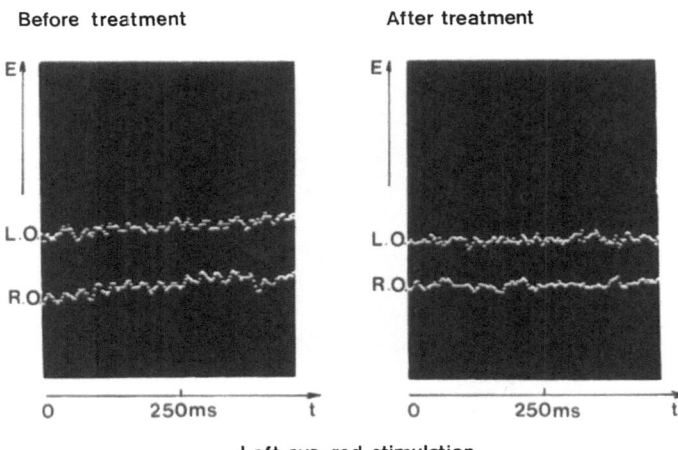

Left eye : red stimulation

III . VISUAL ACUITY

Before treatment   After treatment

R.E. : $\frac{5}{10}$; P.2   R.E. : $\frac{5}{10}$; P.2

L.E.: L.P.   L.E.: L.P.

Fig. 2. Central retinal artery obstruction: visual evoked potentials and visual acuity. E: potential; t: time; R.O.: right occiput; L.O.: left occiput; R.E.: right eye; L.E.: left eye; P.: Parinaud; L.P.: light perception.

Prognostic conclusion

All of the tests improved after treatment except for VEP and visual acuity demonstrating the loss of macular function, although there was a definite improvement of retinal vascularization.

Case 2

A 42-year-old man with a central retinal vein obstruction in his right eye, was treated without much success three weeks after the occurrence of the disease.

ERG (Fig. 5: I)

It shows, in the right eye, a very marked decrease of the amplitude of b_1-wave that partly increases after treatment, hence, R reaches +189% demonstrating a partial recanalization of the bipolar cells layer of the retina.

VEP (Fig. 6: II)

37

IV. ANGIOGRAPHY

Before treatment

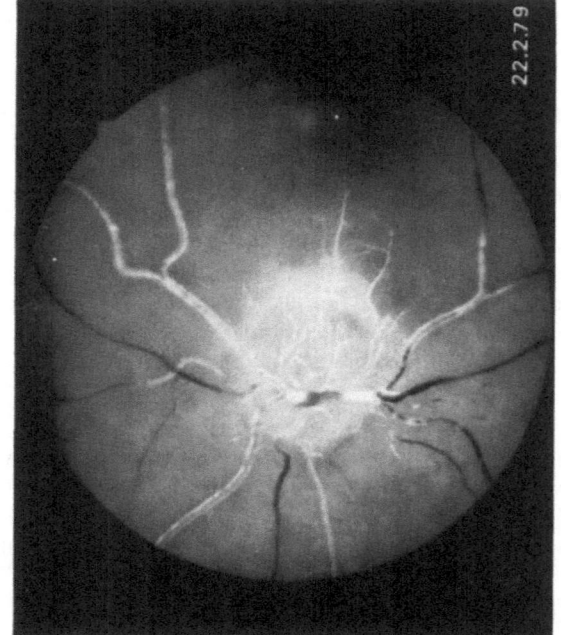

After treatment

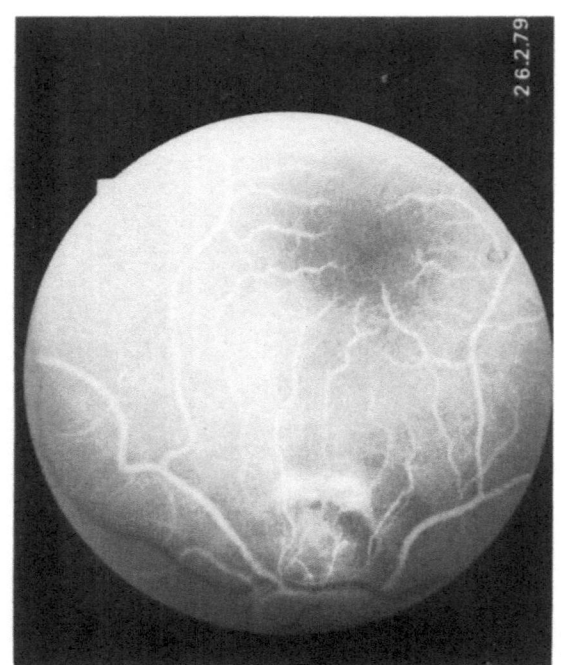

Fig. 3. Central retinal artery obstruction: angiography.

Ⅴ. TRANSIT TIMES

Before treatment	After treatment
T1:　259 s	T1:　21 s
T2:　>319 s	T2:　36 s
T3:　—	T3:　70s

Ⅵ. VESSEL WIDTH

Before treatment

	w
Artery	2.2　a.u.
Vein	1.0　a.u.

After treatment

	w˙	$\frac{w'-w}{w} \times 100 = W\%$
Artery	1.6 a.u.	− 27%
Vein	2.2 a.u.	+ 120%

Fig. 4. Central retinal artery obstruction: transit time and vessel width. T2–T1: capillary transit time; T3–T2: venous transit time; a.u.: arbitrary unit.

On the contrary, recordable before treatment with a low amplitude, it remains unchanged. This demonstrates a persisting macular impairment.

Visual acuity (Fig. 6: III)
After treatment, improvement in the right eye is negligible, corroborating the VEP results.

Angiography (Fig. 7: IV)
After treatment, it demonstrates in the periphery as well as in the posterior pole, the persisting ischemic lesions that underlay the hemorrhages and the ensudates observed in the initial stage. This explains that ERG recovery should only be partial and that the VEP should stay unchanged.

Angiographic transit times measurement (Fig. 8: V)
Before treatment, the capillary transit time T2−T1 reaches 10 s; after treatment it improves and reaches 6 s. This shortening is in good accordance with ERG results.

Vessels lumen width measurement (Fig. 8: VI)
After treatment, the relative variation is nearly null, in the artery as well as in the vein (W = ±1%).

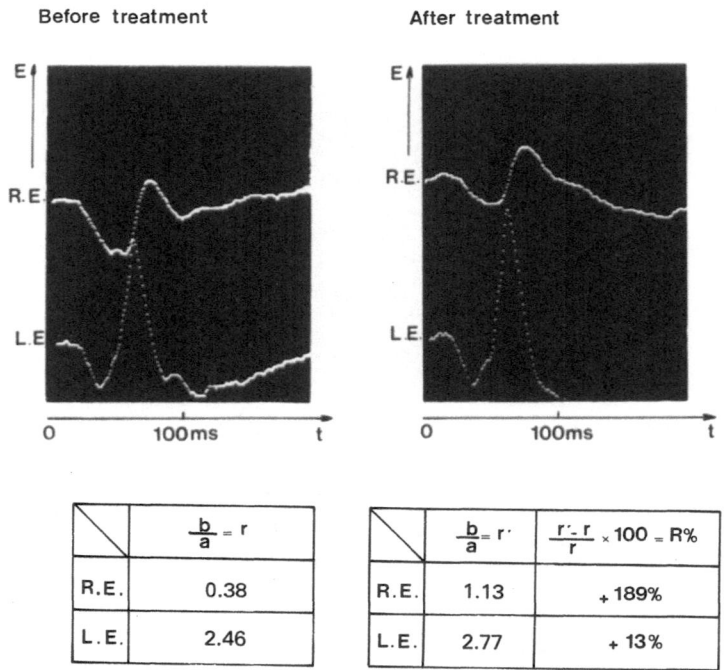

Fig. 5. Central retinal vein obstruction: electroretinogram. E: potential; t: time; R.E.: right eye; L.E.: left eye.

Prognostic conclusion
Only ERG and angiographic transit times were slightly modified after treatment, demonstrating a slight improvement in vascular flow, with yet, a persisting impairment of macular function.

Case 3

A 63-year-old man with an upper temporal branch vein obstruction associated with a lower temporal little branch artery obstruction in his right eye, was successfully treated 24 hours after the occurrence of the disease.
ERG (Fig. 9: I)
It shows, in the right eye, an important decrease of the amplitude of b_1-wave that increases slightly after treatment, hence R reaches only +51%; this demonstrates a partial recanalization of the bipolar cells layers of the retina.
VEP (Fig. 10: II)
Practically normal as from the beginning, it shows that macular sensorial function is not severely injured.

II. VISUAL EVOKED POTENTIALS

Before treatment

After treatment

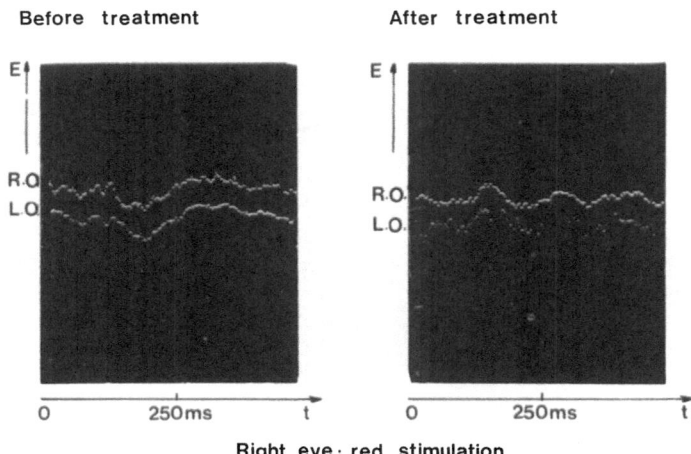

Right eye: red stimulation

III. VISUAL ACUITY

Before treatment

R.E.: $\frac{1}{20}$; < P. 14

L.E.: $\frac{10}{10}$; P. 1.5

After treatment

R.E.: $\frac{1}{20}$; < P. 14 → $\frac{1}{10}$; P. 10

L.E.: $\frac{10}{10}$; P. 1.5

Fig. 6. Central retinal vein obstruction: visual evoked potentials and visual acuity. E: potential; t: time; R.O.: right occiput; L.O.: left occiput; R.E.: right eye; L.E.: left eye; P.: Parinaud; L.P.: light perception.

Visual acuity (Fig. 10: III)
After treatment, there is an excellent recovery in the right eye, and this corroborates VEP results.
Angiography (Fig. 11: IV)
After treatment, it shows, at the level of the vein obstruction, as well as at the level of the arterial obstruction a localized ischemia. This is in accordance with the relative low value of R observed in ERG.
Angiographic transit times measurement (Fig. 12: V)
Before treatment, the capillary transit time T2−T1 reaches 18 s in the drainage area of the superior temporal vein. After treatment it improves and reaches 10 s. This shortening is in good concordance with the ERG results. It is worth noting that the capillary transit times is not modified in the sound area of the inferior temporal vessels (8 s before and after treatment).
Vessels lumen width measurement (Fig. 12: VI)
After treatment, the relative variations are coherent as well in the artery

41

IV. ANGIOGRAPHY

After treatment

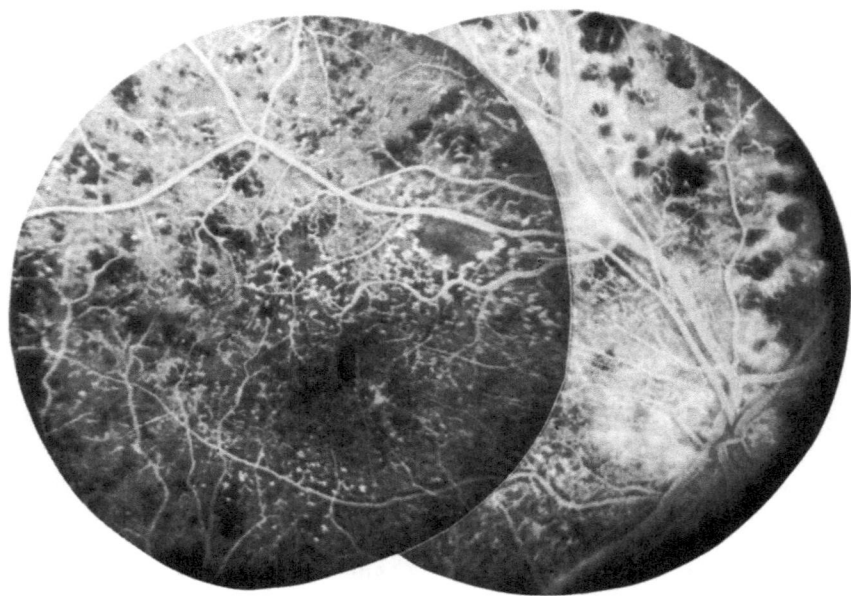

Fig. 7. Central retinal vein obstruction: angiography.

(W = +23%) where the positive value demonstrates a better filling, as well as in the vein (W = −43%) where the negative value demonstrates a better drainage.

Prognostic conclusion

All of the tests improved, after treatment, but in a lower range in ERG and angiography. This demonstrates the persistence of ischemic areas.

DISCUSSION

Whatever the type of vascular obstruction, comparison between electrophysiological and circulatory parameters shows obviously a nearly perfect parallel from a clinical level (diagnosis and prognosis); a few divergences can be explained from a methodological level (accuracy of measures and modalities of therapy).

Clinical level

Diagnosis

In all retinal vascular troubles, it is worth noting a decrease, even a disappearance, of b_1-wave. In correlation, during the course of the disease, R will be as

Ⅴ. TRANSIT TIMES

Before treatment	After treatment
T1: 11 s	T1: 14 s
T2: 21 s	T2: 20 s
T3: 24 s	T3: 32 s

Ⅵ. VESSEL WIDTH

Before treatment

	w
Artery	29.8 a.u.
Vein	70.2 a.u.

After treatment

	w'	$\frac{w'-w}{w} \times 100 = W\%$
Artery	29.6 a.u.	+ 1%
Vein	71.0 a.u.	_ 1%

Fig. 8. Central retinal vein obstruction: transit times and vessel width. T2–T1: capillary transit time; T3–T2: venous transit time; a.u.: arbitrary unit.

much higher as vascularization will be greatly improved, as can be followed on the circulatory parameters (perfusion recovery on angiographic pictures, capillary transit time shortening, coherent variations of vessels lumen width).

Prognosis
A VEP disturbance, as from the initial stage is an unfavorable prognosis element; indeed, it often demonstrates a lesion (here of ischemic origin) of the macular cells, and/or of the macular fibers bundle. In spite of a recanalization, shown in ERG, cells will remain destroyed, and therefore this explains the absence of function recovery. In this case, circulatory parameters confirm this hypothesis (angiographic aspects of the posterior pole).

Methodological level

Accuracy of measures
(a) R. In the sound right eye, in case 1, R reaches −26%. In the same way, in the sound left eye, in case 2, R reaches +13%. Lastly, in the sound left eye, in case 3, R reaches 33%. Now, in a sound eye, the theoretical value would

ⅠＴ . ELECTRORETINOGRAM

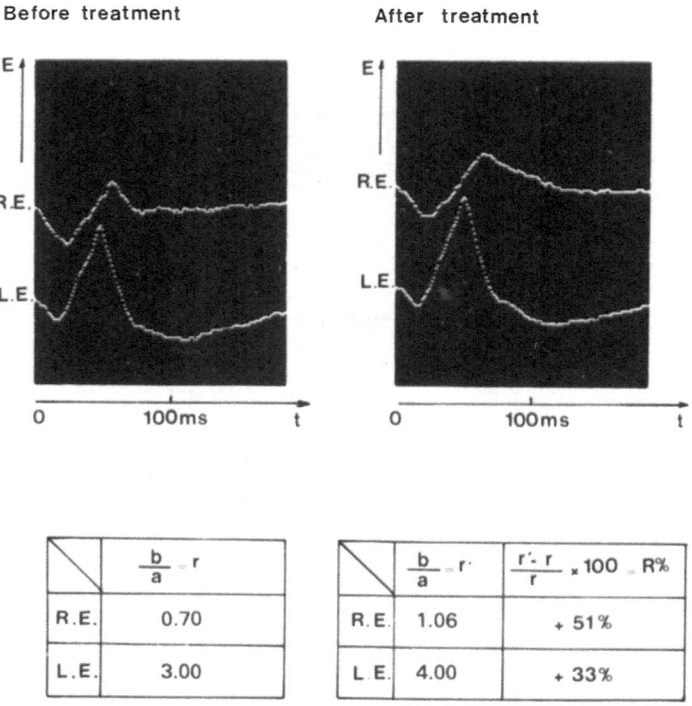

Before treatment

After treatment

	$\dfrac{b}{a} = r$
R.E.	0.70
L.E.	3.00

	$\dfrac{b}{a} = r\cdot$	$\dfrac{r\cdot - r}{r} \times 100 = R\%$
R.E.	1.06	+ 51%
L.E.	4.00	+ 33%

Fig. 9. Retinal branch vein and branch artery obstruction: electroretinogram. E: potential; t: time; R.E.: right eye; L.E.: left eye.

be 0%. In fact, the inaccuracy 1 mm range) in measurement of a- and b_1-wave amplitude can bring an absolute error in R up to 40%: R values obtained in sound eyes are hence coherent.

(b) T1, T2, T3. The frame counter inaccuracy brings in angiographic transit times a relative error up to 20%. Therefore, we shall only consider the variation when interpreting T2 − T1 capilary transit time values.

(c) W. Inaccuracy in aiming explains the uncoherent value (in the sign) observed in arterial W in case 1.

Modalities of therapy
Early treatment seems to be necessary to obtain a favorable result (case 1 and 3), however, one can not deduce this condition to be sufficient, for the efficiency of this fibrinolytic therapy postulates, *a priori*, a vascular obstruction to be due to a coagulation phenomenon (Coscas and Dhermy, 1978).

II. VISUAL EVOKED POTENTIALS

Before treatment   **After treatment**

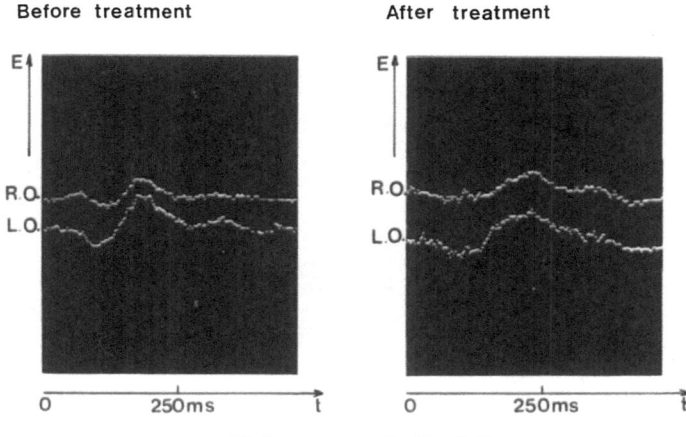

Right eye : red stimulation

III. VISUAL ACUITY

Before treatment   After treatment

R.E.: $\dfrac{1}{20}$; P.14   R.E.: $\dfrac{1}{20}$; P.10 → $\dfrac{8}{10}$; P.2

L.E.: $\dfrac{9}{10}$; P.2   L.E.: $\dfrac{9}{10}$; P.2

Fig. 10. Retinal branch vein and branch artery obstruction: visual evoked potentials and visual acuity. E: potential; t: time; R.O.: right occiput; L.O.: left occiput; R. E.: right eye; L.E.: left eye; P.: Parinaud; L.P.: light perception.

ACKNOWLEDGMENTS

We would like to express our thanks to Misses M. Maussan, S. Roux and C. Reynaud, and to Messrs J.-M. Giraud, P. Heydel and G. Rouaisnel for their friendly assistance. In addition, vessels lumen width measurements were performed in the Laboratory of corpuscular Physics (Professor D. Isabelle), University of Clermont II; and the protocol of urokinase therapy was realised by Professor J. Ponsonnaille in the Department of Cardiology (Professor H. Gras), St Jacques Hospital, University of Clermont I. Finally K. Isaacson and D. Singleton reviewed the translation.

45

IV. ANGIOGRAPHY

After treatment

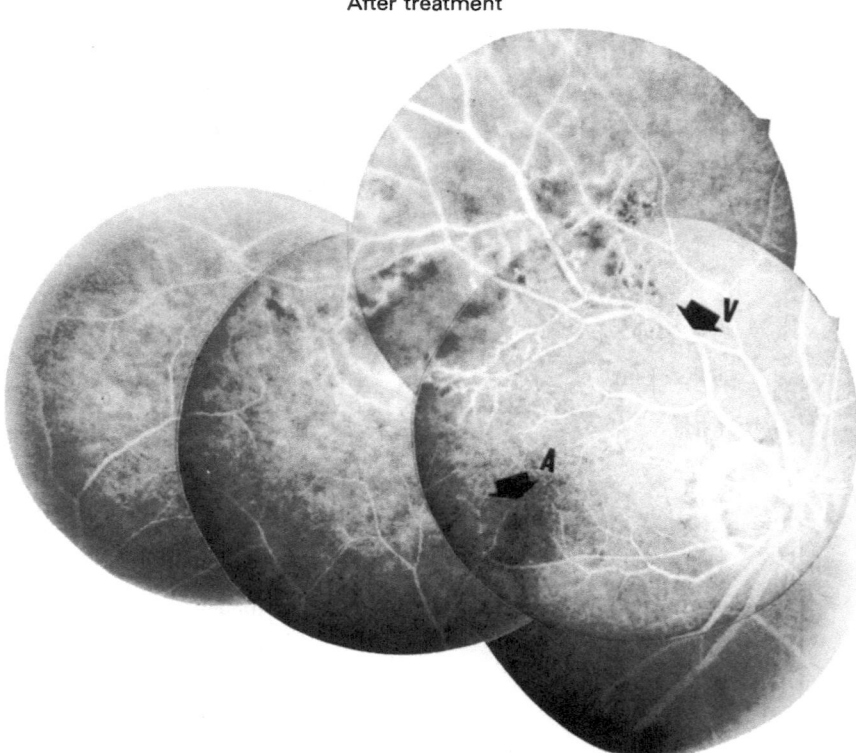

Fig. 11. Retinal branch vein and branch artery obstruction: angiography. V: venous obstruction; A: ischemic edema from arterial obstruction.

REFERENCES

Alfieri, R. & P. Solé. Exploration électrophysiologique fonctionnelle, sectorielle et stratigraphique de la fonction visuelle. *J. Fr. Biophys. Méd. Nucl.* 3: *63–75* (1979).

Brunel, J.-M. Téléchrono-angiographie fluorescéinique oculaire. Thèse de Médecine, Clermont-Ferrand, 1975.

Coscas, G. & P. Dhermy. Occlusions veineuses rétiniennes. Masson, Paris, 1978.

Flower, R.W., P. Speros & K.R. Kenyon. Electroretingographic changes and choroidal defects in a case of central retinal artery occlusion. *Am. J. Ophthalmol.* 83: *451–459* (1977).

François, J., A. De Rouck & E. Cambie. Electrophysiological aspects in retinal venous thrombosis. In: Pearlman, J.T. (ed.). 10th I.S.C.E.R.G. Symposium, Los Angeles 1972. *Doc. Ophthalmol. Proc. Series* 2: *43–56* (1973).

François, J., A. De Rouck, E. Cambie & A. Zanen. L'électro-diagnostic des affections rétiniennes (Etude des potentiels de repos et d'action rétiniens). *Bull. Soc. Belge Ophtalmol.* 166: *353–358* (1974).

Henkes, H. E. Electroretinography in circulatory disturbançes of the retina. I. Elec-

Ⅴ. TRANSIT TIMES

Before treatment	After treatment

Before treatment

T1 :   24 s

T2 $\begin{cases} \text{u.v.} : 42 \text{ s} \\ \text{l.v.} : 32 \text{ s} \end{cases}$

T3 $\begin{cases} \text{u.v.} : 55 \text{ s} \\ \text{l.v.} : 47 \text{ s} \end{cases}$

After treatment

T1 :   16 s

T2 $\begin{cases} \text{u.v.} : 26 \text{ s} \\ \text{l.v.} : 24 \text{ s} \end{cases}$

T3 $\begin{cases} \text{u.v.} : 30 \text{ s} \\ \text{l.v.} : 30 \text{ s} \end{cases}$

Ⅵ. VESSEL WIDTH

Before treatment

	w
Artery	23.4 a.u.
Vein	38.9 a.u.

After treatment

	w'	$\frac{w'-w}{w} \times 100 = W\%$
Artery	28.7 a.u.	$+23\%$
Vein	22.0 au	-43%

Fig. 12. Retinal branch vein and branch artery obstruction: transit times and vessel width. T2–T1: capillary transit time; T3–T2: venous transit time; a.u.: arbitrary unit.

troretinography in cases of occlusion of central retinal vein or one of its branches. *Arch. Ophthalmol.* 49: *190–201* (1953).

Henkes, H. E. Advances in electro-ophthalmology. Its use in retinal vascular diseases. In: Deutman, A.F. (ed.). New developments in ophthalmology, Nijmegen 1975. *Doc. Ophthalmol. Proc. Series* 7: *181–186* (1976).

Henkes, H.E. & M.K. Th. van Mierlobensteijn. Electro-ophthalmology and circulatory disturbances of retina, choroid and optic nervehead. In: François, J. (ed.). 5th Congress of the European Society of Ophthalmology, Hamburg 1976. Enke, Stuttgart, pp. 68–71, 1978.

Jayle, G.E., R.L. Boyer & J.B. Saracco. L'électrorétinographie. Bases physiologiques et données cliniques. Masson, Paris, 1965.

Letrone, S. Aspects électrophysiologiques des occlusions des branches de la veine centrale de la rétine. Thèse de Médecine, Paris Val-de-Marne, 1977.

Solé, P., R. Alfieri, F. Bacin, B. Kantelip & M. Bussière. Epithéliopathie expérimentale: corrélations anatomo-cliniques et fonctionnelles chez le lapin. In: Shimizu, K. (ed.). XXIII Concilium ophthalmologicum, Kyoto 1978. Excerpta medica, Amsterdam, vol. 2, pp. 1662–1665, 1979.

Vilaire, M. Angiographie cinématographique fluorescéinique couleur. Thèse de Médecine, Clermont-Ferrand, 1973.

Authors' addresses:
P. Solé & F. Bacin
Dept of Ophthalmology
Faculty of Medicine
P.O. Box 38
63001 Clermont-Ferrand CEDEX
France

R. Alfieri
Dept of Biomathematics
(As above)

48

Docum. Ophthal. Proc. Series, Vol. 23

ERG AND EOG IN CAROTID ARTERY OCCLUSION DISEASE

W.-D. ULRICH, CH. ULRICH, R. KÄSTNER AND J. REIMANN

(Berlin, G.D.R.)

ABSTRACT

ERG changes during occlusion of the carotid have repeatedly been reported in the literature. This paper presents typical electrophysiological findings obtained during occlusion processes in the carotid area. A comparison is made with data obtained by cerebral angiography, ophthalmodynamometry/ophthalmodynamography as well as ultrasonic Doppler measurements. The meaning of the results of ophthalmological electrodiagnostics is discussed.

INTRODUCTION

Occlusion of the carotid artery system often results in ocular ischaemia, though in different degrees; changes in the ERG, however, have been observed only in part of the cases (Kriz 1955, Krill, Diamond and Ilser 1962). Wulfing (1963), therefore, suggested an i.o. pressure load test to detect the side differences in the ERG. This procedure, which he called ERDG, was improved by the introduction of the suction cup method (Henkes, Usami and van Lith 1967; Ch. Ulrich 1970).

The object of this paper is to find out why ERG changes occur in one part of the cases of carotid artery occlusion disease, and not in the other. For this purpose, electrodiagnostic results (ERG and EOG) are compared with haemodynamic data obtained with ophthalmodynamometry (ODM), ophthalmodynamography (ODG), temporalisdynamography (TDG), Dopplersonography, and cerebral angiography.

MATERIAL AND METHODS

ERGs were taken simultaneously from both eyes using silver electrode contact lenses according to Henkes. The recordings were made by means of a multiple direct recorder (Schwarzer, Munich).

The amplifier time constant was 5.0 s, the upper frequency limit 200 Hz. The stimulator used was a stroboscope FS4 (VEB TUR, Dresden). The intensity of the light stimuli was raised in 8 steps: 0.2; 0.4; 0.6; 2; 7; 26; 50; 92 Ws. ERGs were derived in maximum mydriasis and after 30 minutes dark adaptation. The amplitudes of the a- and b-waves were measured relative to the footpoint of the a-wave.

EOGs were taken according to Arden, Barrada and Kelsey (1962), *ODM*, *ODG*, and *TDG* performed and evaluated as described in earlier papers (Ulrich, W.-D. 1976; Ulrich, Ch. 1979).

Doppler sonography was performed in some cases to establish the direction of flow in the ophthalmic artery. Our results are based on 47 cases out of 169 patients who had been examined for symptoms of cerebro-vascular insufficiency.

For each of the 47 patients, an ERG and EOG were made, and in addition to ODM and ODG, cerebral angiography was performed (*i.e.* an angiographic representation of the aortic arch and all cervico-vascular arteries). Based on the characteristic ODM, ODG, TDG and Doppler sonographic results as compared with the angiographic picture series, the respective prevailing collateral circulation could be evaluated.

RESULTS

The changes in the extracranial cerebral arteries found in the 47 patients are shown in Table 1.

Typical electrodiagnostic and haemodynamic results for stenosis or occlusion of the proximal part of the internal carotid artery with collateral circulation via the external carotid artery and reversed blood flow through the ophthalmic artery are shown in Fig. 1. In all 7 cases, a marked reduction of the ERG b-wave amplitude can be seen. The a-wave has also changed, but not so much

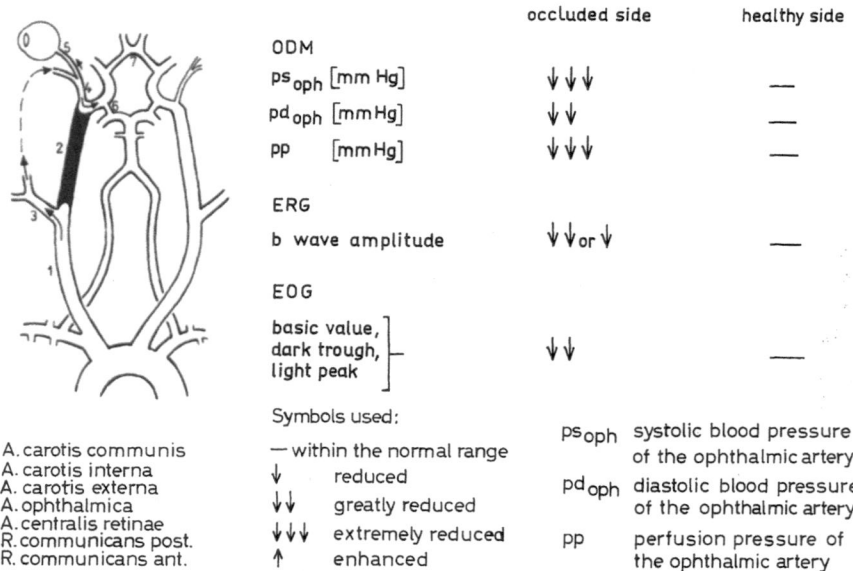

	occluded side	healthy side
ODM		
ps$_{oph}$ [mm Hg]	↓↓↓	—
pd$_{oph}$ [mmHg]	↓↓	—
pp [mmHg]	↓↓↓	—
ERG		
b wave amplitude	↓↓ or ↓	—
EOG		
basic value, dark trough, light peak	↓↓	—

1 A. carotis communis
2 A. carotis interna
3 A. carotis externa
4 A. ophthalmica
5 A. centralis retinae
6 R. communicans post.
7 R. communicans ant.

Symbols used:
— within the normal range
↓ reduced
↓↓ greatly reduced
↓↓↓ extremely reduced
↑ enhanced

ps$_{oph}$ systolic blood pressure of the ophthalmic artery
pd$_{oph}$ diastolic blood pressure of the ophthalmic artery
pp perfusion pressure of the ophthalmic artery

Fig. 1. Occlusion of the proximal part of the internal carotid artery with collateral circulation via the external carotid artery and reversed flow through the ophthalmic artery

Table 1. Summary of angiographic findings and results of ERG and EOG recordings.

	Number of cases	Results in ERG and EOG
Stenosis or occlusion of the distal part of the internal carotid artery	1	Amplitudes of the ERG a- and b-waves are unchanged
Stenosis or occlusion of the proximal internal carotid artery with collateral circulation via ophthalmic artery	7	In all cases ERG a- and b-wave amplitude and EOG amplitude diminished. EOG dark and light responses are present
Stenosis or occlusion of the proximal internal carotid artery with collateral circulation and cross flow via the anterior cerebral artery and/or via the vertebro-basilar arterial system	13	diminished ERG a- and b-waves and EOG amplitudes in 4 cases. No significant changes in 9 cases.
Stenosis or occlusion of the common carotid artery	1	ERG a- and b-wave amplitudes diminished. Low EOG-basic value, and depressed dark and light responses
Stenosis or occlusion of the brachiocephalic truncus	1	ERG a- and b-wave amplitudes diminished. Low EOG basic value, and depressed dark and light responses
Stenosis or occlusion of vertebral artery	9	No significant ERG and EOG side differences
Stenosis or occlusion of the A. subclavia with subclavian steal syndrome	1	No significant ERG and EOG side differences
Multiple stenosis and/or occlusion of the cervicovascular arteries	14	In severe cases ERG a- and b-wave amplitudes and EOG basic value extremely diminished, mostly on both sides. EOG dark and light responses depressed.

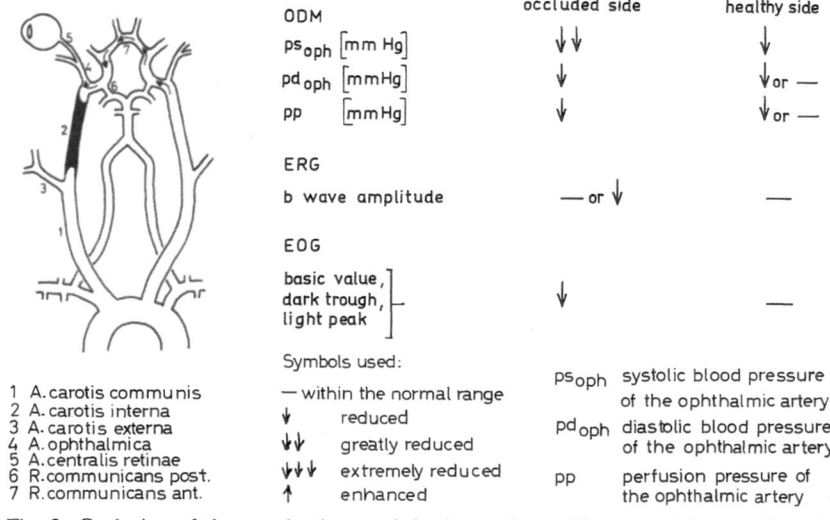

	ODM	occluded side	healthy side
	ps_{oph} [mm Hg]	↓↓	↓
	pd_{oph} [mmHg]	↓	↓ or —
	pp [mmHg]	↓	↓ or —
	ERG		
	b wave amplitude	— or ↓	—
	EOG		
	basic value, dark trough, light peak	↓	—

Symbols used:

1 A.carotis communis	— within the normal range	ps_{oph} systolic blood pressure of the ophthalmic artery
2 A.carotis interna	↓ reduced	
3 A.carotis externa	↓↓ greatly reduced	pd_{oph} diastolic blood pressure of the ophthalmic artery
4 A.ophthalmica		
5 A.centralis retinae	↓↓↓ extremely reduced	pp perfusion pressure of
6 R.communicans post.	↑ enhanced	the ophthalmic artery
7 R.communicans ant.		

Fig. 2. Occlusion of the proximal part of the internal carotid artery with cross flow via the anterior communciating artery

as the b-wave, which is more sensitive to ischaemia. In the EOG, the basic value is strongly reduced, but the EOG changes due to dark and light adaptation are maintained.

Occlusion of the proximal part of the internal carotid artery with collateral circulation through the circle of Willis and cross flow via the anterior communicating artery (Fig. 2) and/or the vertebro-basilar system will seldom yield

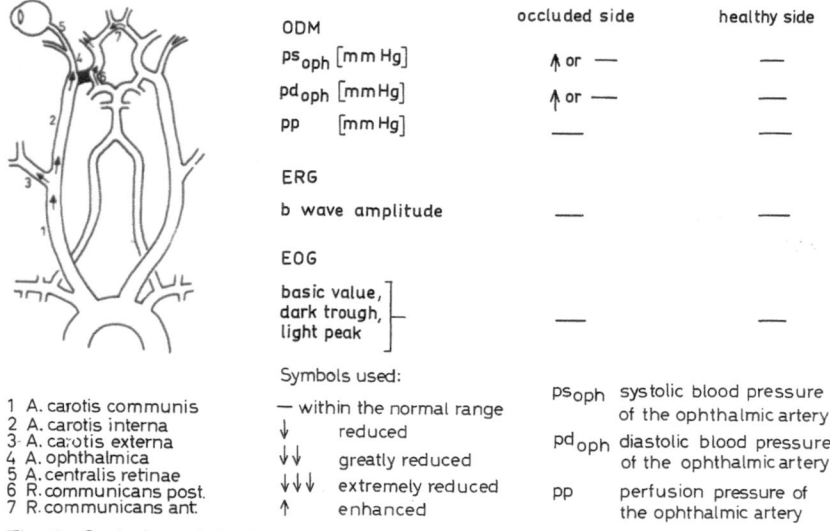

	ODM	occluded side	healthy side
	ps_{oph} [mm Hg]	↑ or —	—
	pd_{oph} [mmHg]	↑ or —	—
	pp [mmHg]	—	—
	ERG		
	b wave amplitude	—	—
	EOG		
	basic value, dark trough, light peak	—	—

Symbols used:

1 A.carotis communis	— within the normal range	ps_{oph} systolic blood pressure of the ophthalmic artery
2 A.carotis interna	↓ reduced	
3 A.carotis externa	↓↓ greatly reduced	pd_{oph} diastolic blood pressure of the ophthalmic artery
4 A.ophthalmica		
5 A.centralis retinae	↓↓↓ extremely reduced	pp perfusion pressure of
6 R.communicans post.	↑ enhanced	the ophthalmic artery
7 R.communicans ant.		

Fig. 3. Occlusion of the internal carotid artery distal to the origin of the ophthalmic artery

clearly distinguishable side differences in ERGs and EOGs. Significant ERG and EOG changes were found in only 4 cases out of 13.

Occlusion of the internal carotid artery distal to the origin of the ophthalmic artery (Fig. 3) leaves the ERG and EOG unchanged.

Stenosis or occlusion of the common carotid artery or the brachio-cephalic trunk exert a distinct influence on the ERG and EOG.

Since arteriosclerosis is a general disease of the vascular system, stenosive and occlusive processes are often bilateral and multiple. In such processes of the extracranial cerebral vessels one rarely finds any side difference in the ERG and EOGs. In severe multiple occlusion processes, however, ERG potentials and EOG basic value are often extremely reduced on both sides. Contrary to isolated occlusion processes of the carotid artery, the dark and light responses in the EOG are strongly depressed.

DISCUSSION

An important way of supplying blood from the homolateral external carotid artery to the internal carotid artery in cases of proximal occlusion of the internal carotid artery is via the collateral ophthalmic artery (Fig. 4). The

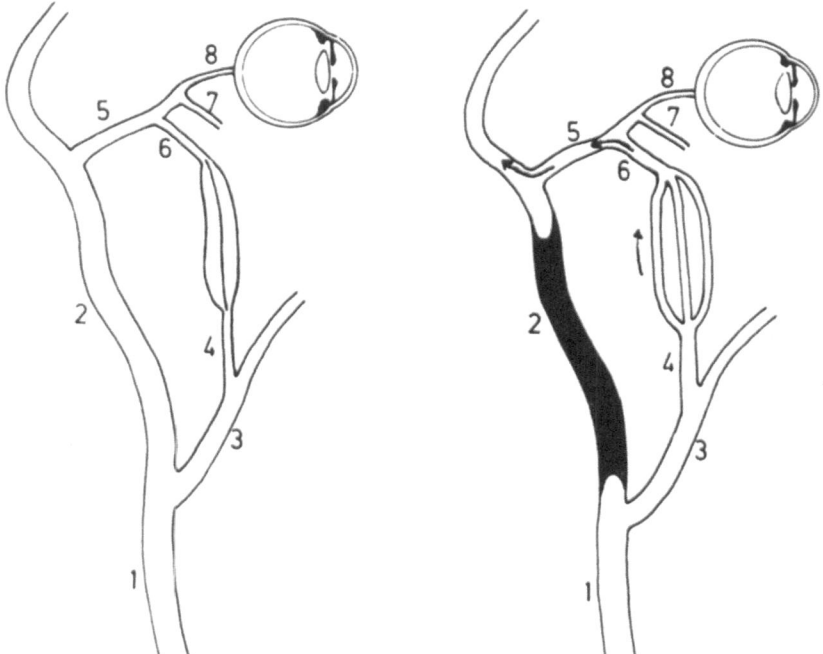

Fig. 4. Reversed flow through the ophthalmic artery in occlusion of the proximal part of the internal carotid artery. 1. A. carotis communis, 2. A. carotis interna, 3. A. carotis externa, 4. Branches of the external carotid artery with anastomoses to the ophthalmic artery, 5. A. ophthalmica, 6. Branches of the ophthalmic artery with anastomoses to the external carotid artery, 7. Branches of the ophthalmic artery without anastomoses to the external carotid artery, 8. A. centralis retinae

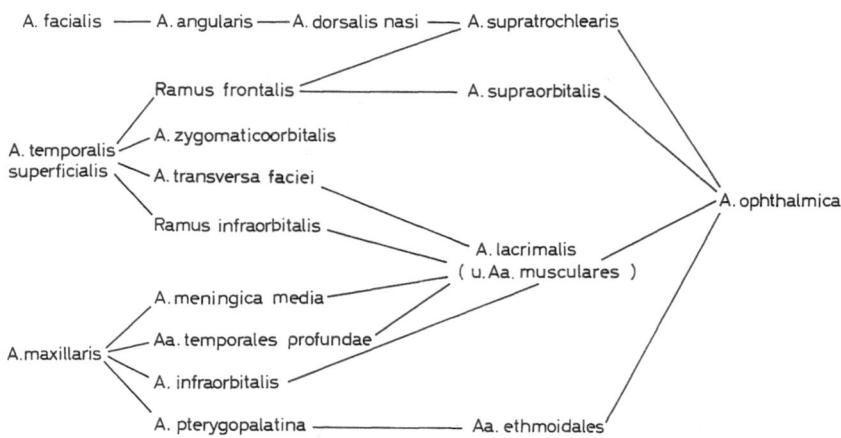

Fig. 5. The collateral anastomoses between the internal and external carotid arteries

collateral anastomoses bètween the internal and external carotid arteries (Fig. 5) are of particular importance in this respect. The external carotid artery and its dominating branch, and the ophthalmic artery become cerebral arteries. In the ophthalmic artery, the direction of blood flow is reversed, and high pressure gradients will result in a high velocity of blood flow.

Reversed direction of flow and high velocity of flow result in a haemodynamic situation which is quite unfavourable to the eye. With normal direction of flow, the central retinal artery and the ciliary arteries branch off from the ophthalmic truncus at acute angles. In the case of carotid occlusion, with the collateral ophthalmic artery still functioning, they become insignificant side branches.

1. After reversal of flow direction in the ophthalmic artery, the central retinal artery and the ciliary arteries branch off at obtuse angles to the flow direction.
2. The velocity of flow in the ophthalmic artery remains distinctly increased even after morphologic changes and widening of the vessels.
3. The ophthalmic blood pressure is greatly reduced.

Haemodynamic examination (Ulrich, Ch. 1979) shows why ERGs and EOGs are greatly reduced in cases of isolated occlusion of the internal carotid artery with circulation via the collateral ophthalmic artery and reversal of flow direction. They correspond to the greatly reduced perfusion pressure in the central retinal artery.

In cases of collateral circulation mainly via the circle of Willis, the side differences of perfusion pressure in the ophthalmic arteries are not so marked, which explains why side-different electrodiagnostic findings are rare. Occlusion of the common carotid artery and the truncus, however, affects the blood flow in the orbital region considerably and result in ERG and EOG changes. Severe multiple extracranial cerebral occlusion processes mostly reduce the ERG a- and b-waves from both eyes. The EOG also shows a reduction in the basic value and a depression of the dark and light responses from both eyes.

CONCLUSION

1. The one and only one typical electrodiagnostic finding in carotid artery occlusion disease does not exist. The electrodiagnostic results will depend, firstly, on the respective collateral circulation that has developed, and, secondly, on whether we have to do with an isolated arterial occlusion or multiple occlusive vascular processes.
2. Therefore electrodiagnostic examination by itself does not suffice to exclude the presence of an occlusive process in the carotid system.
3. If, however, the side difference in ERGs and EOGs cannot be explained otherwise, one should think of possible occlusive processes and investigate the haemodynamics of the carotid artery system using noninvasive methods such as ODM, ODG, TDG, Dopplersonography, ERDG. So ERG and EOG appear to be valuable adjuncts in the diagnosis of carotid artery occlusion disease.

REFERENCES

Henkes, H.E. und G.H.M. van Lith. Flicker-Electro-Retino-Dynamography. Sixth ISCERG-Symp., Erfurt, 1967. In: Advances in Electro-physiology and -pathology of the visual System. VEB Georg Thieme Verlag, Leipzig p. 391, 1968.

Henkes, H.E. & E. Usami. The clinical application of Flicker-Electro-Retino-Dynamography. *Jap. J. Ophth.* 12: 2 (1968).

Krill, A.E., M. Diamond & G. Isler. The electroretinogram in carotid artery disease. *A. M. A. Arch. Ophth.* 68: *42–51* (1962).

Kriz, K. Vyznam elektroretinografie pri trombose arteria carotis interna. *Cesk. Ofth.* 11: *307–311* (1955).

Ulrich, Ch. 1970. in Ulrich, W.-D.: Grundlagen und Methodik der Ophthalmo-dynamometrie, Ophthalmodynamographie, Temporalisdynamographie. Abhandlungen aus dem Gebiete der Augenheilkunde, Sammlung von Monographien, Band 44, VEB Georg Thieme Verlag, Leipzig, 1976.

Ulrich, Ch. Klinik und Praxis der Ophthalmodynamometrie, Ophthalmodynamographie, Temporalisdynamographie. Ein Beitrag zur neuroophthalmologischen Kreislaufdiagnostik. Abhandlungen aus dem Gebiete der Augenheilkunde, Sammlung von Monographien, Band 46, VEB Georg Thieme Verlag, Leipzig, 1980.

Ulrich, W.-D. Grundlagen und Methodik der Ophthalmodynamometrie, Ophthalmodynamographie, Temporalisdynamographie. Abhandlungen aus dem Gebiete der Augenheilkunde, Sammlung von Monographien, Band 44, VEB Georg Thieme Verlag, Leipzig, 1976.

Wulfing, B. Clinical Electro Retino Dynamography. A Diagnostic Aid in Occlusive Carotid Artery Disease. *Acta Ophthalmologica* (Kbh.) 73 (1963).

Author's address:
Dr. sc. med. W.-D. Ulrich
Abteilung für Elektrophysiologie und Elektrodiagnostik
Augenklinik-Charité der Humboldt-Universität zu Berlin
Ziegelstraße 5/12
DDR-104 Berlin

Docum. Ophthal. Proc. Series, Vol. 23

ELECTRORETINOGRAPHIC FINDINGS IN RETINAL VASCULAR OBSTRUCTIONS

J. EICHLER AND J. STAVE

(*Rostock, G.D.R.*)

ABSTRACT

Fifty patients (aged 23 to 75 years) affected with retinal vein occlusion were examined. The ERG has been studied by comparing affected and unaffected eyes in the course of recovery. During the time of observation the a-wave amplitude of the unaffected eye has slightly increased while that of the affected one has decreased to some extent on the average. This behaviour became more obvious in the b-wave amplitudes. No agreement between the clinical course and the ERG could be stated. The authors discuss some facilities which are helpful to improve the results.

Eighteen years ago – on the occasion of the 1st ISCERG symposium held in Stockholm – Karpe and Germanis reported in an extensive study on the prognostic value of the electroretinogram in cases of retinal vein occlusion.

Our investigations follows up the course of the electroretinogram in this disease and give an answer to the question concerning the prognostic value.

Whereas the retinal damage in cases of retinal artery occlusions, that is to say the complete central artery obstruction in their electrophysiological correlation, can be determined comparatively accurately, the problem involved in vein occlusion, however, is by far more complex for the evaluation of the results obtained. According to the expansion, dimension and localisation of the obstruction the damage to the retinal elements, and the success obtained in the recovery might vary widely. In general it is to be expected that the damage occurred has mainly affected the inner layers of the retina due to an insufficient retinal circulation. From this it can be deduced that in the electroretinogram the a-wave is reduced, the b-wave and the oscillatory potentials are much more affected.

In addition, the clinical course and electroretinographic characteristics are of complex correlation because the clinical success of recovery, in general, is expressed by visual acuity, the latter being dependent on a fairly small retinal area. Accordingly, the routine ERG is an inadequate aid inasmuch as their is no isolation of phototic and scotopic potentials unless a local ERG is used.

MATERIALS AND METHODS

Fifty patients (aged 23 to 75) affected with retinal vein occlusion were examined. There were 21 men and 20 women. In 23 cases a central vein occlusion (CVO) and in 27 cases a branch vein occlusion (VBO) happened to take place. Only those patients were chosen whose unaffected eyes were being considered healthy.

On the occasion of the first clinical examination the recording of the ERG was carried out, then again after 1 month and again after 6 months, and repeatedly in a great number of these cases. At the time of the first clinical examination the occlusion on the average lasted 23 days (minimum 1 day, maximum 6 months). All patients had been treated with vasoprotective drugs, corticosteroids or photocoagulation.

The first ERG was recorded after dark adaptation of 20 minutes. The stimulator used by us was a xeon-flash-lamp (white light at a different intensity ranging from 0.2 to 2.0 J). Recently, we have applied the ganzfeld stimulation in order to isolate scotopic and photopic potentials (in blue light stimulation of from 0.01 to 1.0 J), and in red light (0.4 to 10.0 J) after blue preadaptation.

The a- and b-waves were measured starting out from the iso-electric line, the results of the disordered eyes were compared to those eyes that can be considered healthy.

RESULTS

In Fig. 1 the average percentages in the comparison of the a-wave of affected and unaffected eyes are represented. As expected, there is no statistically significant difference of amplitudes within the different intensity ranges. However, during the time of observation it became apparent that the amplitude of the unaffected eye has slightly increased while that of the affected one was somewhat decreasing.

Figure 2 shows the behaviour of the b-wave amplitude. Here the differences in the comparison made become more distinct. In all ranges of intensity the

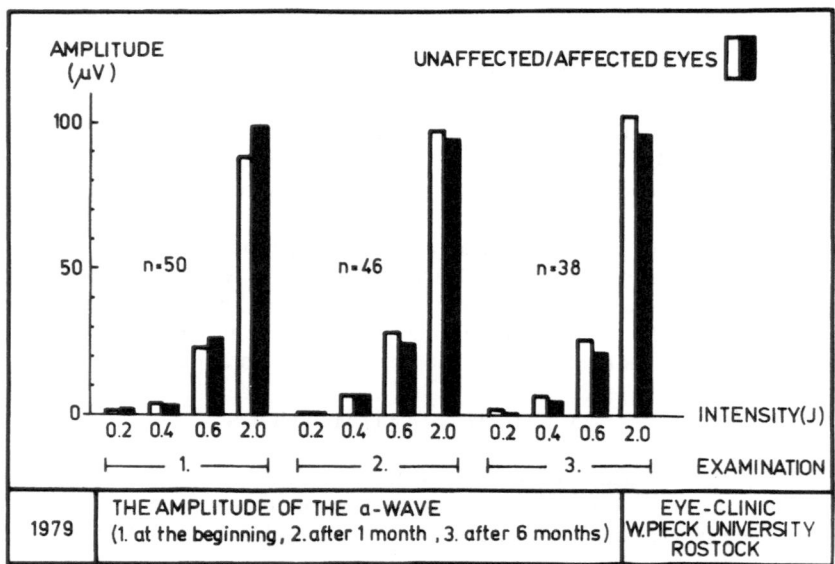

Fig. 1

58

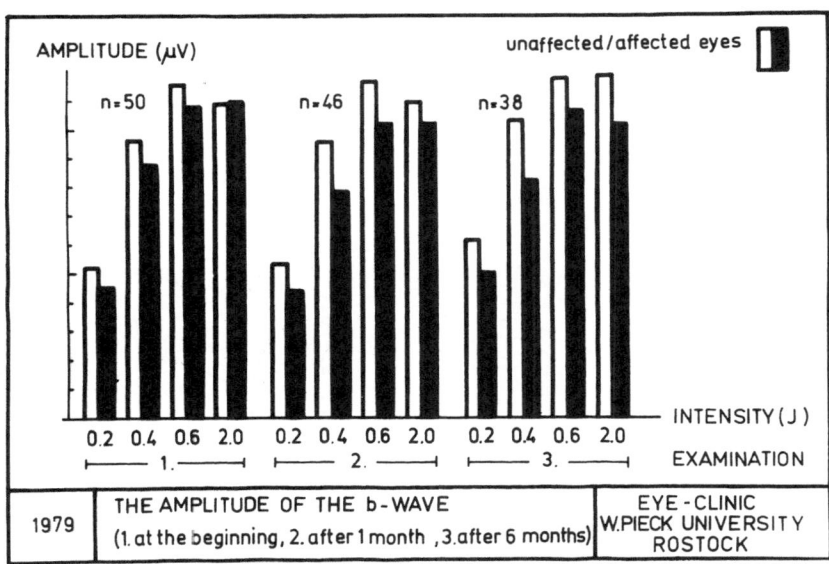

Fig. 2

amplitude of the affected eye is below that of the unaffected one. In some cases there are statistically significant differences.

Figure 3 represents the comparison made between the two eyes, and shows the course of the averaged a- and b-wave amplitudes at the time of observation. The potentials of the healthy eyes are points of reference (= 100 p.c.).

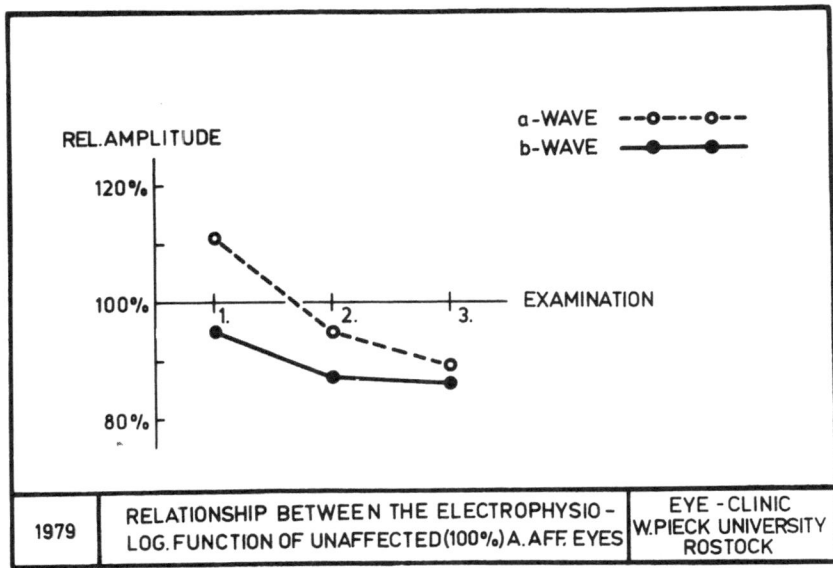

Fig. 3

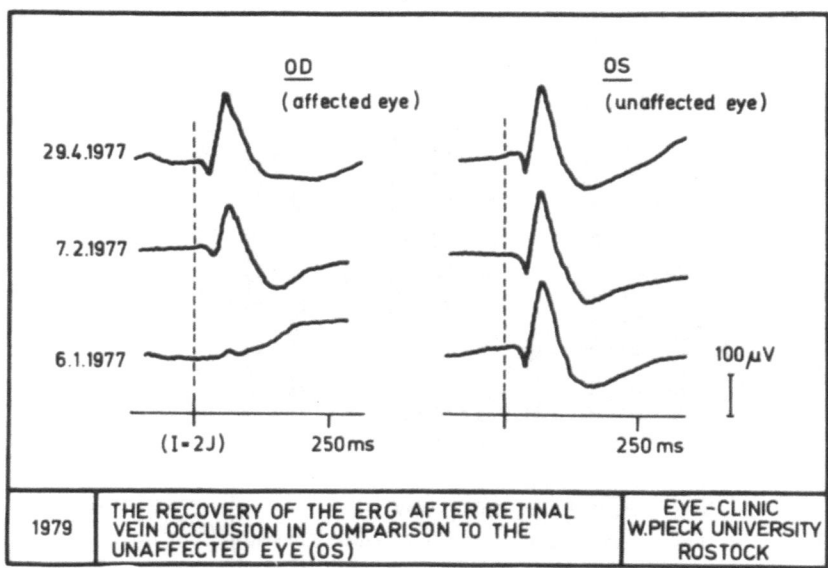

| OD | OS |
| (affected eye) | (unaffected eye) |

29.4.1977

7.2.1977

6.1.1977

100 μV

(I-2J)   250 ms   250 ms

| 1979 | THE RECOVERY OF THE ERG AFTER RETINAL VEIN OCCLUSION IN COMPARISON TO THE UNAFFECTED EYE (OS) | EYE-CLINIC W.PIECK UNIVERSITY ROSTOCK |

Fig. 4

Figure 4 represents the original recordings. On the left side first the extinguished ERG of the affected eye and then the recovery almost brought to an end are shown. The functional findings were unvarying during the whole period of observation at a visual acuity of 0.3 – which is an absolute contradiction.

DISCUSSION

By application of the ERG it is almost impossible or even doubtful that a clinical prognosis can be made in the course of retinal venous occlusion as this is evidenced by our results. In viewing all our cases, no agreement between the clinical course and the ERG can be stated. The last figure gives the extreme values.

The causes that make a prognosis of vein occlusion so difficult, when investigating electrophysiologically, are as follows:

1st. The highly intra- and interindividual variation of the human ERG, though the conditions of recording are constant.

2nd. The examination of the visual acuity as a test of therapeutical success. Logic, but practically not feasible, would be the comparison between an exact, quantitative perimetry of the overall retina and the ERG in terms of an electrophysiological correlation.

By isolating certain components of the ERG, especially when using the local ERG, the photopic ERG and the oscillatory potentials, the facilities would have been improved to a fairly high degree. The test has been changed now to the effect that the photopic ERG and the oscillatory potentials could be evaluated by far better. In our investigation, described above, we did not dispose of these facilities.

REFERENCE

Karpe, G. & M. Germanis. The prognostic value of the electroretinogram in thrombosis of the retinal veins. *Acta Ophthal.* (Kbh.), Suppl. 70; *202–229*, (1962).

Author's address:
Dr. J. Eichler
Augenklinik der Wilhelm-Pieck-Universität Rostock
Doberaner Str. 140
DDR-25 Rostock
German Democratic Republic

Docum. Ophthal. Proc. Series, Vol. 23

ELECTRORETINOGRAPHY AND CHRONOPERIMETRY IN TREATMENT OF DIABETIC RETINOPATHY BY DRUGS AND LIGHT COAGULATION

H.J. NEMTSEEV, N.A. MIKHAILOVA, N.V. MAKARSKAYA, L.A. KATSNELSON, T.I. FOROFONOVA AND G.F. SABAEVA
(*Moscow, U.S.S.R.*)

ABSTRACT

Express dynamic electroretinography (EDERG) and chronoperimetry (CP) were performed before and after the treatment in patients at a proliferative stage of diabetic retinopathy. Laser coagulation or Peritol therapy were used in the treatment. Since the therapeutic effect was found in relation to the ERG type, the authors concluded that ERG might help in prognosis and in the selection of the therapy methods.

Laser coagulation is frequently used in the treatment of diabetic retinopathy. Recently, medicamentous treatment with serotonin antagonists (Peritol, EGYT, Hungary) was initiated, for in this disease excessive accumulation of serotonin takes place on the retina (Quickel, 1971). As can be read from the relevant publications, the ERG amplitude after laser coagulation is reduced. The influence of limited laser coagulation on the functional state of retinal regions, not previously submitted to coagulation and on the optic nerve fibers conduction is not clear, the same as the beneficial effect of laser coagulation in diabetic retinopathy (Apple *et al.*, 1976). And there is still little known about the influence of the antiserotonin line of drugs such as Peritol. In this paper we shall try to answer these questions with the help of some new adequate methods of investigation.

METHODS

In order to evaluate the effect of both laser coagulation and Peritol in the treatment of diabetic retinopathy it is necessary to apply functional tests, selectively sensitive to changes in retinal blood circulation and nerve fiber conduction. Such tests, previously developed, were express dynamic electroretinography (EDERG) and chronoperimetry (CP).

Express dynamic electroretinography, other than the one-time routine ERG registration, is a repeated scotopic ERG record, 7–8 times at an interval of 3 seconds and at a relatively high stimulus intensity – 36 J (Nemtseev, 1974). It was found that "a" and "b" ERG wave amplitudes change in response to repeated light stimulation other than in one-time ERG recording, especially in retinal blood circulation disorders.

Chronoperimetry (Nemtseev, 1973) is a simultaneous testing of both the visual field boundary lines and visual motor reaction time at these boundary lines. This is provided by automatically moving the target at constant and known speed from the visual field center towards the periphery and vice versa with the later determination of reaction time by the difference between boundary line markings. It helps locally determining the first preclinical stage of optic nerve parabiosis – delayed conduction – even though visual field boundary lines remain still normal, *i.e.* due to the prolonged reaction time. This stage was already determined in electrophysiologic studies. In 1967, at the 6th ISCERG symposium, we mentioned, that in patients with optic nerve diseases retino-cortical time prolongation may be determined prior to visual function disorders, and in this case it indicates the first symptom of the disease. At a later date it was confirmed by other authors (Halliday *et al.*, 1972; Huber, 1978; Ikeda *et al.*, 1978). We, however, decided for CP in this study, as it permits to test locally visual field areas in the periphery of from 30 to 60°, which can hardly be accomplished in electrophysiologic retino-cortical time determination. CP was done under photopic conditions (the background bowl luminance 14 nt) with II/3 object in 12 meridians.

RESULTS

EDERG and CP were performed before and after the treatment in patients at a proliferative stage of diabetic retinopathy (45 observations). The patients were grouped in two, one of the groups was treated by laser coagulation (25 observations), the other one by Peritol (20 observations). EDERG and CP were done a day before/after laser coagulation or a day before/after the beginning or termination of the Peritol treatment. Coagulation, mainly paravenous and sectorial, was performed by an argon laser on limited retinal regions (10–30% of the surface, mean 400 burns). 4 mg of Peritol were given 4 times a day, the whole course lasting from 1 to 3 months.

Before the treatment in the EDERG recording wave amplitude, especially "b", appeared to be reduced as compared to normal values after the first and subsequent stimuli (amplitudes were measured from the isoelectric line). As a result, the ERG, on the whole, approached a negative form, especially after the first stimulus, when the mean difference "b-a" was negative (wave "a" amplitude was higher in value, than that if "b" in 43.9% of the patients). In subsequent flashes "b-a" almost remained unchanged; in the norm, however, the amplitude increases (Table 1). This amplitude indicates insufficiency in retinal blood circulation (Nemtseev, 1974). In CP studies we noticed constriction of the visual field from the temporal side by 12° on the average and visual motor reaction time prolongation mainly on these boundary lines by 87% as compared to the norm.

On the whole, after the treatment of diabetic retinopathy patients with Peritol the wave "b" amplitude did not substantially change, remaining reduced, but dynamics of wave amplitude changes approached the norm in repeated stimulation. Wave "a" amplitude decreased. As a result, the ratio of b:a amplitude was: in healthy persons 1.21; in diabetic retinopathy patients before Peritol treatment 1.09, after – 1.52. Thus minus-negative ERG type became subnormal after the treatment (Table 1). Positive effect (visual field improvement) was noticed in 58.3%, negative – in 33.3%, uncertain – in 8.4%.

Table 1. Express dynamic ERG data in healthy persons and diabetic retinopathy patients before and after the Peritol treatment and laser coagulation (mean amplitude values in mcv).

ERG wave	Group	Number of stimuli							
		1	2	3	4	5	6	7	8
a	healthy persons	171	123	121	115	113	116	115	109
	before Peritol treatment	104	91	96	85	82	91	93	78
	after Peritol treatment	82	52	62	71	71	62	73	54
	before laser-coagulation	137	108	103	98	101	95	97	93
	after laser-coagulation	125	102	91	99	97	93	98	103
b	healthy persons	207	174	180	192	196	197	199	194
	before Peritol treatment	113	128	127	124	114	141	126	171
	after Peritol treatment	125	129	120	115	107	110	121	122
	before laser-coagulation	118	158	137	132	138	128	140	109
	after laser-coagulation	109	140	122	120	124	135	122	129

The positive effect was noticed mainly in patients with a positive ERG type (mean b:a ratio 1.16), negative mainly in negative ERG type (mean b:a ratio 0.71). Visual field boundary lines and reaction time relative to such variables showed no substantial changes on the whole.

After laser coagulation within the restricted areas of retina (10–30% of the surface) the patients suffering from diabetic retinopathy have shown reduction in the ERG amplitude – wave "b" from 57% to 52%, wave "a" from 80% to 73% of the norm. The b:a ratio did not change, so that after laser coagulation we mainly observed the negative ERG type. Wave "a" and "b" amplitudes did not show any noticeable changes in repeated stimulation (Table 1). Positive effect (visual field improvement) was observed in 31.6%, negative – in 36.9%, uncertain – in 31.5%. A positive effect was noticed mainly in patients with the negative ERG type (mean b:a ratio 0.96), negative (deterioration) and uncertain effects – in patients with positive ERG type (mean b:a ratio 1.29 and 1.32 accordingly). On the whole, the mean value of the visual field boundary line and visual motor reaction time did not substantially change.

DISCUSSION AND CONCLUSION

In patients with diabetic retinopathy we observed ERG amplitude reduction. In many of them the ERG has approached the negative type. In repeated stimulation "b-a" difference did not increase, which also points to insufficient retinal blood circulation. Constriction of the visual field and visual motor reaction time prolongation on these boundary lines, mainly from the temporal side denote a higher frequency of diabetic neuropathies, than this is presumed in general.

The positive effect (visual field improvement) in laser coagulation only in patients with the negative ERG type and in Peritol treatment–only in patients at a mainly normal b : a ratio,–denote that these methods of therapy have different mechanisms. It gives hope that ERG will help in prognosis and in the selection of the therapy methods.

The limited argon laser coagulation and peritol treatment do not affect substantially optic nerve fibers conduction.

REFERENCES

Apple, D, G. Wyhinny & M. Goldberg. Experimental argon laser photocoagulation. I. Effects in retinal nerve fiber layer. *Arch. Ophth.* (Chicago). 94: N I, *137–147* (1976).

Halliday, A., W. McDonald & J. Mushin. Delayed visual evoked responses in optic neuritis. *Lancet.* VI: *982* (1972).

Huber, C. Stimulation, spezifische V.E.R.-Untersuchungen in der Klinik. *Klin. Mbl. Augenheilk.* 172: *496–499* (1978).

Ikeda, H., K. Tremain & M. Sanders. Neurophysiological investigation in optic nerve disease; combined assessment of the visual evoked response and electroretinogram. *Brit. J. Ophthalmol.* 62: *227–239* (1978).

Nemtseev, H.J. Chronoperimetry – The new test for the visual functions explorations. Proc. 4th Congress Opthalmol. of USSR, Kiev (pp. 126–129), 1973 (in Russian).

Nemtseev, H.J. Express dynamic electroretinography in retinal blood circulation disorders. 2nd Conf. on use of the electrophysiological tests in opthalmology. Abstracts of papers, Moscow (pp. 120–124), 1974 (in Russian).

Nemtseev, H.J. Diagnostic significance of retino-cortical time and optic perception time in the optic nerve diseases. In: Schmöger, E. (ed.) Advances in electrophysiology and -pathology of the visual system. Proc. 6th ISCERG Symposium 1967. Georg Thieme, Leipzig. (pp. 179–186), 1968.

Quickel, K. Enhasement of insulin secretion in adult onset diabetes by methysergide maleate. *J. Clin. Endorcrinol. Metabol.* 33: *877–881* (1971).

Author's address:
H.J. Nemtseev, M.D.
Helmholtz Institute of Ophthalmology
Sadovo-Chernogriasskaya 14/19
103064 Moscow
USSR

Docum. Ophthal. Proc. Series, Vol. 23

ERGs IN STREPTOZOTOCIN-DIABETIC RATS UNDER DIFFERENT INSULIN REGIMENS*

L.G. DENEAULT, W.M. KOZAK AND T.S. DANOWSKI

(*Pittsburgh, Pa., U.S.A.*)

ABSTRACT

It is generally hoped but not proved that good control of diabetes mellitus will delay the onset or stay the progression of diabetic retinopathy (DR). In order to obtain a better insight into this problem, we have tested the effects of different insulin injection regimens upon the development of retinopathy in Streptozotocin-diabetic female albino rats. Electroretinograms (ERGs) which are known to change in DR, were tested every two weeks in four groups of rats: 1. Normals; 2. Diabetic, no treatment; 3. Diabetic, treated with once-a-day injections of regular insulin, 10 units/kilogram (u/kg) body weight; and 4. Diabetic, treated with three 3.3 u/kg insulin injections every eight hours. Blood glucose, urine glucose and ketone levels, body weight and water intake were measured in all groups every two weeks. Animals were kept in semi-darkness, with food and water *ad libitum*. During four months following Streptozotocin injections in groups 2.–4., the diabetic (No. 2) no-insulin group behaved similarly to the diabetic (No. 3) once-a-day group of rats with respect to various ERG parameters and to other bodily assays. The normal (No. 1) and the thrice-a-day (No. 4) groups behaved similarly, with respect to both the ERG parameters and other assays. There were, however, highly statistically-significant (p < 0.001) differences between the joint No. 2 and No. 3 groups on the one hand, and the joint No. 1 and No. 4 groups, on the other. In conclusion, the multiple-dose daily insulin therapy is far superior to the conventional therapy. A correlation of these results with the ongoing clinical trial of multiple-dose insulin therapy in human patients is discussed.

INTRODUCTION

There are strong indications that Electroretinograms (ERGs) can serve as a prognostic tool in early detection of diabetic retinopathy. Thus, Simonsen (1968, 1969, 1974), Kojima *et al.* (1966), Wang and Heath (1968), Ohtsubo (1970) and Yonemura *et al.* (1972) have shown that ERG changes precede visible microangiopathy of the retina. On the other hand, there are strong arguments for the beneficial effects of good control of blood glucose levels on diabetic microangiopathy including retinopathy (Bloodworth and Engerman, 1973; Mauer *et al.*, 1975; Job *et al.*, 1976; Cahill *et al.*, 1976a, b; Buzney *et al.*, 1977).

A direct action, or lack thereof, of insulin on the electrical properties of the retinal cell membranes (Honda, 1971; Kozak *et al.*, 1979; Abel and Kozak, 1979) may be responsible for the ERG changes in diabetic retinopathy.

* Supported by the Juvenile Diabetes Foundation.

67

There exist objections to the contention that good control of blood glucose will prevent the development of the diabetic vascular disease (Siperstein et al., 1977).

In the present paper we have tested the hypothesis that a precise control of diabetes mellitus by multiple-daily injections of regular insulin will defer or minimize the development of diabetic retinopathy as tested by electroretinography.

MATERIALS AND METHODS

Forty eight female albino rats (Wistar), about 260 g body weight, were randomly assigned to four groups of twelve animals each: 1. Normal, and 2., 3., 4. – Diabetic. The animals of the three latter groups were rendered diabetic by intravenous injections of Streptozotocin (Upjohn, 70 mg/kg), freshly prepared according to the manufacturers' stipulations. The diabetic animals of group 2. were not treated at all. Group 3. rats received regular insulin (Lilly, 10 u/kg) subcutaneously once-a-day, using the Lo-dose 0.5 ml syringes. The treatment started 24 hrs after Streptozotocin injections. Group 4. rats received the same average daily dose of insulin (10 u/kg) as the group 3. rats, but divided into three equal doses injected once every eight hrs. All rats (groups 1.–4.) were maintained in semi-darkness and fed ordinary rat food (Wayne Lab-Blox) and water ad libitum. Their body weight, water intake, blood and urine glucose, urine ketones and electroretinograms were tested every two weeks. Blood glucose was assayed in capillary blood using the Eyetone Reflectance Meter (Ames Co.). Urine glucose and ketone bodies were assayed by the Ames Keto-Diastix methods in freshly collected urine.

Electroretinograms were recorded in dark-adapted (1 hr.) animals under light ether anesthesia, after pupillary dilation with ophthalmic Atropine and 2.5% Neosynephrine and corneal anesthesia by Proparacaine 0.5%. Cotton wick–platinum wire corneal electrode and platinum wire formed into an eyelid retractor were used for ERG recording. The animal and a battery-operated preamplifier (Grass P 15B) were placed inside of a shielded enclosure. Flashes from a Grass PS-2 Photostimulator were delivered every 1 min. via a ULGM-5 fiber optics cable (American Optical). The electrode and eyelid rectractor assembly was attached to the end of the fiber optics cable to provide standardized conditions for recording while illuminating the retina along the eye's optic axis. The variability between single ERG waveforms taken from the one animal was within 1%, and variability between animals of the same group was typically 5%. Statistical significance of differences between means of various parameters tested was evaluated using the two-tail t-test.

The ERG waveforms were amplified 1000X using a band pass of 0.3–1000 Hz and subsequently stored on FM magnetic tape (Bell & Howell VR-6400) together with a synchronous flash signal and verbal description. The waveforms were analysed off-line on a Nova 830 (Data General) computer. Four consecutive ERGs obtained under identical conditions were digitized (12 bit at 1000 Hz) and averaged in time domain. Subsequently, a smooth curve was fitted to the ERG b-wave using a polynomial-fitting program (Kozak et al., 1979). The initial fifth-degree polynomial was fitted between the lowest point of the a-wave and the middle of the rising slope of the b-wave. A second 5th degree polynomial was fitted to the remaining part of the b-wave. Then the combined a- and b-waves were subtracted from the original averaged ERG waveform in order to obtain the wavelets (oscillatory potentials) in separation. The average amplitudes and latencies of the principal ERG components were subsequently calculated.

RESULTS

The *weight* of normal rats progressively increased from about 260 g to about 380 g in four months. The group 4. rats (3X-a-day-insulin), after an initial post-Streptozotocin weight loss by an average of -10 g, have resumed their growth at about the same rate as normals. Four months later, they did not significantly differ from normals. The rats of groups 2. and 3. had lost weight within two weeks after Streptozotocin (average -48 g) and maintained a steady weight for two months thereafter. A month later both these groups had increased their weights by an average $+13$ g (Fig. 1).

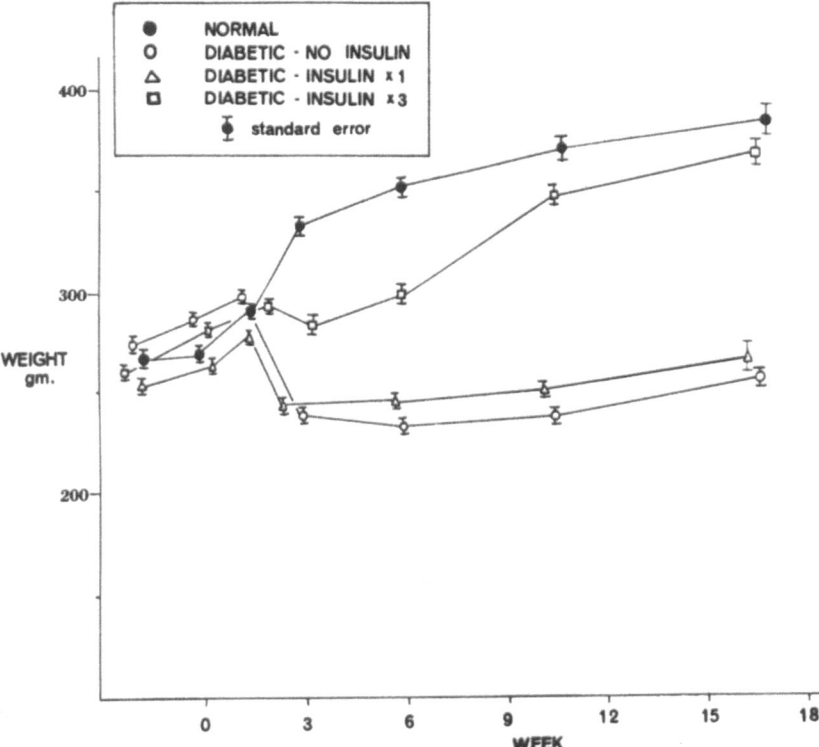

Fig. 1. Body weight of rats before and after injections of Streptozotocin. The difference between the larger categories (normals and diabetics injected 3X a-day, versus diabetics treated 1X a-day or not treated at all) is significant by t-test ($p < 0.001$) from the tenth post-Streptozotocin week onwards.

The *blood glucose* levels had increased to over 500 mg% following Strep-tozotocin in all diabetic groups (2., 3. and 4.). Three months later, these levels were still over 500 mg% in groups 2. and 3., whereas the blood glucose level has slowly decreased to 190 mg% in group 4. rats (3X-a-day-insulin) and continues to decrease. Normal rats (group 1.) have maintained their glucose levels close to 90 mg% (Fig. 2).

The *urine glucose* levels had increased to 1000–2000 mg% in all diabetic rat groups during the first month following Streptozotocin. Subsequently, in group

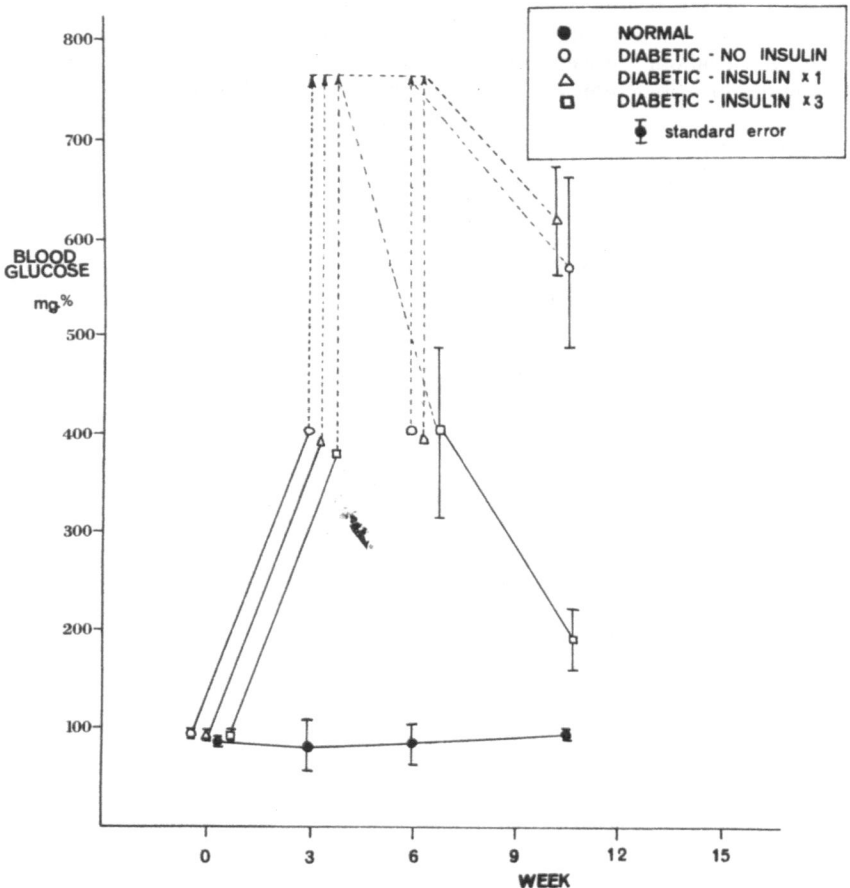

Fig. 2. Blood glucose levels of rats before and after Streptozotocin. The blood glucose increased about 7-fold in all diabetic groups. Three months later, the no-insulin and the 1X a-day insulin rats still had very high, and virtually identical, blood glucose levels. The thrice-a-day-insulin rats showed a marked decrease of blood glucose in comparison with the once-a-day-insulin rats. The difference between these groups was significant by t-test (p < 0.001). The dashed arrows indicate that the levels exceeded the range of the measuring instrument.

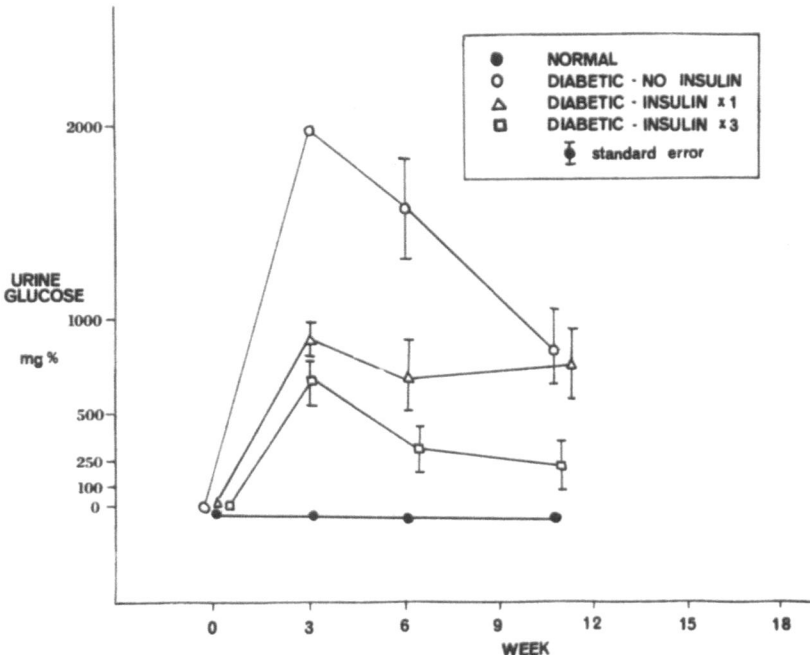

Fig. 3. Urine glucose levels of rats before and after Streptozotocin. Three months after injections, the no-insulin and the once-a-day-insulin rats had identical urine glucose levels, statistically higher than the thrice-a-day-insulin rats (t-test, $p < 0.001$).

2. and 3. rats, these levels have dropped somewhat and are maintained at about 800 mg% level. On the other hand, the urine glucose has either disappeared altogether, or has been maintained at a low (0–250 mg%) level in the group 4. rats (Fig. 3).

The *ketone bodies* had initially appeared in the urine of all diabetic rat groups (+ or ++ by the Keto-Diastix method). Subsequently, they have disappeared from the urine of group 4. rats within six weeks. Some rats with severe ketonuria had died within 1 to 12 weeks following Streptozotocin.

Water intake has sharply increased in all diabetic rat groups from about 20 ml/12 hrs. up to about 120 ml/12 hrs. It has remained to be that high in groups 2. and 3. However, in group 4. rats the water intake has since decreased to about 70 ml/12 hrs. and tends to decrease further.

The *Electroretinograms* underwent characteristic changes. In normals and in group 4. diabetic rats, the ERG *amplitudes* had initially increased by about 200 μV and have remained high. The ERG *latencies*, as measured from the flash to the intersection of the b-wave with the iso-electric line, have shortened by about 3.5 ms and have remained so. On the contrary, in the diabetic rat groups 2. and 3., the ERG amplitudes decreased by about 100 μV and the ERG latencies had initially increased by about 3 ms and, subsequently, have been maintained at that level. At the end of the three-month period, there

71

were no significant differences between the normal group and the diabetic group 4. (3X-a-day insulin). No significant differences were observed at the same time between the rat groups 2. and 3. either. However, the differences between these two combined categories are highly statistically significant (Figs. 4 and 5). Figures 6 and 7 show examples of computer-processed ERGs of four rats: A, B, C and D. Rats A and B (Fig. 6) belong to group 4., whereas rats C and D (Fig. 7) belong to group 3. The ERGs marked A, B, C, D were taken prior to Streptozotocin, and ERGs marked a, b, c, d were recorded three months after Streptozotocin. We can notice that there are very small differences between the ERGs of group 4. rats (A vs. a; B vs. b) before and after Streptozotocin. Similar results (not shown) were obtained with normal rats.

On the other hand, the differences between ERGs of group 3. rats (C vs. c; D vs. d) are quite obvious: the latencies (lengths of dashed lines) are longer, and the amplitudes of the wavelets, shown on the right side, are smaller after

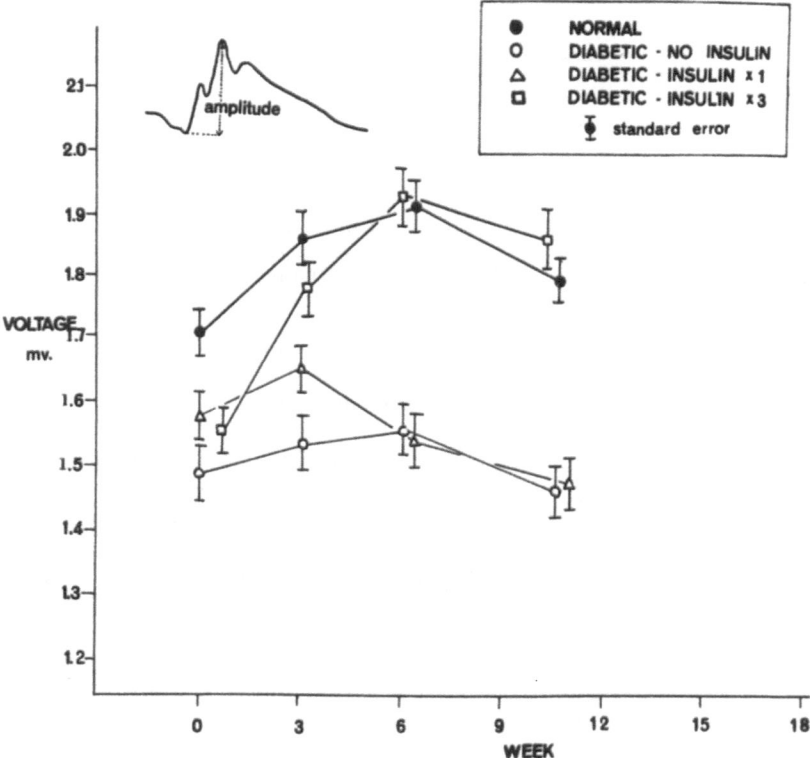

Fig. 4. Electroretinogram amplitudes of rats before and after Streptozotocin. The peak-to-peak ERG amplitudes (see inset) were virtually the same in the normal and in the 3X a-day-insulin groups. However, the no-insulin and the 1X a-day-insulin rats had significantly (t-test, $p < 0.02$) lower ERG amplitudes, starting from the 6th week after Streptozotocin injections.

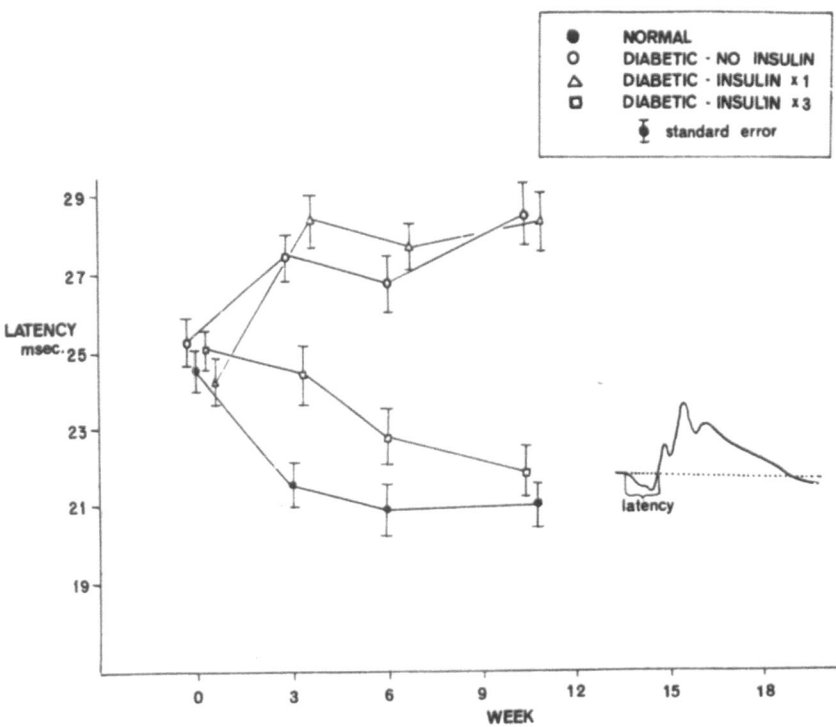

Fig. 5. Electroretinogram latencies of the b-wave intersection point with the iso-electric line (see inset), before and after Streptozotocin. These latencies have lengthened significantly in both the no-insulin and the 1X a-day-insulin groups. The latencies have shortened significantly in the normal and the 3X a-day-insulin groups. Three months after Streptozotocin, the difference between these larger categories was highly significant by t-test ($p < 0.001$).

Streptozotocin than before. Similar results (not shown) were obtained with diabetic rats maintained without insulin (group 2).

CONCLUSIONS

There are little differences between the no-insulin and the once-a-day-insulin diabetic rats with respect to a variety of indices, such as their body weight, water intake, blood glucose, urine glucose and ketones, amplitude and latency of electroretinograms. On the other hand, there are small differences between the normal and the thrice-a-day-insulin rats with respect to the same indices. However, the differences between the first and the second combined categories are highly statistically significant (see legends to Figs. 1–5). To sum up, the once-a-day-insulin therapy is no better than no therapy at all. On the contrary, the thrice-a-day-insulin therapy, with the same total daily insulin dosage as in the once-a-day group, brings the diabetic animal close to a normal healthy

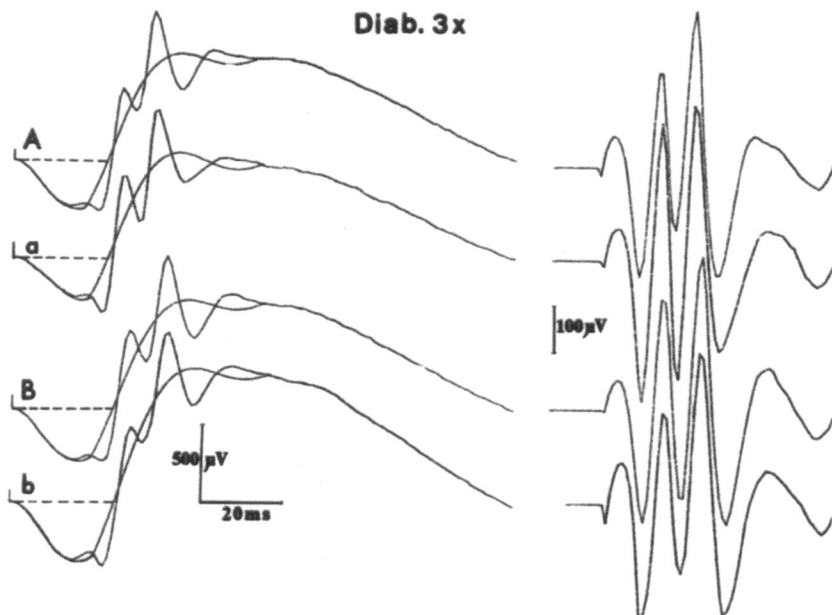

Diab. 3x

Fig. 6. Computer-processed electroretinograms of two diabetic rats before and after three months of thrice-a-day treatment with regular insulin; average daily dosage was 10 units/kg. A, B.: before, and a, b; after treatment. Each ERG waveform is an average of four individual ERGs. The smooth curve of the b-wave is the fitted spline function composed of two fifth-order polynomials (see methods). The curves on the right are the ERG wavelets (oscillatory potentials) obtained in separation by subtraction of the a- and b-waves from the entire averaged ERG waveform on the left. Note the higher gain on the right side. There are no significant differences between the electroretinograms recorded before and those taken after Streptozotocin followed by the thrice-a-day-insulin treatment.

state within three months, and prevents a deterioration of the retina as assayed by electroretinography.

DISCUSSION

Our studies in human patients with diabetes mellitus (Kozak *et al.*, 1979) have shown that insulin restores subnormal ERGs towards a normal pattern in some patients with or without diabetic retinopathy. We have found that persons who manifested an improvement in the ERG either had only the initial stages of retinopathy or none at all. The changes in the ERG were not correlated with the levels of blood glucose.

A regimen of multiple injections of insulin, *i.e.*, intermediate insulin at night and regular insulin before meals, is now undergoing clinical trials in this clinic (Danowski and Sunder, 1978a, b). Preliminary data indicate that the electroretinograms of these patients show an increase in the size of various

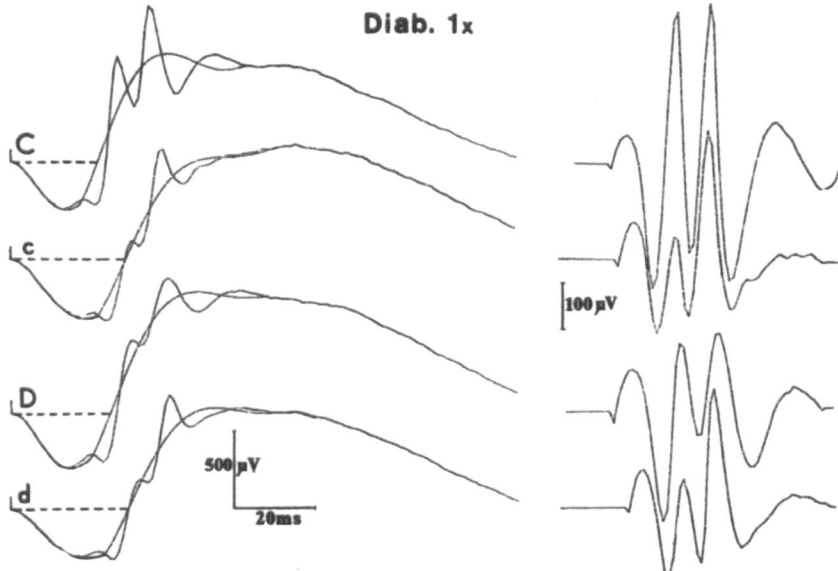

Fig. 7. As in Fig. 6., but these rats were treated once-a-day with regular insulin, 10 units/kg per day. C, D: before, and c, d: after treatment, three months later. Note the lengthened b-wave latency (dashed lines) in c and d, and the decreased amplitudes of the wavelets in c and d (right side), indicating a general deterioration of the ERGs after Streptozotocin followed by the once-a-day-insulin treatment.

components one to two years following introduction of this insulin injection regimen (Kozak *et al.*, 1979).

The thrice-a-day-insulin rats (group 4.), reported here, approach normal healthy animals in many respects. On the other hand, the once-a-day (group 3) diabetic rats deteriorate with time, in par with the no-insulin diabetic group 2. Our results thus confirm and enlarge the results obtained with human diabetics undergoing the clinical trial and present a new hope to those millions of diabetics who would otherwise face an inevitable diabetic retinopathy and other angiopathic complications despite their conventional insulin treatment.

ACKNOWLEDGEMENTS

We are very indebted to the Upjohn Company for their gift of Streptozotocin.

REFERENCES

Abel, L.A. & W.M. Kozak. Effect of insulin on electroretinograms in the isolated retina of the rat. In preparation (1979).

Bloodworth, J.M.B. Jr. & R.L. Engerman. Diabetic microangiopathy in the experimentally-diabetic dog and its prevention by careful control with insulin. *Diabetes* 22: *290* (1973).

Buzney, S.M., R.N. Frank, S.D. Varma, T. Tanishima & K.H. Gabay. Aldose reductase in retinal mural cells. *Invest. Ophthal.* 16: *329–396* (1977).

Cahill, G.F. Jr., D.D. Etzwiler & N. Freinkel. Blood glucose control in diabetes. *Diabetes* 25: *237–239* (1976a).

Cahill, G.F. Jr., D.D. Etzwiler & N. Freinkel. "Control" and diabetes. *New Engl. J. Med.* 294: *1004–1005* (1976b).

Danowski, T.S. & J.H. Sunder. Jet injection of insulin during self-monitoring of blood glucose. *Diabetes Care* 1: *27–33* (1978a).

Danowski, T.S. & J.H. Sunder. Precise control of insulin-dependent diabetes by self-monitoring of blood glucose and four jet injections of insulin. J. D. F. Bulletin, Oct. 1978, pp. 1–5 (1978b).

Honda, Y. The mode of action of insulin upon the electrical activity of mammalian retinas *in vitro. Experientia* 27: *395–396* (1971).

Job, D., E. Eschwege, C. Guyot-Argenton & G. Tchobroutsky. Effect of multiple daily insulin injections on the course of diabetic retinopathy. *Diabetes* 25: *463–469* (1976).

Kojima, K., Y. Sugita, I. Watanabe, K. Niimi, F. Ando, F. Yato & H. Nozaki. ERG in diabetes. Proc. 4th I.S.C.E.R.G. Symp. Tokyo. *Jap. J. Ophthal.* 10 *Suppl.:* *120–127* (1966).

Kozak, W.M., T.S. Danowski, E.K. Vey & J. Segen. Changes of Electroretinograms induced by Insulin in Diabetes mellitus. Proc. 16 I.S.C.E.V. Symp. Morioka. *Jap. J. Ophthal. Suppl.:* *181–194* (1979).

Mauer, S.M., M.W. Steffes & D.E.R. Sutherland. Studies of the rate of regression of the glomerular lesions in diabetic rats treated with pancreatic islet transplantation. *Diabetes* 24: *280–285* (1975).

Ohtsubo, S. Clinical and experimental study of electroretinogram in diabetic state. *Jap. J. Ophthal.* 14: *278–290* (1970).

Simonsen, S.E. ERG in diabetics. Pp. 403–412, in: The clinical value of the electroretinography. I.S.C.E.R.G. Symp. Ghent, 1966. Basel: Karger (1968).

Simonsen, S.E. ERG in juvenile diabetics: A prognostic study. Chap. 56, in: Symp. on the treatment of diabetic retinopathy (M. F.Goldberg & S.L. Fine, eds.), Warrenton, VA., 1968, U.S. Publ. Health Service Publ. No. 1890: pp. 681–689 (1969).

Simonsen, S.E. Prognostic value of the ERG (oscillatory potential) in juvenile diabetics. *Acta Ophthal.* (Copenhagen) *Suppl.* 123: *223–224* (1974).

Siperstein, M.D., D.W. Foster, H.C. Knowles, Jr. R. Levine, L.L. Madison & J. Roth. Control of blood glucose and diabetic vascular disease. *New Engl. J. Med.* 296: *1060–1063* (1977).

Wang, M.K. & H. Heath. Effect of β,β-iminodiproprionitrile and related compounds on the electroretinogram and the retinal vascular system in the rat. *Exper. Eye Res.* 7: *56–61* (1968).

Yonemura, D., K. Kawasaki, M. Kunita *et al.* A statistical study of the oscillatory potential of the ERG in Diabetes mellitus. *Folia Ophthal. Jap.* 23: *93–96* (1972).

Author's address:
Dr W.M. Kozak
Biomed. Engin Program, Science Hall 1325
Carnegie-Mellon University
5000 Forbes Avenue
Pittsburgh, PA. 15213
U.S.A.

Docum. Ophthal. Proc. Series, Vol. 23

THE SIGNIFICANCE OF SOME ELECTROPHYSIOLOGICAL METHODS IN THE DIAGNOSIS OF THE DIABETIC RETINOPATHY

M.C. MÀRQUEZ, R. SANTIESTEBAN, A. CASTRO, E. NENINGER AND A.M. SHAMSHINOWA

ABSTRACT

ERG, oscillatory potentials (OP) and EOG were investigated in 50 persons, who suffered from diabetes or were being suspected to develop diabetes. A group of 30 healthy persons served as a control group. These electrophysiological methods, especially the OPs and the EOG, proved early diagnosis of diabetic retinopathy since the changes appeared prior to clinical manifestation. The findings in healthy sons of diabetic parents were essential.

The early diagnosis and prognosis of the diabetic retinopathy must be considered as a serious problem. Since only a few methods are available for the functional test of the retina we made choice of the electrophysiological methods and confront the results in order to establish its usefulness.

MATERIAL AND METHODS

Out of a group of 50 persons of both sexes, aged from 25 to 55 years, the electroretinogramm (ERG), the oscillatory potentials (OP) and the electrooculogramm (EOG) have been recorded. In order to evaluate the results a control group of 30 healthy people has been studied.

The 50 examined subjects were divided into 3 groups: 13 were healthy sons of diabetic parents, 12 diabetics without retinopathy and 25 with diabetic retinopathy of different stages. All of them were endocrinologically examined in the "Instituto de Endocrinologia y Enfermedades Metaboliscas des la Habana". For the registration of the ERG and OP the retinograph Handaya was used. Light stimulation of 5 and 20 Joules, 16 responses were being averaged. The EOG was registrated by applying the "Arden" method using the electroencephalograph Nihon-Koden (135-D), the time constant being 1.5 s.

RESULTS

In the first group changes were found by applying the three methods, most changes, however become discernable in the OP registration. In most of the healthy sons of diabetic parents OPs with diminished amplitudes, and a reduced number of waves were registered, whereas the ERG and EOG were normal. Several patients showed disturbances in the ERG and EOG of subnormal and supernormal character.

In the second group the changes in the OP and EOG were more pronounced and more frequent, in the ERG the b-wave changes were dominating. In the third group the data of ERG, OP and EOG showed greatest changes as a function of the stage of diabetic retinopathy as compared to the first and second group. The OP were reduced (60%) or absent (32%), the ERG had a subnormal or supernormal character, the EOG was flattened in light and darkness, but we did not find any reduction in the basic value.

CONCLUSIONS

The electrophysiological methods are useful in the early diagnosis of diabetic retinopathy since the changes appear prior to the clinical manifestation. Analogous to Yonemura (1962) we found that the OP and EOG alterations appear earlier than the ERG alterations. The most important fact is that in the healthy sons of diabetic parents modifications appear in the OP, ERG and EOG. These data are probably an expression of initial phases of disturbances caused by the metabolic alterations. Comparing the percentage of alteration in the three groups it is shown that the alterations of the OP, ERG and EOG were according to the development of the disease, detecting early functional changes in the retina layers (Imaizumi 1966, Gliem 1971, Okano 1973).

The results obtained in our research are useful for the diagnosis and knowledge of the disease stage, and they represent a basis for further investigations in the early diagnosis and evaluation of the therapeutic results in diabetic retinopathy.

REFERENCES

Gliem, H. *et al.* Die Bioelektrische Aktivität der Netzhaut bei der diabetischen Retinopathie. *Acta Ophthal. (Kbh.)* 49 : *353–363* (1971).

Imaizumi, K. *et al.* The study of the existence of the primary unilateral pigmentary degeneration of the retina. *Jap. J. Clin. Ophthal.* 20 : *736–742* (1966).

Yonemura, D. *et al.* Clinical importance of the oscillatory potential in the human ERG. Proc. 1st ISCERG Symp. Stockholm 1961, *Acta ophthal. (Kbh), Suppl.* 70: *115ff* (1962).

Author's address:

Dra. Melba Màrquez Fernandez
Instituto de Neurologia y Neurocirurgia
29 Y D Vedado
Ciudad Habana
Cuba

Docum. Ophthal. Proc. Series, Vol. 23

WHY DO CORTICOSTEROIDS INCREASE THE ERG AMPLITUDE? AN EXPERIMENTAL STUDY IN RABBITS

AKIRA NEGI, YOSHIHITO HONDA AND SHIN-ICHIRO KAWANO

(Kyoto, Japan)

ABSTRACT

Effects of betamethasone and dexamethasone (which have no mineralocorticoid action) on the visual function of adult albino rabbits were studied in *in vitro* and *in vivo*. In *in vitro* study, betamethasone and dexamethasone had no effects on ERG at a concentration of 4×10^{-5} g/ml or below. Concentration of 8×10^{-5} g/ml increases the amplitudes of *in vitro* ERGs, but the concentration was considered too high to be a possible level *in vivo*. An intravenous injection (single shot) of betamethasone 0.5 mg/kg body weight did not change ERGs and VECPs within 5 hours observations. In chronic *in vivo* study (daily intravenous injections of betamethasone 0.1 mg/kg and 0.3 mg/kg body weight for 15 days), ERGs did not change so much.

Based on these observations, we concluded that glucocorticoids have no direct effect on the visual functions of rabbits, and that the increase of ERG amplitude previously reported might be secondary to any environmental change.

INTRODUCTION

Patients suffering from adrenocortical diseases sometimes show various psychoneural symptoms, suggesting that adrenocortical hormones have some effect on the central nervous system. In 1967, Wirth *et al.* (Wirth and Tota, 1968) reported that patients with Conn's and Cushing's disease showed supernormal ERGs and that the b-wave amplitude of normal rabbits increased to an extent of about 145% after an intravenous injection of aldosterone. They concluded that the ERG enhancement was secondary to changes of sodium-potassium balance induced by steroid.

In 1973, Zimmerman *et al.* (Zimmerman, Dawson and Fitzgerald, 1973a) revealed a significant increase of ERG amplitude in normal subjects receiving a glucocorticoid. However, analysing the ERGs of patients from renal dialysis unit, they could find no relationship between ERG amplitude and serum sodium and potassium concentrations of patients. They concluded that glucocorticoids among adrenocortical hormones have a direct neural effect. (Zimmerman, Dawson and Cade, 1973b). In this study, effects of betamethasone and dexamethasone, which have no mineralocorticoid action, on rabbit's visual function were investigated.

MATERIALS AND METHODS

(1) *in vitro* experiment;
Thirty five eyes of adult albino rabbits, weighing about 3 kilograms each, were

used as experimental materials. The excision and perfusion methods were essentially the same as those described previously. (Honda, 1969a) A pair of cotton wicks of Zn-$ZnSO_4$ electrodes were immersed in chambers on both sides of retina as active and reference electrodes. After getting a response of a constant amplitude under intermittent photostimuli, the time courses of ERG amplitude were followed. Betamethasone (betamethasone disodium phosphate, Rinderon), and dexamethasone (dexamethasone sodium phosphate, Decadron) were administered by perfusion from the vitreous side of the retina. pH (8.9) and temperature (35°C) were constant throughout experiments.

The principle of photo stimulator employed in this study was the same as previously reported. (Honda, 1969a; Honda, 1969b) Stimulus intensity was varied by neutral density filters. The electrodes were connected to an universal dual beam oscilloscope (VC-7, Nihon Kohden Kogyo. Co. Japan) through preamplifiers. The time constant of the amplifying system was 0.3 sec. In some parts of recordings, responses were summed by an averaging computer (Signal Processor 7S06, Sanei Sokki Co. Ltd.). The amplitude of the b-wave was measured from the baseline.

(2) *in vivo* experiment;

(A) acute experiment: Three adult albino rabbits, weighing 3.0–3.3 kilograms each, were used. The active electrode for recording the VECP was embedded in the cranium over the visual cortex of the contralateral side according to the topographic brain atlas by Sawyer *et al.* (Sawyer *et al.*, 1954). The detailed methods were reported previously (Honda *et al.*, 1979). A week or more after the implantation, the rabbits were secured for recording under Urethane anaesthesia (1.0 g/kg body weight). The pupil of the stimulated eye was maximally dilated. A contact lens electrode was used as an active electrode for ERG and a cotton wick of Zn-$ZnSO_4$ electrode was attached to an ear as reference electrode. After the amplitudes were equilibrated, the time courses of ERG and VECP from the contralateral side were followed. Betamethasone of 0.5 mg/kg body weight was injected intravenously (a single shot).

(B) chronic experiment: Seven adult albino rabbits, weighing 2.6–3.3 kilograms each, were used. Pupils were dilated by a mydriatic. As a control study, ERG amplitudes were measured for 5 days prior to administration. Then, 4 of the rabbits were injected by betamethasone of 0.1 mg/kg body weight intravenously, and the others were injected by betamethasone of 0.3 mg/kg body weight, every 24 hours for 15 days. ERGs were recorded every 2 days after starting a series of injections, and also in the 2nd and 5th day after stopping injections. Body weights of the rabbits did not change in 3 materials and reduced in 4 materials (100–300g) in the 15th day after starting the injection.

RESULTS

(1) *in vitro* experiment;

The time courses of ERG amplitude after administration of betamethasone of 1×10^{-5} g/ml, 2×10^{-5} g/ml and 4×10^{-5} g/ml into the perfusate are shown in Fig. 1 by three series of recordings. In Fig. 2, excerpts of ERGs photographed

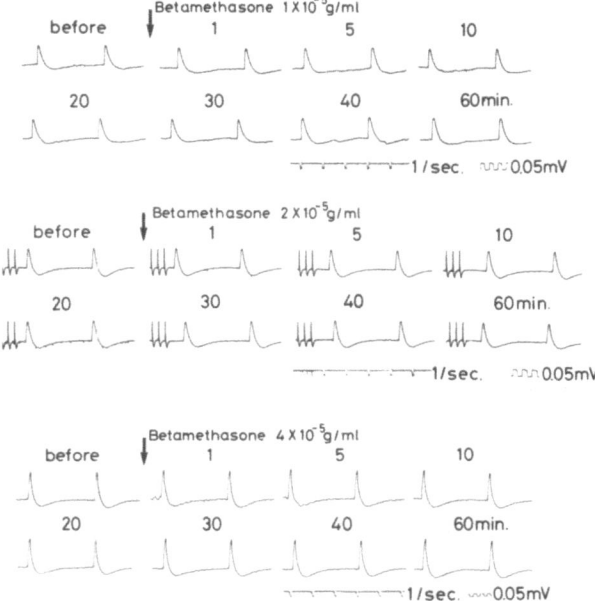

Fig. 1. Three series of *in vitro* experiments showing the effect of betamethasone of 1×10^{-5} g/ml, 2×10^{-5} g/ml and 4×10^{-5} g/ml, administrated into the perfusate. Figures on the top of recordings indicate lapsing time in minutes.

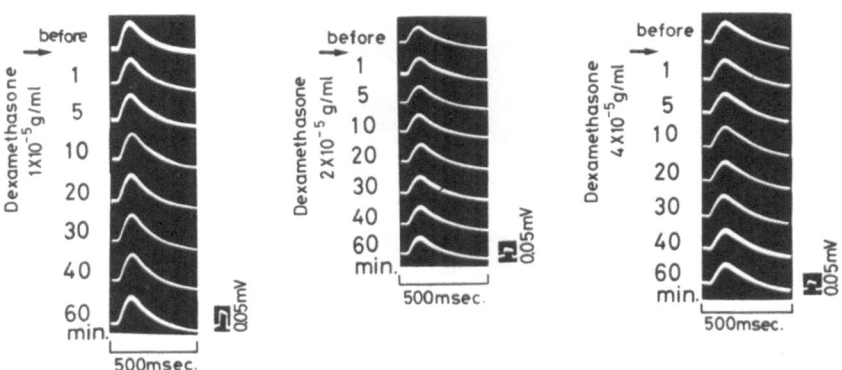

Fig. 2. Excerpts of *in vitro* ERGs after dexamethasone of 1×10^{-5} g/ml, 2×10^{-5} g/ml and 4×10^{-5} g/ml was administrated into the perfusate.

from oscilloscope after administration of the same concentration of dexamethasone were shown. In each concentration, changes of the b-wave amplitudes were within an extent of 5% of the preadministrating level. The implicit time of the b-wave did not change within 60 minutes incubation. Betamethasone and dexamethasone below 4×10^{-5} g/ml had no effect on *in vitro* ERG.

81

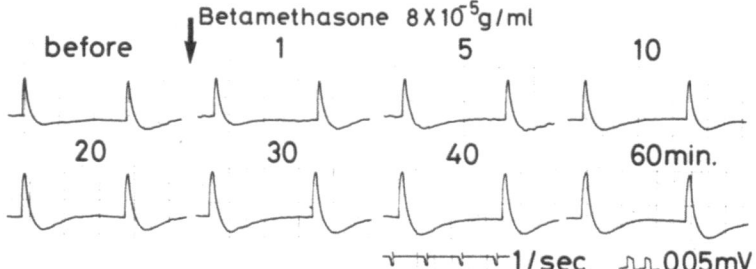

Fig. 3. *In vitro* ERGs showing an effect of betamethasone administrated to the perfusate at a concentration of 8×10^{-5} g/ml.

As shown in Fig. 3, the b-wave amplitude increased gradually from 20 minutes after administration of 8×10^{-5} g/ml betamethasone, and in 60 minutes reached to an extent of 130% of the preadministrating level. The same tendency was also observed by administration of dexamethasone of 8×10^{-5} g/ml (Fig. 4). The implicit time of the b-wave increased gradually and in

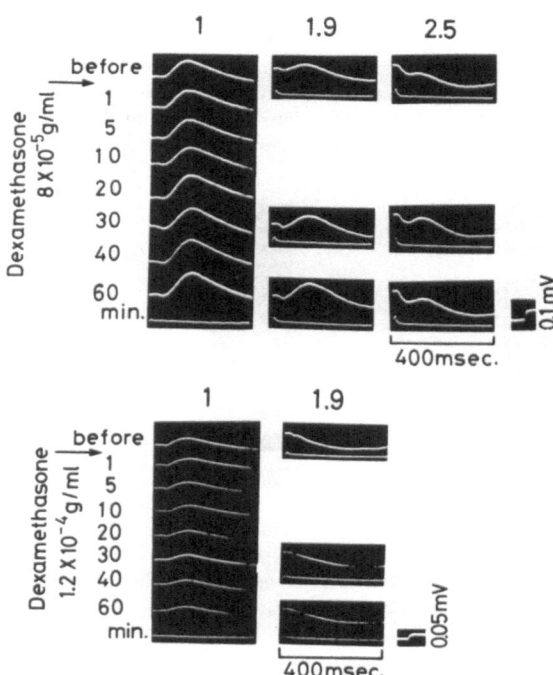

Fig. 4. *In vitro* ERGs showing an effect of dexamethasone, administrated at a concentration of 8×10^{-5} g/ml (top), and 1.2×10^{-4} g/ml (bottom). Stimulus intensity was shown at the top of each column in the logarithmic scale.

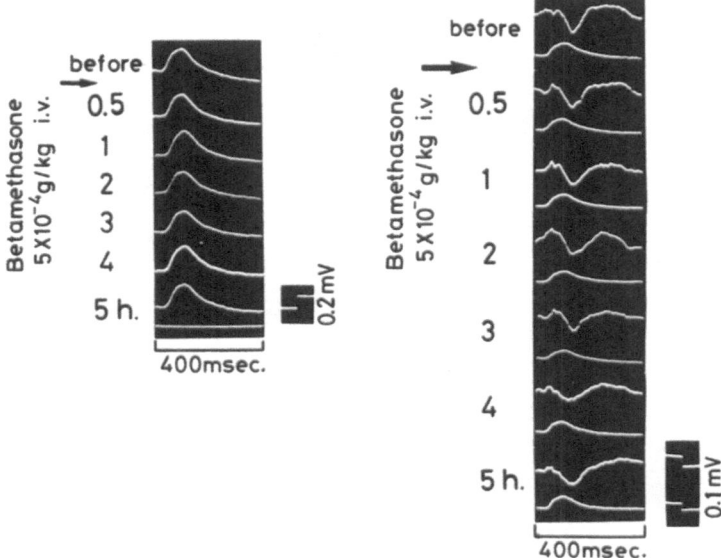

Fig. 5. Excerpts of *in vivo* ERGs showing an effect of intravenous injections of betamethasone (0.5 mg/kg body weight). Figures on the left side represent lapsing time in hours. In the right column, the upper trace of a pair of recording represents VECP, simultaneously recorded from the contralateral side.

60 minutes, was prolonged to 180 msec, (preadministration: 140 msec). By increasing the stimulus intensity, the a-wave amplitude was also increased. Immediately after administration of 1.2×10^{-4} g/ml dexamethasone, the implicit time of the b-wave was prolonged suddenly, resulting in attenuation of response.

(2) *in vivo* experiment;

In Fig. 5, excerpts of ERGs after an intravenous injection of betamethasone (0.5 mg/kg body weight) were shown. During 5 hours, no change was observed in the b-wave amplitude and implicit time, and also the VECP, simultaneously recorded, did not change much. In Fig. 6, changes of the b-wave amplitude by a series of intravenous injection of betamethasone (0.1 mg/kg body weight and 0.3 mg/kg body weight, every 24 hours for 15 days) were shown. Averages of the b-wave from the right eye and the left eye were plotted to elapsing days. In both concentrations, the b-wave amplitude did not increase so much, and stopping the injection also did not affect on the responses. The mean value of b-wave amplitudes in control was 268 ± 34 (1 SD) microV and that in the 15th day was 288 ± 17 microV in materials of 0.1 mg/kg body weight injections. In materials of 0.3 mg/kg body weight injections, the mean values were 286 ± 29 microV (control) and 293 ± 8 microV (15th day), respectively.

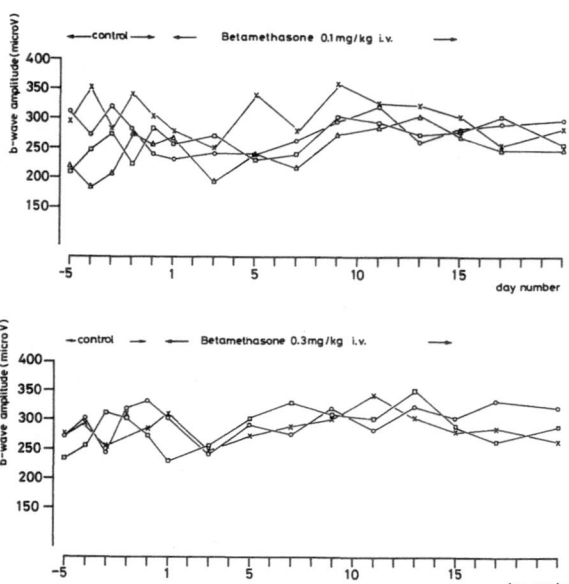

Fig. 6. Time courses of b-wave amplitudes after intravenous injection of betamethasone of 0.1 mg/kg body weight (upper chart, in 4 materials) and 0.3 mg/kg body weight (lower chart, in 3 materials) every 24 hours for 15 days were shown. Before starting a series of injections, the b-wave amplitude of materials was measured daily as control for 5 days. Responses were recorded every two days and in the 2nd and 5th day after stopping the injection. In each material, the average of the b-wave amplitude recorded from the right and the left eye was plotted to elapsing time in days.

DISCUSSION

There are some reports suggesting that glucocorticoids have more marked effects on the central nervous system than mineralocorticoid. For example, glucocorticoid therapy in patients with untreated adrenocortical insufficiency decreased the latency of visual evoked responses, while by mineralocorticoid therapy such a change could not be observed (Ojemann and Henkin, 1967). In Addison's disease, a characteristic pattern of brain signals was not restored by mineralocorticoid therapy, but they recovered slowly by glucocorticoid therapy. (Hoffman, Lewis and Thorn, 1942; Nishitani, 1962).

Studying the in vivo effect of a glucocorticoid, Zimmerman et al. (1973b) suggested it might have any direct neural effect on the visual function. If glucocorticoids have such a function, some changes on ERG and VECP should be observed by increasing glucocorticoid level in the retina. In this study, glucocorticoids, betamethasone and dexamethasone, which are considered to have no mineralocorticoid action, were administrated. As O'Malley et al. said, the molecular weights of steroid hormones are roughly the same as that of common table sugar, so they pass through the plasma membrane. (O'Malley and Schrader, 1976) Similarly, in our *in vitro* study, betamethasone or dexamethasone, administered in the vitreous side of perfusate, is expected easily to reach to the reactive site in the retina.

However, betamethasone and dexamethasone showed no effect at a concentration of 4×10^{-5} g/ml or below. Indeed, concentrations of 8×10^{-5} g/ml or more changed ERGs. But, such concentrations were too high to consider that the effect was induced by physiological action of steroid. Besides, an intravenous injection of high doses of betamethasone (0.5 mg/kg body weight) induced no change on ERGs and VECPs within 5 hours. In chronic *in vivo* study (daily intravenous injection of betamethasone 0.1 mg/kg body weight and 0.3 mg/kg body weight for 15 days), the ERGs did not change so much. Difference of hormonal secretion, hormonal sensitivity or feed back mechanisms between human and rabbits seems to be related to results. Based on these observations, we concluded that glucocorticoids have no direct effects on the visual function of albino rabbits and the increase of ERGs previously reported was secondary to environmental changes.

REFERENCES

Hoffman, W.C., Lewis, R.A. & G.W. Thorn. The electro-encephalogram in Addison's disease. *Bull. Johns Hopkins Hosp.* 70: *335*, (1942).

Honda, Y. Studies on electrical activities of mammalian retina and optic nerve *in vitro*. (1) Factors affecting activities of the retina. *Acta Soc. Ophthalm. Jap.* 73: *1865–1899*, (1969a).

Honda, Y.: Rhythmic wavelets recorded from an *in vitro* preparation of mammalian retina. *Experientia* 25: *551*, (1969b).

Honda, Y., Kawano, S., Mitsuyu, M. & A. Negi. Vulnerability of the rabbit eye to axial torsion – a functional study, monitored by ERG and VECP. *Acta Soc. Ophthalm. Jap.* 83: *113–117*, (1979).

Nishitani, H. Electroencephalogram in endrocrine diseases, Part 2. adrenal diseases. *Jap. Arch. Intern. Med.* 9: *413–428*, (1962).

Ojemann, G.A. & R.I. Henkin. Steroid dependent changes in human visual evoked potentials. *Life Sci.* 6: *327–334*, (1967).

O'Malley, B.W. & W.T. Schrader. The receptors of steroid hormones. *Scientific American* 234: *32–43*, (1976).

Sawyer, C.H., Everett, J.W. & J.D. Green. The rabbit diencephalon in stereotaxic coordinates. *J. comp. Neurol.* 101: *801–823*, (1954).

Wirth, A. & G. Tota. Electroretinogram and adrenal cortical function. Advances in Electrophysiology and Pathology of the Visual System. Ed. Schmöger, E. 6th. IS-CERG Symposium Erfurt, 1967. Leipzig, Georg Thieme Verlag, *347–350*, (1968).

Zimmerman, T.J., Dawson, W.W. & C.R. Fitzgerald. ERG in human eyes following oral adrenocorticoids. *Invest. Ophthalmol.* 12: *777–779*, (1973a).

Zimmerman, T.J., Dawson, W.W. & J.R. Cade. Electroretinographic changes: pre- and postrenal dialysis. *Ann Ophthal.* 5: *769–772*, (1973b).

Author's address:
A. Negi, M.D.
Department of Ophthalmology
Faculty of Medicine,
Kyoto University
Sakyo-ku Kyoto 606
Japan

Docum. Ophthal. Proc. Series, Vol. 23

THE EFFECTS OF ALDOSTERONE ON THE C-WAVE OF THE RABBIT

M. PEROSSINI AND G. TOTA

(*Pisa, Italy*)

ABSTRACT

The Authors have studied the changes of c-wave induced in the rabbit by intravenously administred aldosterone. A rapid decrease of this ERG component was found. Since this hormone also increases the b-wave, the way in which aldosterone, by producing ionic changes, varies electroretinographic potentials is discussed.

It is known that changes of ERG can be of remarkable interest in endocrinology since the ERG is a sensitive tool in some dysfunctions like thyrotoxicosis (Wirth and Stirpe 1965) and primary aldosteronism (Tota and Cavallacci 1967). These clinical observations were supported by some experiments which showed that different hormones may alter the ERG (Nagata 1956, Yamane 1958, 1959). Having demonstrated in a previous paper that aldosterone induces an increase of the b-wave (Tota and Cavallacci, 1968) within a few minutes (Fig. 1), we have considered it interesting to extend the study to the c-wave.

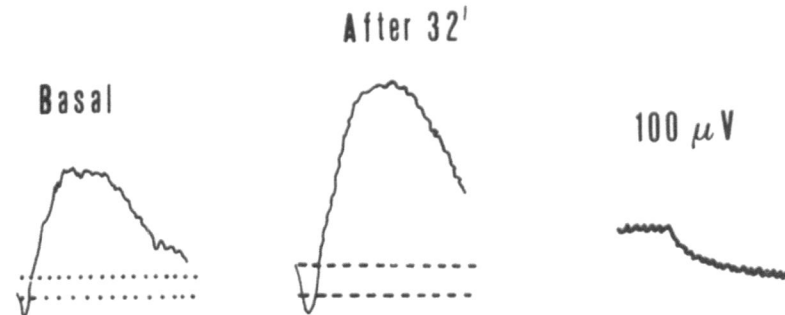

After 32'

Basal

100 μV

Fig. 1. Variations of b-wave induced by aldosterone.

MATERIAL AND METHOD

Experiments have been performed on 15 rabbits of both sexes, weighing between 1500 and 2000 gr, three–four months of age. After the recording in general anesthesia (ct 1341 0,75 ml/Kg†) of the basal c-wave, we slowly injected aldosterone (0,5 mgr‡) intravenously and we followed the changes of

† Althesin, Glaxo
‡ Aldocorten, Ciba.

the tracing for at least two hours. According to our usual technique the active electrode was a small Ag-Cl silver ring kept in contact with the corneal surface by a blepharostate made of plexiglass, the indifferent electrode being a needle inserted in the ear skin. The potentials were taken to a high impedence differential preamplifier of 10 second time-constant connected with a Tektronix oscillograph model 502 A. The sweep was synchronised with the light stimulus by means of a photodiode: the stimulus was emitted by a 8 volt-50 watt Philips lamp type 131/3 c/04 and conveyed to the cornea by a fiber optic bundle.

Stimulus duration: 1 second.

Intensity: 1150 lux measured at the cornea.

RESULTS AND DISCUSSION

When the aldosterone is injected in the rabbit intravenously at the dose we used, a decrease of the c-wave and even a transient extinction is observed. Such a decrease is only transient and after having been reached within 20 minutes 46% of the basal value (Fig. 2), it vanishes completely within 90 minutes.

It is difficult to explain the mechanism by which aldosterone interferes with the behaviour of the c-wave, but according to the status of the knowledge of the origin of the slow retinal potentials we have to admit that changes of the c-wave depend upon variations of bioelectric activity of the pigment epithelium like those which are found with other substances: sodium iodate (Noell, 1953), dithizone (Wirth, Quaranta and Chistoni, 1957), rifampicin (Knave, Persson, Calissendorff and Nilsson, 1973), barbiturates and ethanol (Knave, Persson

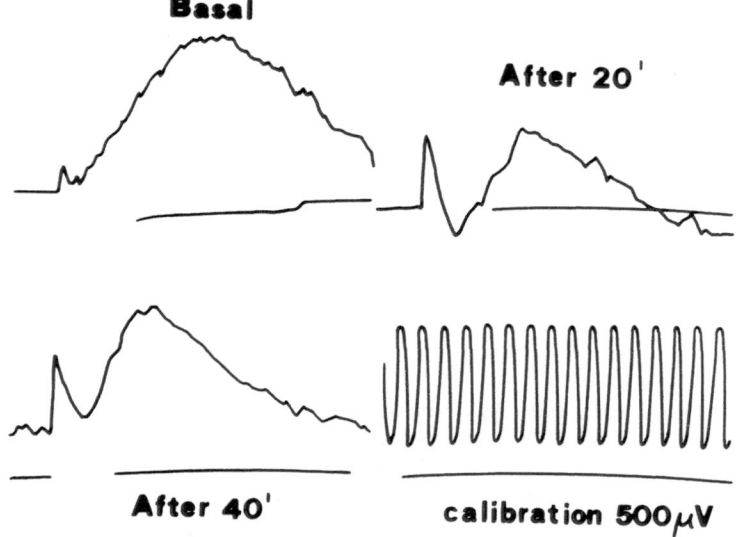

Fig. 2. Variations of c-wave induced by aldosterone.

and Nilsson, 1974), chloroquine and chloropromazine (Calissendorff 1976), cysteine (Shibata, 1975; Yonemura, Kawasaki and Kawaguchi 1977).

Noell (1953) showed undoubtedly that the origin of the c-wave is in the pigment epithelium and recently the intracellular recordings by Steinberg, Schmidt and Brown (1970) have correlated the response of the pigment epithelium with the parameters of the c-wave, thereby confirming that the c-wave is strictly dependent upon the light stimulation of the rods and is generated by active transport of ions across the pigment epithelium membrane (Miller and Steinberg 1975). These results have stressed the importance of the pigment from a metabolic point of view, because being situated between the choroidal vascular bed and the neuro-retina it constitutes a barrier between two chemically different compartments. In vertebrates the exchanges of electrolytes and other molecules between blood and retina is through this barrier and the pigment epithelium is functionally very important not only for the nutrition of the photoreceptors and the regeneration of visual pigment (Hubbard and Wald, 1951), but also in phagocytosis needed for the renewal of the outer segment of the photoreceptors (Young and Bok 1969).

As far as our research is concerned it seems plausible to suggest that aldosterone, by determining cellullar sodium retention and potassium depletion, alters the electrolytic and water-omeostasis at retinal level and produces changes of membrane potentials from which the components of the ERG take their origin. We know that the photocurrents may be reversibly influenced by ionic changes of the intra and extracellular fluids and since the pigment epithelium is in close contact with the rich choroidal vascular bed, one can easily understand why the c-wave could be altered before the b-wave which (see Table 1) has its origin in cellular structures which are affected later and perhaps indirectly by these ionic changes.

The reason why aldosterone influences the b and c-waves in opposite directions lies in the fact that the ERG is a polyphasic response made of different components of differing origin and significance. In fact the a and b waves are present in all the species, whereas the c-wave is an important phenomenon but not closely related to the overall image of the retinal action currents. Since the different components of the ERG may react independently to the same stimulus, it seems reasonable to conclude that a complete picture of the several electrical phenomena is needed if one wants to obtain all the information that the ERG test can give.

Table 1. b-wave (average $\pm \sigma$) before and after injection of aldosterone.

Rabbits	b wave Before	(average $\pm \sigma$) After 32'	$\Delta + \%$
28	90 ± 23	125 ± 20	39
15	c wave Before 625 ± 137	(average $\pm \sigma$) After 20' 333 ± 116	$\Delta - \%$ 46

REFERENCES

Calissendorff B. Melanotropic drugs and retinal functions. I. Effects of quinine and chloroquine on the sheep ERG. *Acta ophthal.* 54: *109–117* (1976).

Hubbard R. & G. Wald. The mechanism of rhodopsin synthesis. *Proc. nat. Acad. Sci. (Wash.)* 37: *69–79* (1951).

Knave B., Persson H.E., Calissendorff B. & S.E.G. Nilsson. Selective effect of a new antituberculous drug, rifampicin, on the c-wave of the sheep electroretinogram. *Acta ophthal.* 51: *371–374* (1973).

Knave B., Persson H.E. & S.E.G. Nilsson. A comparative study on the effects of barbiturate and ethyl alcohol on retinal functions with special reference to the c-wave of the electroretinogram and the standing potential of the sheep eye. *Acta ophthal.* 52: *254–259* (1974).

Miller S.S. & R.H. Steinberg. An electrophysiological analysis of the frog retinal pigment epithelium. Spring Meeting *Assoc. Res. Vision Ophthalm.* p. 5, 1975.

Nagata M. Experimental studies on the influence of pituitary hormones and thiamine on the retinal action current. Report II. *Acta Soc. Ophthal. Jap.* 60: *690–695* (1956).

Noell W.K. Studies on the Electrophysiology and the Metabolism of the Retina. USAF School of Aviation Medicine, Randolph Field, Texas, 1–122 (1953).

Shibata N. Effects of L-cysteine on the rabbit ERG. *Acta Soc. Ophthal. Jap.* 79: *1163–1166* (1975).

Steinberg R.H., Schmidt R. & K.T. Brown. Intracellular responses to light from cat pigment epithelium: origin of the electroretinogram c-wave. *Nature* (Lond.) 227: *728–730* (1970).

Tota G. & G. Cavallacci. Il quadro oftalmoscopico ed elettroretinografico dell'aldosteronismo primario (Sindrome di Conn). *Folia Endocrinologica* 20: *324–330* (1967).

Tota G. & G. Cavallacci. Gli effetti prodotti dall'aldosterone sull'elettroretinogramma. *Ann. di Ottalm.* 94: *427–434* (1968).

Wirth A., Quaranta C.A. & G. Chistoni. The effect of dithizone on the electroretinogram of the rabbit. Elektroretinographie, Hamburger Symposium 1956. *Bibl. Ophthal.* 48: *66–73;* S. Karger, Basel/New York 1957.

Wirth A. & M. Stirpe. The electroretinogram in thyroid disfunction. Current topics in Thyroid research. Acad. Press, New York 711 (1965).

Yamane T. Experimental studies on the influences of adreno cortical hormone and adrenocortitropic hormone on the electroretinogram. I: The influences of ACTH on the ERG of the rabbits. *Acta Soc. Ophthal. Jap* 62: *938–945* (1958).

Yamane T. Experimental studies on the influences of adreno cortical hormone and adrenocortitropic hormone on the electroretinogram. III. The influences of intramuscolar injection of adrenal cortical hormone on the ERG of the rabbit. *Acta Soc. Ophthal. Jap.* 63: *3563–3570* (1959).

Yonemura D., Kawasaki K. & H. Kawaguchi. Enhancement of the electroretinographic c-wave with cysteine. *Acta Soc. Ophthalmol. Japn.* 81: *268–274* (1977).

Young R.W. & D. Bok. Participation of the retinal pigment epithelium in the rod outer segment renewal process. *J. Cell. Biol.* 42: *392–403* (1969).

Authors' address:

Istituto di Clinica Oculistica
della Università di Pisa
Pisa
Italy

Docum. Ophthal. Proc. Series, Vol. 23

ERG OF BEHÇET'S DISEASE AND ITS DIAGNOSTIC SIGNIFICANCE

YASUO KUBOTA AND SHUKUKO KUBOTA

(*Toyama, Japan*)

ABSTRACT

Behçet's disease is seen most frequently in Japan. About 20 per cent of uveitis cases are Behçet's disease. Sometimes the differentiation of Behçet's disease from other types of uveitis is difficult.

Recently electroretinographic evaluation was carried out on 26 cases of Behçet's disease and the diagnostic significance of abnormalities of the ERG were studied.

CASE REPORT

Case 1. A 34-year-old man with a chief complaint of asthenopia. The visual acuity of both eyes was 1.2. Retinoscopic examination revealed only slight oedema of the retina. Past history revealed that he had been suffering from ulcers of the mouth and scrotum. Based on these findings, the patient was diagnosed as having Behçet's disease.

Despite minimal ocular changes, the abnormalities of the ERG were marked. As shown in Fig. 1, the oscillatory potentials of the ERG were markedly reduced. The amplitudes of the a- and b-wave were normal.

Case 2. A 37-year-old man who suffered from frequent attacks of uveitis during the past 2 years. The patient also complained of an ulcer of the mouth and the erythema of the lower extremities. He was diagnosed as having Behçet's disease prior to his first visit to our clinic.

The visual acuity of the right eye was 0.2 and that of the left eye was 0.1. Slitlamp examination revealed an aqueous flare in the anterior chamber and precipitates on the surface of the lens. Ophthalmoscopic examination revealed severe oedema of the retina.

The changes of the ERG in these cases were more marked than in Case 1. Oscillatory potentials were almost absent, and the amplitudes of the a- and b-wave were reduced. The peak time of the b-wave was prolonged (Fig. 2).

Case 3. A 54-year-old man who had suffered frequent attacks of uveitis during the past 5 years. This case was also diagnosed as Behçet's disease with typical mucocutaneous syndrome. The disk of the fundus was pale. The vessels of the retina were extremely thin and contained no blood. The ERG of this case was almost non recordable, only an extremely reduced a-wave was seen.

CASE 1   NORMAL

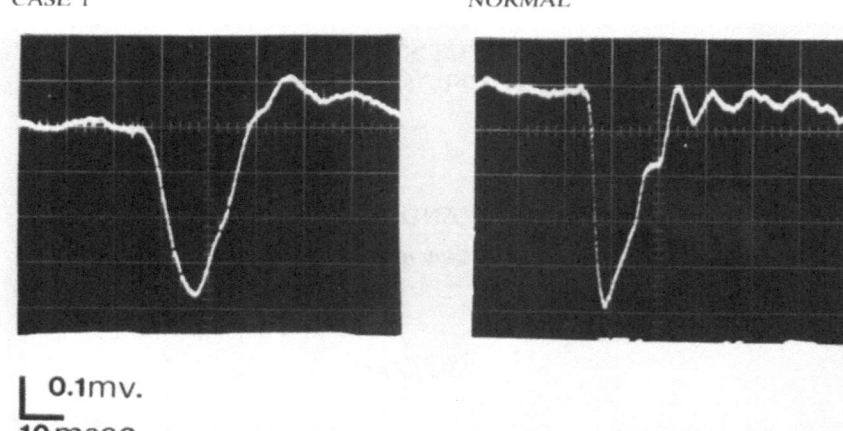

| 0.1mv.
10msec.

Fig. 1. The ERG of Case 1. Oscillatory potential of the ERG were markedly reduced.

CASE 2   NORMAL

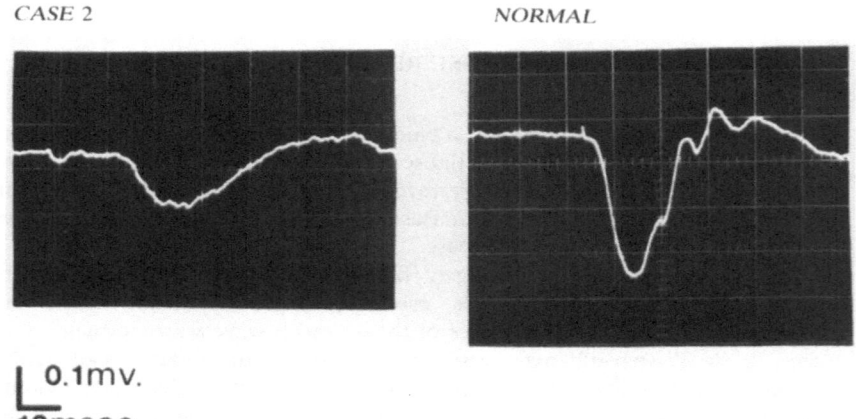

| 0.1mv.
10msec.

Fig. 2. The ERG of Case 2. The amplitudes of a- and b-wave were reduced. Oscillatory
potential disappeared.

DISCUSSION

Studies on the ERG of Behçet's disease have already been reported by Hirata
(1967) and Kubota (1971). These authors reported that the oscillatory potentials of the ERG of this disease are often diminished or absent.

In our study, as described above, it was found that the abnormalities of the
ERG in Behçet's disease may be marked even if ocular changes were minimal.
Loss or diminution of the oscillatory potentials was observed in the early stage
of this disease. Therefore, the evaluation of the ERG, especially oscillatory

potentials, is very important for early diagnosis of this disease. The other components of the ERG (a- and b-wave) decreased with progression of this disease. In the far advanced stage of this disease the ERG is often non recordable.

By ERG examination it is also possible to estimate the damage to the retina in cases in which funduscopic examination is impossible because of complicated cataract. In cases with markedly reduced ERG the prognosis of an operation on the complicated cataract will be poor.

SUMMARY

ERG examination was made on cases of Behçet's disease. It was found that the abnormalities of the ERG were marked even if ocular changes were minimal. Loss or diminution of oscillatory potentials of the ERG were often seen in the early stage of the disease. This has proven very important in differentiating this disease from other causes of uveitis.

REFERENCES

Hirata, Y. Clinical investigation of EOG, practical application of EOG for early diagnosis of Behçet's disease *Folia Ophthalm. Jap.* 18: *841–847* (1967).
Kubota, Y. The ERG of Behçet's disease. *Folia Ophthalm. Jap.* 22 *395–397* (1971).

Authors' address:
Department of Ophthalmology
Toyama Medical and Pharmaceutical University
Toyama-shi 930–01
Japan

Docum. Ophthal. Proc. Series, Vol. 23

STUDIES ON THE EARLY RECEPTOR POTENTIAL IN THE HUMAN EYE VIII. ERP IN BEHÇET'S DISEASE

AKIHIKO TAMAI AND KAZUNORI TANAKA

(*Yonago, Japan*)

ABSTRACT

In 22 cases of Behçet's disease (43 eyes, one eye with corneal staphyloma being excluded) manifesting ocular symptoms in the complete form, abnormal changes in the amplitude of the early receptor potential (ERP) were noted at the first consultation in 51.2% of the eyes examined as compared with 53.3% with abnormal areal indices (ΣA) of the oscillatory potential and 39.5% with abnormal amplitudes of the b-wave in the ERG. Almost the same detection rate of abnormalities as in the ΣA of the oscillatory potential was obtained with respect to the ERP amplitude. The ERP and the b-wave were either reduced in their amplitude or absent in accordance with the grade and duration of this disease. Relatively early disappearance of the oscillatory potential was also noted.

As a result, it was concluded that the concomitant recordings of ERP and ERG are of high clinical value in evaluating the retinochoroidal function in this disorder.

INTRODUCTION

Behçet's disease is a chronic systemic disorder of unknown etiology affecting various parts of the body, the highest incidence of which is found in Japan. Ocular involvement is very frequent, comprising about 25% of all endogenous uveitis (Araki, 1971).

The present study was performed to evaluate clinical applicability of the early receptor potential (ERP) in Behçet's disease, along with the examination results of the concomitantly recorded ERG. The ERP tracings have been reported to show, in certain uveal diseases, characteristic amplitude changes in accordance with the severity of the diseases (Tamai, 1976).

MATERIALS AND METHODS

Twenty-two patients aged 16 to 62 years with Behçet's disease manifesting ocular symptoms in the complete form (43 eyes; one eye with corneal staphyloma was excluded from the study) were examined (For diagnostic criteria of Behçet's disease, see *Jap. J. Ophthal.*, 18: 291–294, 1975). Of the patients, 15 were male and 7 were female. Their pupils reacted well to mydriatics or dim illumination and the funduscopic examination was not difficult even in the presence of haziness of the optic media.

95

ERP examination

The details of the apparatus for measuring the ERP and the method have been fully given elsewhere (Tamai, 1976), and only the main points will be described below.

The first flash ERP was elicited by the xenon flash with a discharge energy of 80 joules presented initially after 15 minutes of dark adaptation. The second flash ERP 2 minutes later was recorded merely to ascertain the reliability of the first flash ERP in this study. The first flash ERP amplitude (referred to hereinafter simply as the amplitude of the ERP or the ERP amplitude) was measured from the peak of the initial cornea-positive phase (R_1) to the peak of the later cornea-negative phase (R_2).

ERG examination

The ERG was recorded 30 minutes after recording the ERP, from each patient using the same apparatus as in the ERP recording under scotopic conditions. The ERG elicited by the second test flash with a discharge energy of 20 joules, presented 30 sec later than the initial one, was adopted as the ERG response for measuring the amplitude of the b-wave and the "wavelet areal index" or the sum of areas (ΣA) of the oscillatory potential surrounded by each tangent line (Fujinaga et al., 1972). The amplifier time constant in the ERG study was 0.3 sec to avoid the b-wave distortion.

For comparative evaluation of the components, the ERP and ERG values were classified, according to the same criteria as in the previous paper (Tamai, 1976), into five graded categories, i.e., supernormal, normal, subnormal, reduced and extinct, referring to the normal mean values reported previously (Fujinaga et al., 1972; Tamai, 1976).

In this study, supernormal ERP and ERG findings were regarded as abnormal.

RESULTS AND DISCUSSION

Table 1 shows the data from the patients with Behçet's disease obtained at the first consultation. At the time, no specific agents which might influence the ERP and ERG responses were being used.

Abnormal changes in the amplitude of the ERP were noted in 22 out of the 43 eyes examined (51.2%) as compared with 23 eyes (53.3%) with abnormal areal indices of the oscillatory potential and 17 eyes (39.5%) with abnormal amplitudes of the b-wave in the ERG; almost the same detection rate of abnormalities as in the ΣA of the oscillatory potential was obtained with respect to the ERP amplitude.

It is conceivable that the abnormal areal indices of the oscillatory potential in Behçet's disease may be due to early deterioration of the neural elements of the inner nuclear layer from which the oscillatory potential arises (Brown, 1968). Such deterioration may be due to diffuse lesions that occur initiallly as a result of retinal angiitis (Ikui et al., 1960; Shimizu, 1973; Colvard et al., 1977). That similar ERP changes are observed in Behçet's disease is quite explicable, even when the principle site of inflammation is the uvea (Shikano, 1960), since the ERP response may be affected by functional and pathological disorders of the choroid side (Tamai, 1976). Also, it may be that the retina need not necessarily be the primary site of affliction.

Very incipient cases may show supernormal b-wave amplitude in the ERG despite the presence of distinct oscillatory potential (Takata, 1962; Kase et al., 1973). Of the 43 eyes, a supernormal b-wave amplitude was obtained in one eye (2.3%) of a patient at an early stage of Behçet's disease, while supernormal ERP findings were observed in two eyes (4.7%) of two patients (one of them is shown in Fig. 1) at the same stage of the disease in the present series (Table 1).

It was inferred, from these eyes being unaffected, that altered hemodynamics of the choroid might possibly bring about some functional impairment (or in some instances metabolic disorder) of the outer layer of the retina, thereby giving rise to such characteristic excitation even in the ERP originating from the receptor outer segments (Tamai, 1976).

The following are some observations made in various stages of Behçet's disease:

Figure 1 shows the ERPs and the ERG of a 48-year-old male patient at an early stage of the disease, 7 months after the onset (visual acuity, O.D.: 0.2 (n.c.), O.S.: 1.2). Markedly reduced ERG responses were observed in the right eye with recurrent hypopyon iridocyclitis, but it was noticeably prominent that the first flash ERP in the unaffected left eye showed a supernormal response.

Presented in Fig. 2 are the ERPs and the ERG of a 27-year-old male patient at a relatively early stage of the disease whose ocular conditions have often shown exacerbations over the past 2 years with good visual acuity during remissions (1.2 bilaterally). Amplitudes of the a- and b-waves were normal but

Table 1. Distribution of the number of eyes with Behçet's disease in five graded categories of the ERP and ERG values.

	ERP amp.	ERG amp.	O.P. (ΣA)
Normal	21(48.8*)	26(60.5)	20(46.5)
Abnormal	22(51.2)	17(39.5)	23(53.5)
Supernormal	2(4.7)	1(2.3)	0(0)
Subnormal	13(30.2)	8(18.6)	9(20.9)
Reduced	5(11.6)	5(11.6)	3(7.0)
Extinct	2(4.7)	3(7.0)	11(25.6)
Total	43	43	43

The "ERG amp." represents the amplitude of the b-wave in the ERG. The "O.P. (ΣA)" represents the "wavelet areal index" (ΣA) of the oscillatory potential.
* Percentage of the total of 43 eyes with Behçet's disease.

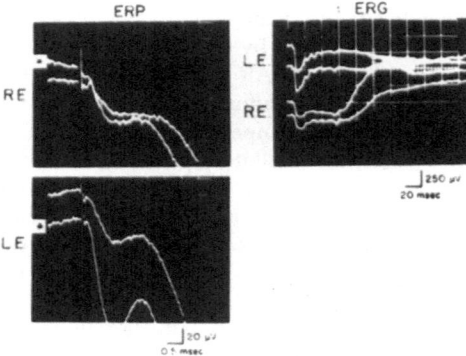

Fig. 1. ERPs and ERG of a 48-year-old male patient with Behçet's disease (early stage). Asterisk in each ERP photograph indicates the first flash ERP. Second trace in each eye in the ERG photograph: second flash ERG 30 sec after the first one. Turbulent waves after the b-wave observed in the ERG traces are artifacts.

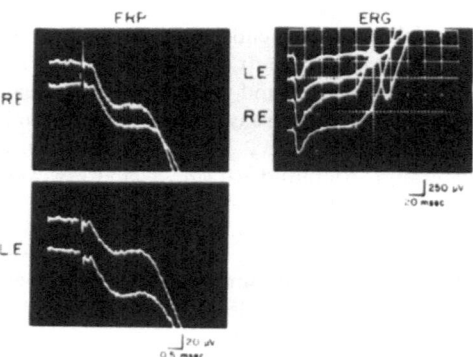

Fig. 2. ERPs and ERG of a 27-year-old male patient with Behçet's disease (relatively early stage). Upper trace in each ERP photograph: first flash ERP. Second trace in each eye in the ERG photograph: second flash ERG 30 sec after the first one. Turbulent waves after the b-wave observed in the ERG traces are artifacts.

the oscillatory potential was absent in both eyes, while the first flash ERP amplitude was subnormal bilaterally even at this stage.

Figure 3 shows the ERPs and ERG of a 31-year-old male patient at a progressing stage of the disease, 8 years after the onset, with a complication of mild cataract in both eyes (visual acuity, O.D.: 0.01 (0.1 with a −13D sph.), O.S.: m.m./20 cm (n.c.)). Considerably reduced ERP and ERG responses were noted in both eyes.

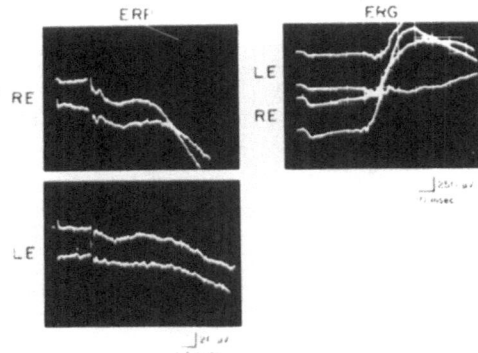

Fig. 3. ERPs and ERG of a 31-year-old male patient with Behçet's disease (progressing stage). Upper trace in each ERP photograph: first flash ERP. Second trace in each eye in the ERG photograph: second flash ERG 30 sec after the first one. Turbulent waves after the b-wave observed in the ERG traces are artifacts.

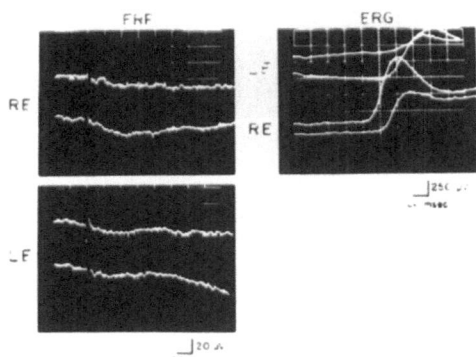

Fig. 4. ERPs and ERG of a 35-year-old male patient with Behçet's disease (advanced stage). Upper trace in each ERP photograph: first flash ERP. Second trace in each eye in the ERG photograph: second flash ERG 30 sec after the first one. Turbulent waves after the b-wave observed in the ERG traces are artifacts.

Figure 4 shows the ERPs and the ERG of a 35-year-old male patient at an advanced stage of the disease, 8 years after the onset, who had bilateral atrophy of the optic nerve (visual acuity, O.D.: n.d./20 cm (n.c.), O.S.: 0.02 (n.c.)). Both ERP and ERG responses were only vestigial in both eyes.

Presented in Fig. 5 are the ERPs and the ERGs of a 25-year-old male patient who was followed up from the initial stage of the disease.

On August 29, 1973, or 3 months after the onset (visual acuity, O.D.: 0.03 (n.c.), O.S.: 1.0), the ERP amplitude and the b-wave amplitude in the ERG

ERP   ERG

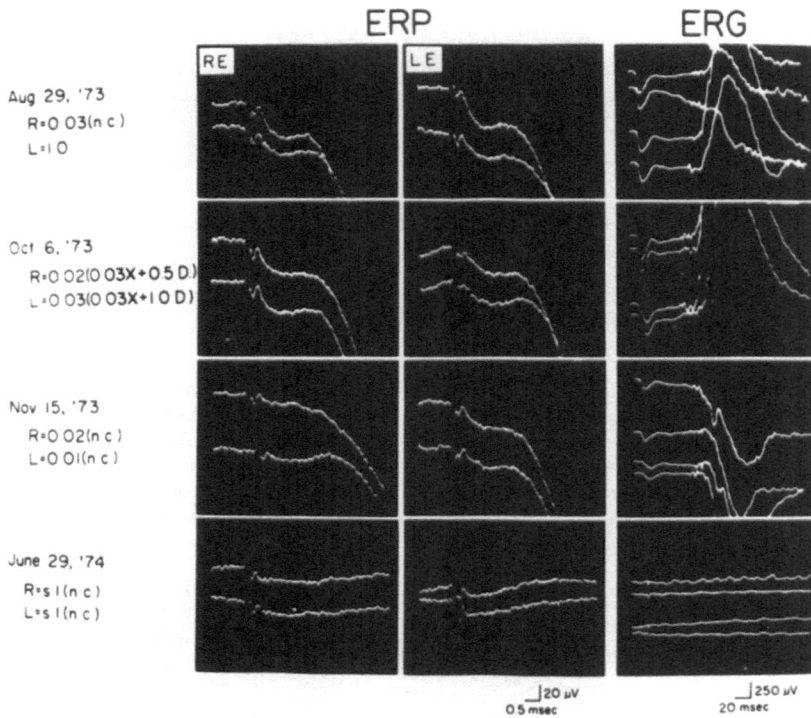

Aug 29, '73
R=0 03(n c)
L=1 0

Oct 6, '73
R=0 02(0 03X+0 5 D)
L=0 03(0 03X+1 0 D)

Nov 15, '73
R=0 02(n c)
L=0 01(n c)

June 29, '74
R=s 1(n c)
L=s 1(n c)

⌐20 μV   ⌐250 μV
0 5 msec   20 msec

Fig. 5. ERPs and ERGs of a 25-year-old male patient with Behçet's disease. Upper trace in each ERP photograph: first flash ERP. Upper two traces in each ERG photograph belong to the left eye and lower two traces to the right eye. Each second trace of both eyes in each ERG photograph: second flash ERG 30 sec after the first one. Turbulent waves after the b-wave observed in the ERG traces are artifacts.

were subnormal with a complete extinction of the oscillatory potential in both eyes. With the subsequent exacerbation of the disease, both ERP and ERG responses progressively decreased in their amplitudes and, on June 29, 1974 (visual acuity, light perception only bilaterally), the ERG became completely extinguished and the ERP vestigial in both eyes.

As may be noted from the findings, the oscillatory potential disappeared in relatively early stages of Behçet's disease and the amplitudes of the ERP and ERG were observed to diminish or became extinct in accordance with the severity of the disease. In cases where these changes could be followed up during the course, a progressive diminution of both ERP and ERG amplitudes to extinction was observed with the exacerbation of the symptoms.

These findings indicate that the retina and the underlying choroid are conspicuously, intensely and extensively affected by this disease as compared with various other types of uveitis (Tamai, 1976). While the ERP showed a tendency to recover in the amplitude with the progressive amelioration in cases of Harada's disease (Tamai, 1976), none of the 22 patients with Behçet's disease showed alleviation and no trend of recovery in the ERP could be observed. The authors would like to further investigate this problem as well as its relation to the central visual acuity in additional series of cases.

In conclusion, the results of the present study further confirm that the ERP is worth measuring, along with ERG evaluation, not only for assessment of the severity of the ocular condition, but also for elucidation of the pathophysiology of Behçet's disease as well.

ACKNOWLEDGMENT

The authors are very grateful to Professor Yutaka Fujinaga for his constant interest and counsel in this investigation.

REFERENCES

Araki, Y. Classified incidence of uveitis (1965–1969). *Acta Soc. Ophthal. Jap.* 75: *389–399* (1971).

Brown, K.T. The electroretinogram. Its components and their origin. *Vision Res.* 8: *633–677* (1968).

Colvard, D.M., D.M. Robertson & J.D. O'Duffy. The ocular manifestations of Behçet's disease. *Arch. Ophthal.* 95: *1813–1817* (1977).

Fujinaga, Y., A. Tamai & T. Setogawa. Quantitative evaluation of the oscillatory potential in diabetic retinopathy. *Yonago Acta Med.* 16: *83–88* (1972).

Ikui, H., Y. Tahara, K. Nakamizo, J. Ueno, S. Iwaki & J. Maeda. Further studies on histopathology of the eyeballs of Bkehçet's disease. *Jap. J. Clin. Ophthal.* 13: *409–420* (1960).

Kase, M., K. Aoki, K. Fujioka & S. Sugiura. Some observations on scotopic ERGs in Behçet's disease. *Acta Soc. Ophthal. Jap.* 77: *400–407* (1973).

Shikano, S. A histopathological study on Behçet's disease. *Acta Soc. Ophthal. Jap.* 64: *2341–2371* (1960).

Shimizu, K. Fluorescein microangiography of the ocular fundus. pp. 100–112, Igaku Shoin, Tokyo, 1973.

Takata, H. Electroretingogram in uveitis. *Folia Ophthal. Jap.* 13: *535–549* (1962).

Tamai, A. Studies on the early receptor potential in the human eye. V. ERP in various types of uveitis. *Jap. J. Ophthal.* 20: *420–437* (1976).

Authors' address:
Department of Ophthalmology
Tottori University, School of Medicine
86 Nishi-cho
Yonago 683
Japan

Docum. Ophthal. Proc. Series, Vol. 23

ELECTRORETINOGRAPHIC, ELECTROOCULOGRAPHIC AND VISUALLY EVOKED RESPONSE FINDINGS IN ADAMANTIADIS–BEHÇET'S DISEASE

M. MOSCHOS, G. PALIMERIS, E. CHIMONIDOU,
G. THEODOSIADIS E. PANAGAKIS AND H. PAGRATIS

ABSTRACT

The authors study the electrophysiological finding in a series of 34 patients suffering from Adamantiadis–Behçet's disease in various stages.

They draw attention to the early disturbances of the EOG in relation to the disturbances of the ERG and stress the diagnostic significance of the VER in cases where the disease appears in the clinical form of optic neuritis.

Adamantiadis–Behçet's disease was first described by Adamantiadis in 1930. The etiology of this condition, which presents a multiplicity of clinical manifestations, is still unknown and should most probably be ascribed to an immunological mechanism.

It is of interest that in Hippocrates' Third Book on epidemics we find a description of disease which in many respects resembles Adamantiadis–Behçet's condition.

The disease is of particular importance since it shows an almost endemic character in the Mediterranean countries and in Japan where 36.8% of uveitis cases are attributed to it (Bietti, 1966; Palimeris, 1973).

Clinically the disease is characterized by a variety of symptoms, such as ulcerations of the oral mucous membranes (98%) and of the external sexual organs (66%), arthritis (59%), hemorrhagic colitis of the rectum, various cutaneous manifestations (88%), thrombophlebitis (20%), symptoms from the central nervous system (20%), pericarditis, pancreatitis and chiefly affections of the eyes, such as iritis with hypopyon, chorioiditis, bleedings from the eye fundus, periphlebitic changes, atrophy of the optic nerve and resultant secondary alterations, such as glaucoma, cataract, retinal detachment, etc.

The symptoms involving the eyes follow a chronic course with recurrences of the disease. The prognosis of the disease, especially of its ophthalmologic aspects, is grave, since it very often leads to blindness. The disease mainly affects males, females being to a lesser extent subject to it.

The purpose of the present investigation is to provide an analysis of the ERG, EOG and VER findings in patients suffering from Adamantiadis–Behçet's disease who have been followed up in the Athens University Eye Clinic since 1967.

Of the 34 patients who have been followed up repeatedly and at different stages of the disease, 26 were male and 8 female. Of the patients who present a multiplicity of symptoms 4 were blind and in 6 only one eye was involved.

MATERIAL

Every patient was in a different stage of the disease. However, in order to facilitate the analysis of the examination results we have classified the patients according to the following 4 stages:

Stage 1	Stage 2	Stage 3	Stage 4	
			a	b
Iritis with or without hypopyon	Recurring attacks of iridocyclitis with or without hypopyon	Multiple recurrences of uveitis and vasculitis	Cataract	Blindness
Aphthae		Secondary alterations such as glaucoma and cataract	Marked alterations of the fundus	
Eye fundus without Changes	Eye fundus: chorioiditic vascular foci and changes, bleedings			
Second eye not involved				
	Aphthae	Manifestations of the skin and mucous membranes	Aphthae	
	Symptoms from other systems	Aphthae		

The examination of cross tissue compatibility in all patients revealed the antigen B_5 positive in 29 patients, i.e. 86%.

For recording the ERG an NT6 apparatus of the MEDELEC Company was used with electronic averager. This apparatus features a bulit-in oscillograph which registers the ERG and a paper-roll device for automatic photography on which the ERG is recorded.

The method employed has been described in previous publications of the authors (Palimeris and Moschos, 1976).

The electrooculographic examination was performed according to the Arden method, in which the L/D ratio is measured, the patient being kept for 12 minutes in the light and for another 12 minutes in the dark.

L/D 180 is considered to be the normal value, while values below L/D 130 are regarded as abnormal.

For VER recording the eyes were stimulated by pattern stimulation.

RESULTS

In all 108 ERG, 48 EOG and 32 VER were carried out at the various stages in the evolution of the disease in a total of 34 patients.

More specifically, the ERG, EOG and VER were performed at the various stages of the disease as follows:

	ERG	EOG	VER
Stage 1	22	8	4
Stage 2	33	16	7
Stage 3	25	15	10
Stage 4	28	9	11

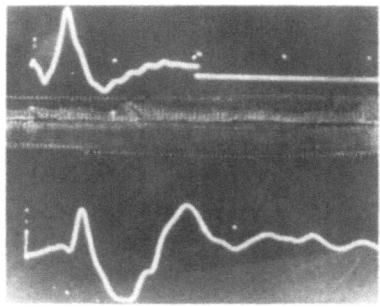

Fig. 1. ERG and VER normal in a case of Stage I of the disease.

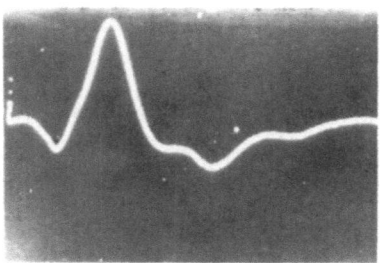

Fig. 2. **ERG Supernormal** in a case of Stage I of the disease.

The results obtained are as follows for each evolutionary stage of the disease:

Stage I

The 19 ERG, the 8 EOG and the 4 VER were normal for both eyes (Fig. 1). In 3 ERG the β-wave was supernormal (Fig. 2), a fact which allows of no clinical interpretation.

Lawill and Wacker (1972) likewise found the b-wave to be supernormal in certain cases of posterior uveitis and attribute this to an irritation of the retina of the affected eye.

Stage II

In 18 cases the ERG was normal, while in 15 it was abnormal with reduced value of the b-wave, the time of appearance of which was delayed.

On the contrary, the EOG was normal in 5 cases and in 11 cases abnormal, a fact which demonstrates the greater sensitivity of the EOG in chorioid alterations, disturbances of pigment metabolism and disorders of the choroid circulation.

In the 11 cases with abnormal EOG the simultaneous examination of the ERG showed that in 6 cases the ERG was abnormal and in 5 cases normal.

One case initially presented a flat ERG in the R.E. and an abnormal ERG and EOG in the L.E. In the course of the follow-up of the patient the ERG of the L.E. progressively diminished until it became completely flat also in the R.E.

Of the 7 VER studied 6 were normal while one was clearly abnormal with increased time of latency, varying between 130–135 ms (Fig. 3). It should be

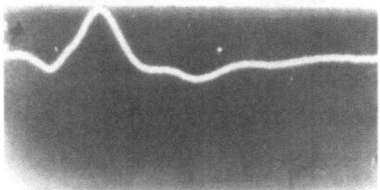

Fig. 3. ERG subnormal in a case of Stage II of the disease.

pointed out that the ERG and the EOG were normal in this case. Clinically the patient presented the picture of a neuroretinitis.

Stage III

In this stage of the 25 ERG 19 were abnormal, of which 6 with totally abolished potentials.

The EOG in all examinations proved abnormal. Of particular significance was one case, in which the patient presented himself with considerably diminished ERG which in the course of the follow-up fell even further off. In this case the EOG followed a parallel course.

Of the 10 VER 7 were normal or almost normal, while the remaining 3 were abnormal or flat.

On the contrary in 2 of the 7 normal VER the ERG was nearly abolished (Fig. 4).

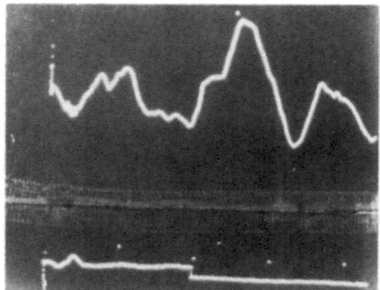

Fig. 4. ERG nearly abolished and VER normal in a case of Stage III of the disease.

Stage IV

In this stage 12 of the ERG were abnormal with reduced electric potentials, while in the remaining 16 they were flat.

The EOG was abnormal in 9 cases and 4 of these there was no reaction to light.

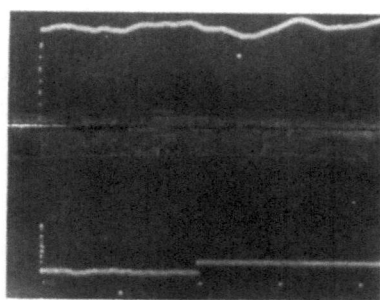

Fig. 5. ERG and VER almost extinguished in a case of Stage IV of the disease.

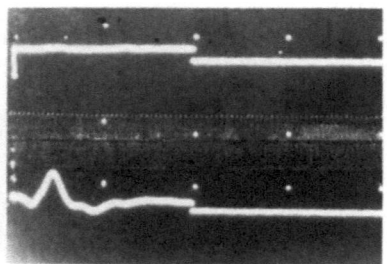

Fig. 6. VER flat, ERG of considerable amplitude in a case of Stage IV of the disease.

In case 5 of the general list the patient who was examined for the first time was found to have both the ERG and the EOG abnormal. In the course of the follow-up the ERG was entirely flat while the EOG became abnormal.

As regards the VER in the 8 cases, these were extinguished (Fig. 5), but in 2 of the cases the ERG was recorded almost satisfactorily, while in 3 of the cases the ERG were of considerable amplitude (Fig. 6).

In 2 of these cases the ERG was recorded, while in 1 case it was almost extinguished.

DISCUSSION

It is an established fact that the development of electrophysiology of the eye has enabled the clinician to gain a better understanding of the phenomena of the sense of vision and to trace the evolution of various pathological conditions of the choroid and of the retina as well as of the visual tract in general.

Thus, while electroretinography is of service in the observation of the progress of such changes as affect the retina in its totality, the electrooculogram constitutes the index of the functional ability of the retinal pigment epithelium and of the choroid.

Finally the visually evoked responses provide information in respect of the conductivity and consequently of the integrity of the remaining visual tract and in particular of the optic nerve.

The existence of potentials in darkness and their variations under light depend on the functional integrity of the choroid, of the pigment epithelium and of the cones and rods.

The combined study of the ERG, the EOG and the VER offers the clinician additional information in respect of chorioretinitis and neuroretinitis, as well as in the present instance concerning Adamantiadis-Behcet's disease.

Already in 1964 Bozin and Dieterle reported that in Behcet's disease electrophysiological disturbances are much in evidence and eventually result in flat ERG.

Thus in 13 cases there was an eventual abolition of the electric potentials in both eyes, visual acuity of which was significantly reduced after the disease had been established for 20 years.

In 3 cases in which the disease had existed but a few years, the electric potentials were found to be reduced.

In a further 3 cases with unilateral involvement, the ERG was perceptibly diminished in the affected eye, whereas in the sound eye it was completely normal.

Hirata (1967) found the L/D value of the EOG subnormal in 5 patients. This value fell even further as the disease progressed. It should also be pointed out that the ERG diminished simultaneously.

This phenomenon was likewise noted by Kozusek (1970) and by Wehner et al. (1970) who observed a progressive diminution of the EOG until its final extinction.

In 1974 Georgiadis et al., who had followed up a series of 30 patients over a period of 23 years, stressed the prognostic significance of the ERG in the study of the disease.

Similarly Hatt and Niemeyer[9] (1976) observed a progressive reduction of the b-wave of the ERG as well as a somewhat earlier and severer impairment of the system of the rods than of the system of the cones.

In our cases both the EOG and the ERG present to an equal degree manifest changes so that in the final stage of the disease the ERG was in most instances completely flat and the L/D value of the EOG extremely low, while in 4 cases there was no reaction whatever to light.

Worthy of special note is the somewhat earlier disturbance of the EOG as compared to that of the ERG: Thus in Stage 2 of the disease of a total of 23 ERG 13 were normal, whereas of 12 EOG only 3 were normal. Similar observations have also been reported by Hirata (1967) and by Bietti *et al.*

Of particular interest is also the study of the VER, seeing that in some instances the disease appears in the form of a neurtis or a neuroretinitis, which have but little effect, if any at all, on the ERG and EOG, at least in the initial stages.

In such cases the VER are perceptibly altered and show little amplitude, the prognosis of the disease being certainly bad despite the relatively satisfactory ERG.

Of such cases we had one each in Stage 2 and Stage 3 of the disease and two in Stage 4.

REFERENCES

Bietti, G. & F. Bruno. An ophthalmic report on Behcet disease. Int. Symposium in Behçet disease. Rome pp 79–110, Karger N.Y. 1966.

Bozin, I. & P. Dieterle. Le comportement de l'ERG dans la maladie de Behçet-Adamantiadis, Bull. et Mémoire S. F. O. *119–122* (1964).

Hat M. & G. Niemeyer. Elektroretinographic bei morbus Behçet. *Albrecht v. Graefes Arch. Klin. exp. Ophtalm.* 189: *113–120* (1976).

Hirata, A. Practical Application of EOG for early diagnosis of Behcet's disease. *Folia Ophthal. Jap.* 18: *840–847* (1967).

Kozusek, V. ERG und Behçet-Uveitis. *Ophthalmologica* 161: *196–201* (1970).

Lawill, T., W. Wacker, & R. MacDonald Jr. The role of electrophysiology in evaluating posterior uveitis. *Am. J. Ophth.* 74: *1086–1093* (1972).

Palimeris, G. & J. Koliopoulos. Adamantiadis–Behçet disease. Acta of panhellenic congress of Dermatology. Athens, *285-288* (1973).

Palimeris G., M. Moschos *et al.* Clinical application of VER in Ophthalmology. *Acta of Hel. Ophth. Soc.* 44: *231–242* (1976).

Wehner, F., E. Alexandridis, & F. Bettinger. Elektrooculographische Befunde bei Uveitis. *Bericht. d. Ophthalmol. Ges.* LXX: *161–165*.

Author's address:
Michael Mochos, M.D.
Athens University Eye Clinic
National Ophthalmologic Center
170, Messoghion Ave.
Cholargos – Athens, Greece

SOME CHARACTERISTICS OF VISUAL EVOKED POTENTIALS IN PATIENTS WITH PERIODIC DISEASE

E.D. BLAVATSKAYA, L.G. BARSEGHIAN, D.S. MELKONIAN
AND S.G. ADAMIAN

(*Yerevan, Armenian SSR, U.S.S.R.*)

ABSTRACT

ERG and VER recordings were carried out in patients suffering from a so-called periodic disease (periodic fever, paroxismal peritonitis, cyclic neutropenia, intermittent arthralgia etc.). Electrodiagnostic findings were normal in cases with normal eye functions, irrespective of the presence of eyeground changes. Neuro-uveitis and neuro-retinopathy in ERG and even more in VER provide pathologic signs. Changes became discernible during the attacks and in the state of cessation.

INTRODUCTION

The periodic disease, which is widespread mainly among Armenians, Jews and Arabs, is not widely known in medical circles. As a systemic disease with all its varied manifestations (periodic fever, paroxismal peritoitis, cyclic neutropenia, intermittent arthrylgia and others) (Reinmann, 1949) the periodic disease in some cases must be considered the cause of visual systemic pathologies (Vinogradova, 1973). There is no statement in this field that could be assumed sufficient and without contradiction, dealing with colloid bodies of an eyeground, neuro-retinitis, neuro-uveitis, neuritis of the optic nerve, retinal apoplexy, *etc.* In the literature we did not find any data on the alectrophysiological investigations of the retina in patients suffering from a periodic disease.

Electroretinography and VEP recording were carried out in patients suffering from a periodic disease, both in those who did not show any retinal changes and functional distortions, and in those suffering from neuroretinopathy and uveopathy.

METHODS

ERG and VEP were recorded in all the patients under investigation. ERG recording had been carried out using a skin electrode on a spectacle-frame. The VEB registration was carried out with the aid of a monopolar connection with an active electrode arranged on a middle line at 2.5 cm above the inion. During the investigation the patient with one eye covered was accommodated in a dark sound-proof chamber. Photostimulation of an eye was performed by means of a light flash of 4.5 Joules and over a period of 2.5 msec. The bandpass of the amplifier ranged from 2 to 700 Hz. Averaging was done upon

109

a segment at 512 msec at a discrete step of 1 msec. (512 channel averager NTA-512M). The registered data were displayed on the X-Y plotter and digital pointer.

Computerization of the ERG and VEP curves was effected by applying the digital spectral analysis algorithms according to the principles presented in the previously published paper (Melkonian, 1968). The digital spectral analysis of the ERG was carried out with the aid of an algorithm based on non-uniform ERG samples at exponentially increasing sampling intervals (Melkonian and Saakov, 1971). The brain VEB analysis was carried out with the aid of the equidistant samples using a modified algorithm at higher accuracy in the high frequency range by comparing the classical Discrete Fourier Transform formulae (Melkonian and Gazarian, 1978).

The quantitative parameter S_c was determined by resorting to amplitude frequency characteristics (AFC). This was equal to the enclosed area under the AFC curve as to the values of frequencies $f \geqslant 25$ Hz. In the estimation of the ERG AFC this parameter mainly typifies the functions of the labile system of retinal cones.

MATERIAL

Twenty-four patients, suffering from the periodic disease for 5 to 20 years in a mixed form, were examined. Electrophysiological indices could not be deviated from normal in 8 patients with a normal eyeground and 12 patients with colloid bodies, typical of the periodic disease (Michaelson et al., 1959). Two patients affected with neuro-uveitis (men aged 28 and 32 years) suffering from the periodic disease for 4 and 5 years, and two patients affected with neuro-retinopathy (a woman aged 38 and a man aged 32 years) and suffering from the main disease over a time of 20 years showed significant deviations from the electrophysiological indices.

As an example we can quote the data of the 32-year old patient M.J. who is suffering from neuro-uveitis of both eyes. The course of neuro-uveitis must be considered similar to that of the serofibrinous type with an abundant exudate in the anterior chamber and vitrous body. We interpret this neuro-uveitis as an allergic one. Visual acuity of the right eye is 0.1, the visual field is concentrically constricted, a central relative scotoma being observed. The absolute scotoma is also observed and is quite similar to the arc-shaped scotoma that accompanies the glaucoma. The adaption curve is reduced. Visual acuity of the left eye is 0.6. Changes are similar to those in the right eye, but they are less significant.

The ERG and VEP and the curves computed therefrom by the AFC are represented in Figs. 1 and 2. The functional meaning of variations of the ERG form (decreased amplitudes of the a-waves, "slowed-down" characters of the curves) becomes clear when estimating the S_c parameters for the AFC of the ERG. These parameters mainly describe the functions of the high frequency system of cones. For the left and the right eye it is 1.59 and 1.42 μV, respectively, provided that the norm can be deemed 3.02 ± 0.81 (μV). These data indicate a decrease in the cone system function and, to a certain degree, they outline the greater retina lesion of the right eye. As compared to the

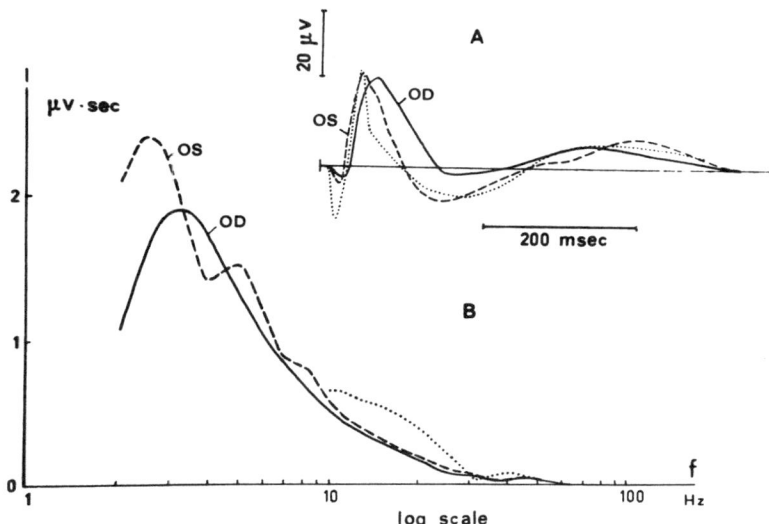

Fig. 1. ERG (A) – and AFC (B) – curves. Dotted curves correspond to healthy eye data, which are within the norm.

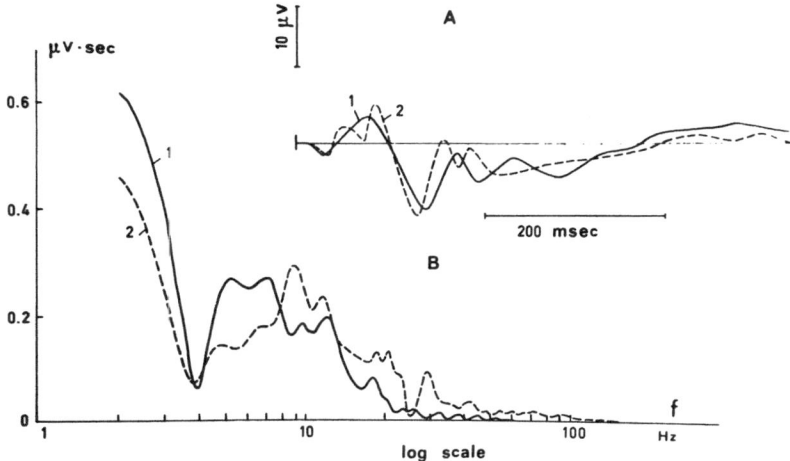

Fig. 2. VEP-curves (A) and corresponding AFC-curves (B), obtained on stimulating the right (curve 1) and left (curve 2) eyes.

norm the VEP curves are reduced more than twice. The values of S_c indicates for the curves 1 and 2 come up to those indicating 0.4 and 1.8 μV. By that an essential asymmetry relative to the high frequency components of the VEP curves is indicated. This can be explained in that the sensory inputs from the retina of the right eye are of an effect that must be considered smaller, and probably is slower.

111

CONCLUSIONS

1. The periodic disease produces both in the case of no eyeground changes and in the presence of colloid bodies, and in the event that no variations of the eye functions can be observed – no deviations of electrophysiological indices from normal.
2. Neuro-uveitis and neuro-retinopathy produce ERG and VEP variations, the VEP variation even being more pronounced. The ERG and VEP analyses by quantitatively estimating their frequency spectra enable to arrive at conclusions regarding the lesion character and dissemination of the pathologic process.
3. Variations of the electrophysiological indices in patients suffering from the periodic disease and showing changes of the eyeground become discernible during the attacks and in the state of cessation.

REFERENCES

Melkonian, D.S. Frequency response analysis of evoked potentials of the visual system based on the operator representation of its structures. In: Adv. in electrophys. and -pathology of vis. syst. (6 ISCERG Symp.) VEB Georg, Leipzig. pp. *203–211*. (1968).

Melkonian, D.S. & A.A. Gazarian. Investigation of some machine algorithms for data digital spectral analysis (In Russian). *Isvestija Acad. Nauk. Arm. SSR*, serie techn. sci. 31: *64* (1978).

Melkonian, D.S. & V.I. Saakov. Computation of transient and frequency-responses of linear systems using Fourier transforms (In Russian). Ibid. 24: *24* (1971).

Michaelson, I., Eliakim, M., Ehrenfeld, E. & M. Rachmilewitz. Fundal changes resembling colloid bodies in recurrent poliserositis. *Arch. Ophthalmol.* 62: *1* (1959).

Reinman, H. Periodic disease. *J.A.M.A.* 141: *172* Vinogradova O.M. Periodic disease. "Medizina". Moscow (1949), (1973).

Author's address:
Prof. Dr. med. E.D. Blavatskaya
Rue Toumanian 9, app. 49
Yerevan 375001
U.S.S.R.

VISUAL EVOKED POTENTIALS AND PATHOLOGY IN RELAPSING EXPERIMENTAL ALLERGIC ENCEPHALOMYELITIS

A.A. LIDSKY, H.M. WISNIEWSKI, R.E. MADRID
AND H. LASSMANN

(*Staten Island, N.Y., U.S.A.*)

ABSTRACT

Guinea pigs with chronically implanted skull electrodes were repeatedly tested for flash evoked responses, in the awake state, before and up to ten months, following a single sensitization with homologous spinal cord in Freund's adjuvant. This method of sensitization leads to chronic relapsing EAE, which has been characterized by Lassmann and Wisniewski (1978 Acta Neuropath.), and proposed as a model of human demyelinating disease – particularly multiple sclerosis. In the present study R–EAE affected the visual systems in a pilot group of animals, with plaque formations in optic nerves, tracts, and white matter of occipital lobes. Changes in amplitudes and latencies of early evoked response components, P1, N1 and P2, from occipital-frontal leads, were found to precede or vary with clinical ratings of disease, and with observations of demyelination. Amplitude reductions in the P1–N1 component generally preceded lengthening of latencies or appearance of clinical changes in the intact animals. Reliable latency delays were usually confined to a severe first attack or more generally to subsequent relapses. One case, with recovery of latencies to preinoculation levels during a clinical relapse, showed up to 50% *remyelination* in optic nerve fibers near the disc. Work in progress will explore the effects of age at sensitization, and relative contributions of central inflammation reactions, parenchyma infiltration, and extent of demyelination on various components of the visual evoked responses.

INTRODUCTION

Clinically and morphologically the course of chronic relapsing experimental allergic encephalomyelitis (R–EAE) in guinea pigs has been proposed as a model for recurrent demyelinating disease in general and multiple sclerosis in particular (Wisniewski and Kieth, 1977; Lassmann and Wisniewski, 1978, 1979). To test and extend the model we have undertaken a series of studies to assess sensory evoked potentials (EPs) during R–EAE. The value of visual, somatosensory, and auditory EPs has already been demonstrated in diagnosis of human demyelinating disorders (Halliday and McDonald, 1977; Robinson and Rudge, 1977; Namerow, 1978). The present report focuses on initial results with flash-evoked responses, recorded from permanent skull electrodes throughout the course of R–EAE in awake guinea pigs.

METHODS

Twenty-one strain 13 guinea pigs, between age 18 and 60 days, were implanted with stainless steel jeweller's screws bilaterally in occipital and frontal skull.

The single sensitization in experimental animals consisted of 0.1 ml. of a 1 : 1 mixture of guinea pig spinal cord and normal saline, and an equal volume of Complete Freund's adjuvant (CFA) containing 10 mg/ml mycobacterium tuberculosis, injected in the dorsum of each hindfoot. The five control animals received equal volumes of CFA and saline.

Daily clinical ratings were obtained on a scale from 0 to 5. Grade 1 represents abrupt weight loss and slowing of movement; grades 2 and 3 are mild to moderate paraparesis, with abnormal gait and occasional leg dragging, while grade 4 is severe paraparesis with dragging hindlimbs; a moribund animal is rated 5.

VEP Recording

Visual evoked responses (VEPs) were obtained at least twice weekly, commencing before sensitization and continuing through clinical attack, remission, and relapse, until animals either died or were perfused. During each test session the awake animal was restrained in a canvas hammock, facing a Grass photostimulator lamp located 30 cm in front of the animal's nose. Three flash intensities ($I = 1$, 4, and 16), with 50 flashes per condition, were presented binocularly at 1 per sec. A 10 minute dark adaptation period preceded stimulation, and 1–2 min intervened between conditions.

VEPs from O_1–F_1, O_2–F_2, and O_1–O_2 electrodes were amplified on a Grass (model 8) EEG machine, stored on magnetic tape, and processed with a PDP 1134 Computer System. Digitization rate was 1 KHz per data channel, with 250 msec average response curves plotted on a DEC VT55 terminal. Identification of amplitudes and peak latencies of the VEP components was performed by computer, using five-point averages. The data presented here are the P1–N1 amplitudes, and latencies of the P_1, N_1, and P_2 components, derived from the O_1–F_1 leads.

Morphology

Selected animals were sacrificed by intracardiac perfusion fixation with 4% glutaraldehyde in 0.1 M Sorensen's phosphate buffer. The brain and spinal cord of dead animals were fixed in 10% neutral formalin. Sections of optic nerve, chiasm, tract, lateral geniculate body, superior colliculus, occipital lobe, and spinal cord, were embedded in paraffin and stained with H and E and Kluver-PAS for myelin. Optic nerves were divided into 1–2 mm segments, postfixed in 1% Dalton's chrome osmium solution, dehydrated and embedded in Spurr. One micron-thick plastic sections were stained with 1% toluidine blue in borax, and examined by light microscopy. A rating system (Lassmann & Wisniewski, 1978) from 0 to 4 estimated the severity of the inflammatory reaction, parenchyma infiltration, or demyelination present in respective tissues.

RESULTS

Three distinct clinical patterns emerged from the 16 experimental animals; *a*, acute fatal or monophasic EAE; *b*, chronic relapsing EAE; *c*, chronic R–EAE with delayed onset. Each pattern of events is represented by one animal, encompassing repeated evoked potentials and clinical ratings throughout the course of EAE, and the final neuropathological analyses. Individual animals survived from 14 to 303 days P.I. (post inoculation) until death or perfusion.

GDA #17, sensitized at 42 days of age, showed a severe first attack and no recovery. Clinical ratings were zero until day 7; on day 8 the first mild symptoms were rated 1, then 2 on day 12, and from days 13 until the animal died at 21 days P.I. it was rated 4.

On day 5 after sensitization *amplitudes* of the P_1–N_1 component of the VEP dropped substantially, relative to baseline values, while latencies were virtually unchanged. For intensity 16 the amplitude reduction was from 168 μV to 98 μV; at I = 4, from 160 to 88 μV; for I = 1, from 120 to 96 μV. One day 11 P.I., when the clinical rating was only *1* the P_1–N_1 amplitudes were 68, 66, and 46 μV, respectively for I = 16, 4 and 1 – less than 50% of initial values. Amplitudes remained depressed until P.I. day 17, when latencies began to lengthen significantly. On subsequent days the latencies of P_1, N_1 and P_2 were even further delayed at all stimulus intensities. The sequential VEP data for I = 1 only, at selected days P.I., are presented in the left panel of Fig. 1, with corresponding clinical ratings in parentheses.

Histologically, a maximal inflammatory reaction was seen in optic nerve (rated 4); optic tract, cerebellum and spinal cord were rated 2(R = 2). Parenchyma infiltration was similarly greatest in optic nerve (R = 3), with occipital lobe white matter rated 2, and both spinal cord and optic tract sections rated 1. No demyelination was evident in optic tract, cerebellum, lateral geniculate or superior colliculi, while estimated demyelination from paraffin sections of spinal cord was rated only *1* and both optic nerve and occipital lobe were rated 3.

This animal shows early dramatic changes in VEP amplitude and latency that precede or correspond to clinical changes, while neuropathological observations indicated greatest severity of attack in the visual system.

GDA #16 represents a typical chronic R–EAE pattern, with two distinct attacks (minimum clinical rating of 3) and intervening remission (N = 5). The longitudinal course of VEP values, together with clinical ratings, is presented in the center panel of Fig. 1 for the I = 1 flash intensity. Additional values for I = 4 and 16 conditions, beginning before sensitization and continuing to 104 days P.I., when the animal was perfused, are presented in Table 1.

Average preinoculation values from four sessions were consistent, showing greater amplitudes and shorter latencies with higher stimulus intensities. At seven days P.I. the animal appeared clinically healthy, and latencies of P_1, N_1, and P_2 were normal; however, amplitudes of the P_1–N_1 component were reduced by at least 30%. The first clinical attack clearly occurred at 15 days P.I., with altered gait, dragging of hindlimbs and weight loss; clinical ratings (*CR*) of 4 or 3 continued to day 19. The P_1–N_1 amplitudes during this period (day 17) showed further reductions to less than 50% of baseline values;

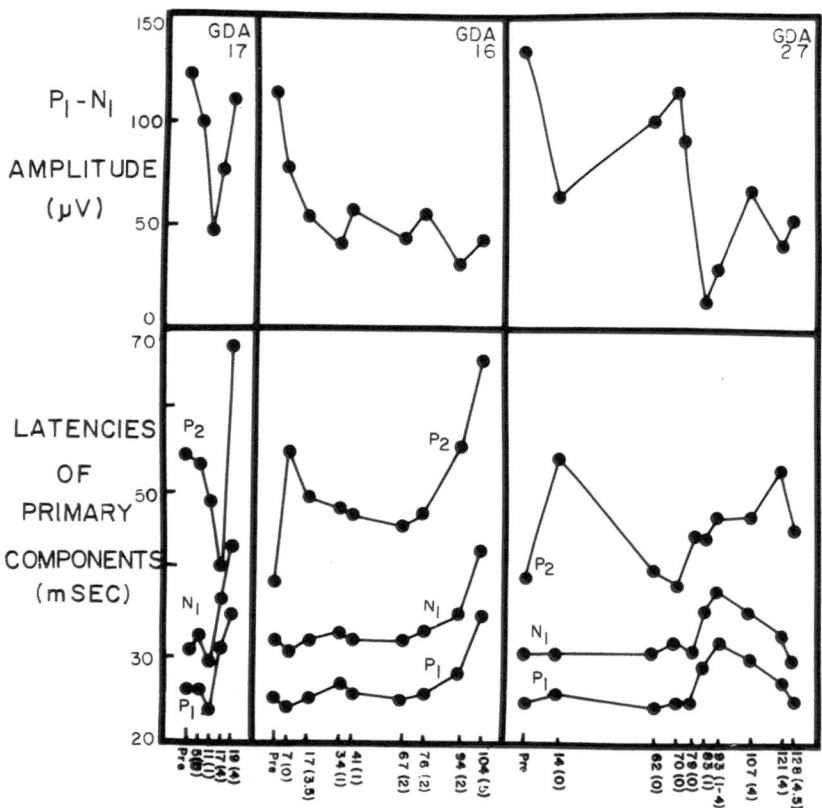

NUMBER OF DAYS POST- INOCULATION
(CORRESPONDING CLINICAL RATING)

Fig. 1. Visual Evoked Responses at Selected Times in the Course of Relapsing EAE in three Representative Guinea pigs. Flash intensity (Grass PS 22) = 1. P_1–N_1–P_2 are successive peaks derived from O_1–F_1 averaged curves.

moreover, the latencies for the I = 4 and 16 conditions began to increase at this time.

A subsequent remission period with CR of 1, throughout days 20 to 64, showed minor changes in VEP parameters which retained differences from baseline values. GDA 16 sustained a relapse at 65 days P.I., progressing from clinical ratings of 2 to 5 until perfusion. Table 1 shows slight further reduction in P_1–N_1 amplitudes, and lengthening of latencies for N_1 in particular on days 76 and 94 P.I. The final two tests on days 103 and 104 show that the longest latencies for P_1, N_1, and P_2 were obtained on the days with highest clinical ratings.

Table 1. Flash-evoked response values during R–EAE: Animal GDA 16

| No. days re Inoculation | Clinical rating | Flash Intensity (Grass PS22)* | | | |
| | | 4 | | 16 | |
		Amplitude P1–N1	Latency P1 N1 P2	Amplitude P1–N1	Latency P1 N1 P2
Pre (4 sessions)	0	122	24 30 37	140	22 28 36
Post					
7	0	80	23 29 45	92	22 28 46
17	3.5	52	25 31 48	68	24 30 48
34	1	58	27 31 45	47	24 30 46
41	1	54	25 31 45	65	23 29 47
76	2	44	26 32 45	50	24 30 45
94	2	50	26 32 45	57	24 30 44
103	4	43	28 36 55	39	27 34 55
104	5	50	33 40 66	57	32 40 60

* See Figure 1 for $I = 1$ values

Pronounced inflammatory reactions were seen in all CNS areas sampled, with parenchyma infiltration also prevalent. *Demyelination* in the visual pathways was confined to optic nerves and occipital white matter $(R = 3)$. Photomicrographs of optic nerves are presented in Fig. 2. Panels 1 and 2 are from a control animal. The optic nerve from GDA 16 in panels 3 and 4 presents a dominant picture of demyelinated axons and perivascular cuffs of inflammatory cells. Sections from thoracic spinal cord revealed substantial myelin debris containing macrophages, as well as de- and remyelinated axons. The presence of both old and recently demyelinated plaques indicate at least two episodes.

GDA #27 illustrates the clinical course of R–EAE with delayed onset $(N = 8)$. It was sensitized at 25 days of age, sustaining a very mild $(CR = 1)$ and brief first attack at 32 days P.I. followed by remission $(CR = 0)$ until 82 days P.I. Thereafter, clinical ratings of 1 continued for 15 days, followed by CR of 4 until day 128 when the animal was perfused.

The parallel VEP data for flash intensity 1 are presented in the right panels of Fig. 1. The *amplitude* panel shows a large reduction in $P_1–N_1$ on day 14 P.I., some recovery until day 70, with major further amplitude reduction from day 79 on. Days 14 and 79 are especially interesting because they precede clinical attacks of EAE by several days, and both attacks were initially very mild (CR 1); moreover, substantial recovery of $P_1–N_1$ amplitude is apparent between these days, during clinical remission.

The *latency* panel for GDA 27 highlights VEP changes and underlying neuropathological changes occurring before and during the relapse (second attack). That is, on day 83 P.I. $(CR = 1)$ latencies commenced dramatic delays which peaked for P_1 and N_1 at 93 days. Thereafter, latencies began to return to normal until the animal was perfused on day 128 P.I. The same pattern of VEP amplitude and latency changes prevailed for all stimulus intensities.

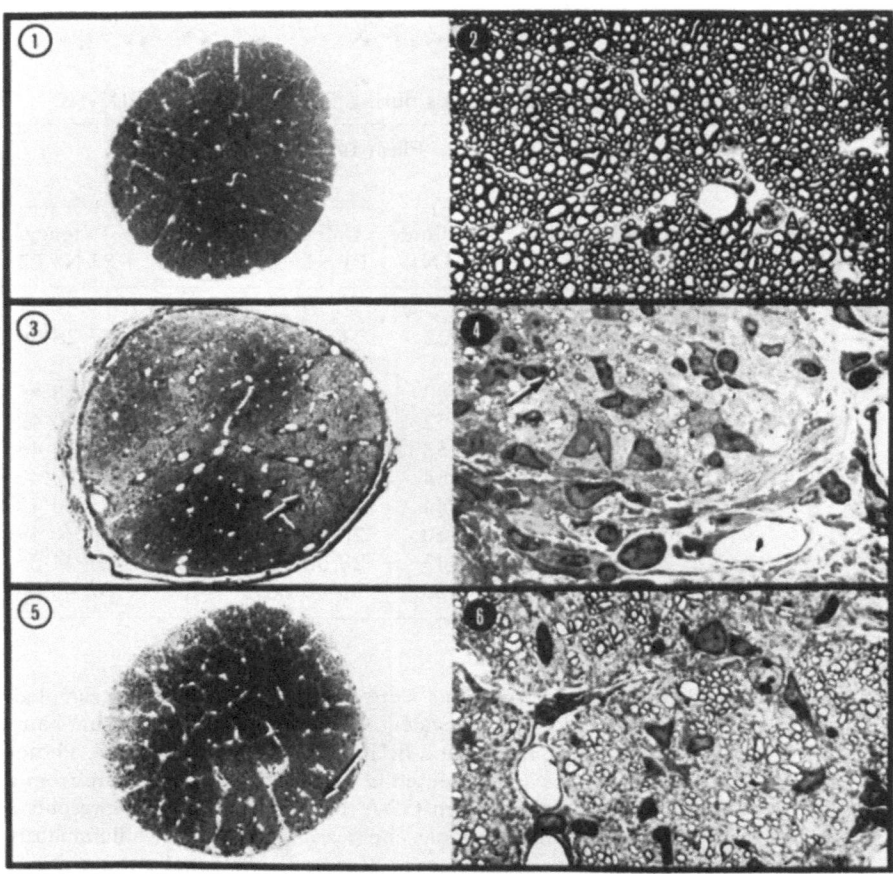

Fig. 2. Optic Nerve Sections from one Control and two R–EAE Guinea pigs. All panels are 1 μm-thick Spurr sections stained with toluidine blue. *1*). Normal control optic nerve near the papillae. The radial distribution of astrocytes at the periphery segregates the myelinated fibers into small bundles and accounts for the subpial palor at this magnification. X81. *2*). High magnification view of Fig. 2–1. Oligodendroglial (O) and astrocytic (A) nuclei among normal myelinated fibers. X1300. *3*). GDA 16, 104 days postinoculation. Most blood vessels are surrounded by cuffs of inflammatory cells. Note presence of parenchymal infiltration (arrow). X95. *4*). High Magnification of Fig. 2–3. Pleomorphic mononuclear cells interspersed with numerous demyelinated axons. Arrow shows few remyelinated fibers. X1300. *5*). GDA 27, 128 days postinoculation. Pale zone involves approximately 50% of optic nerve cross sections at this level. Arrow points to field shown in Fig. 2–6. X81. *6*). High magnification of Fig. 2–5. Large and small axons with abnormally thin myelin sheaths, indicating remyelination. Similar appearance in other pale zones of the nerve. X1300.

Of particular interest in relation to VEP latencies during relapse are the pathology findings for GDA 27, shown in optic nerve sections of Fig. 2, panels 5 and 6. The irregular pale area in panel 5 shows approximately 50% involvement of the optic nerve at this level. Panel 6 shows both large and small axons with abnormally thin myelin sheaths, indicative of *remyelination*. From these and other sections it was concluded that demyelination was maximal

(R = 4) in optic nerve, spinal cord and brain, and that remyelination had occurred in about 50% of optic nerve fibers near the disc and in most fibers near the chiasm. Thus, on the basis of both electrophysiological and morphological findings this animal appeared to be entering a second remission stage.

DISCUSSION

Longitudinal VEPs in awake control guinea pigs, and in experimental animals before sensitization, were reliable and consistent from day to day. The values were similar to those reported by Creel, Dustman, and Beck (1974). In sensitized animals the characteristics of P_1, N_1 and P_2 in the VEP waves showed variations predictive of, and consistent with, clinical and underlying neuropathological events. Initial amplitude reductions tended to occur before or at the onset of the first clinical symptoms, when only inflammatory reactions are present (Lassmann and Wisniewski, 1978). Delayed latencies were most evident in guinea pigs with a severe first attack or during relapse (second attack), and occurred in all animals in which demyelinated plaques were found in the optic nerves. Reduced amplitudes or prolonged latencies of VEPs usually persisted even with clinical remission. In the case (GDA 27) with recovery of latencies to baseline values microscopic examination of the optic nerve revealed considerable repair including remyelination of about 50% of fibers near the optic disc.

Repeated VEP testing in the course of R–EAE with awake guinea pigs has improved the sensitivity of detecting pathology, and extended pathological findings to the visual pathways in R–EAE. The present data are consistent with VEPs obtained in patients with multiple sclerosis, using either flash (e.g. Richey et al, 1971) or checkerboard pattern stimuli (e.g. Halliday and McDonald, 1977), and with the neuropathological observations (e.g. Lumsden, 1970) on demyelination in MS visual systems.

Although delayed VEP latencies were consistently related to demyelination in the visual system in the present R–EAE series some delays also occurred during the first acute episode of EAE. As with amplitude reductions, which consistently yielded the earliest evidence of changes in visual function, the relative contributions of inflammatory reactions, oedema, parenchyma infiltration, etc., remain to be clarified with additional animals.

Acknowledgements

We thank Ms. Barbara Forman and Mr. Leonard Kirsch for capable assistance in various stages of this work.

Abbreviations
VEP   visual evoked potential
$P_1N_1P_2$ successive peaks (P) and troughs (N) in average response curves
P.I.   postinoculation, number of days
CR   clinical rating
R–EAE   relapsing experimental allergic encephalomyelitis

REFERENCES

Creel, D.J., Dustman, R. E., & Beck, E. C. Intensity of flash-illumination and the visually evoked potential of rats, guinea pigs and cats. *Vision Res.*, 14: *725–729* (1974).

Halliday, A.M., & McDonald, W.I. Pathophysiology of demyelinating disease. *Br. Med. Bull.*, 33: *21–27* (1977).

Lassmann, H. & Wisniewski, H. Chronic relapsing EAE: Time course of neurological symptoms and pathology. *Acta Neuropath.* (Berl.), 43: *35–42.* (1978).

Lassmann, H., & Wisniewski, H.M. 1979. Chronic relapsing experimental allergic encephalomyelitis: Clinico-pathological comparison with multiple sclerosis. *Archives of Neurology*, in press.

Lumsden, C. E. The neuropathology of multiple sclerosis. In: *"Handbook of Clinical Neurology,"* P. J. Vinker and G. W. Bruyn (eds.) Amsterdam: North Holland. Vol. 9, *217–309* (1970).

Mamerow, N.S. Evoked potentials in demyelinating disease. In: *"Physiology and Pathobiology of Axons,"* S. G. Waxman (ed.) Raven Press, New York, *421–429* (1978).

Richey, E.T., Kooi, K.A., & Tourtellotte, W.W. Visually evoked responses in multiple sclerosis. *J. Neurol. Neurosurg. Psychiatry*, 34: *275–280* (1971).

Robinson, K., & Rudge, P. Abnormalities of the auditory evoked potentials in patients with multiple sclerosis. *Brain*, 100: *19–40* (1977).

Wisniewski, H. & Keith, A. B. Chronic relapsing experimental allergic encephalomyelitis: An experimental model of multiple sclerosis. *Ann. Neurol.* 1: *144–148* (1977).

Authors' address:
Institute for Basic Research in Mental Retardation
1050 Forest Hill Road
Staten Island, N.Y. 10314
U.S.A.

THE INTEREST OF ELECTRORETINOGRAPHY
IN PARKINSONISM

G. CAVALLACCI, M. PEROSSINI AND A. WIRTH
(Pisa, Italy)

ABSTRACT

The authors have studied the behaviour of the ERG b-wave in humans affected by Parkinsonism during treatment with L-Dopa (Sinemet).

The results obtained lead to the conclusion that a significant decrease of the b-wave amplitude coincides an overdosage on the same line with the comparison of neuropsychiatric side-effects. The authors believe that a routine ERG control in patients affected by parkinsonism during the medical treatment is very useful in order to prevent side-effects from overdosage.

Four dopaminergic loops are known at present: nigro-striatal, hypothalamus-infundibular, meso-limbic, meso-cortical.

Recently other dopaminergic acting neurons have been found in the frontal cortex and in the retina (Costa and Gessa, 1977); in the latter, animal experiments have demonstrated the existence of several neurotransmitters, predominantly dopamine (Starr, 1975). The aim of our work has been to show whether in parkinsonian patients there are, as in the cortex, conductivity changes of the retina nervous structures to be compared with dopamine contents. The ERG seemed to be a useful tool for that purpose.

MATERIAL AND METHOD

In Table 1 the clinical and pharmacological parameters of the 18 subjects studied are reported: none of them was on different neurological therapy, neither had outstanding or post ocular disease. Clinical evaluation of symptomatology, from the neurological point of view, was performed with the aid of the Wechsler Rating Scale (WRS).*

The ERG was recorded in all patients on treatment at variable time from the last given therapy.

Recordings have been made in our laboratory with the conventional technique.

RESULTS

In Table 2 the median values of the b-wave in parkinsonian patients we have examined during treatment are reported. In 11 cases the b-wave did not show

* WRS is an arbitrary scale, which takes into account 10 clinical parameters to measure the parkinsonism symptomatology.

Table 1. Clinical and pharmacological parameters of patients examined

Number of patients	Sex	Age	Neurological status			Treatment			
			Type	Duration of illness (months)	degree** of invalidity	Duration* (months)	SINEMET†	Neurological response	Collateral neuro-psychiatric effects (Number of patients)
18	10♂ 8♀	59 (49–67)	bilateral 10 mixted 9 bradi-cinetic 1 iperci-netic 8	10 (3–48)	10±3	8 (2–19)	from 1 to 3 c	+ + + 2 + + 3 + 13	7

* Mean value
** Average and Ⓖ
† Sinemet, Merck, Sharpe Dohme, 1 bolster is made of Levodopa (250 mg)
+ Carbidopa (25 mg) (inhibitor of dopadecarbossilase).

Table 2. Comparison with variation of b-wave and neuropsychiatric collateral effects

	Number of cases	Patients affected by collateral neuropsychiatric effects
ERG unchanged 220 µV (mean value)	11	0
ERG reduced 147 µV (−30%)	7	7

voltage changes with respect to the values prior to treatment, whereas in 7 cases it appears remarkably decreased ($p < 0.01$): in these cases only are there neuropsychiatric side effects, whereas no significant differences were found between the two groups as far as duration of the disease, pharmacological treatment and clinical picture are concerned.

DISCUSSION

Since the retina, in the words of Ramon y Cayal, is a "true nervous centre" it is reasonable to believe that it should contain almost all the neurotransmitter cells which are present in the brain: especially, it follows that DOPA is the aminoacid predominant among those demonstrated by chemical means (Haggendal and Malmfors, 1965; Laties and Jacobowitz, 1966; Nichols et al., 1967; Ehinger and Falck, 1969; Kramer, 1971).

More recently autoradiographic studies have shown that at the retinal level DOPA is contained in a special group of amacrine cells, the so-called "dopaminergic junctional cells," which stand at the junction between the inner nuclear layer and the inner plexiform layer: they have multiple synaptic connections with a variety of cells and may have thin vertical fibres oriented toward the horizontal cells (Kramer et al., 1971).

The physiological role of dopamine in the retina is still unknown. However, it has been demonstrated that the "dopaminergic junctional cells" are able to store DOPA (Spano et al., 1977) and may also release dopamine after light stimulation of the retina (Kramer, 1971).

It has been suggested that in the retina as in nucleus caudatus (Bloom et al., 1965) the adenilcyclase DA-dependent and DA-receptors are closely related and that the physiological effect of DOPA could be mediated by a cyclic adenosinmonophosphate, cAMP (Spano et al., 1977).

The problem is now to suggest the prospective correlation between dopamine content in the retina and the origin of the changes the ERG (b-wave). It seems reasonable to suppose that in normal conditions, the action of dopamine at synaptic level is not such as to interfere with the cellular structures which according to present views contribute to the generation of the b-wave. According to our experience in parkinsonism there should not be quantitative changes of dopamine at retinal level contrary to what happens at cortical level. It is very interesting to emphasize that a decrease of the b-wave is found only in those cases which present neuropsychiatric side effects (see Table 2). It is our opinion that being in presence of a systemic overdosage, there could be an excess of exogenous dopamine in the retina. Now, if one considers the inhibitory neurotransmitter role of dopamine at the level of the synapses between "junctional cells" and neighbouring cells (Dowling and Ehinger, 1975) it seems reasonable to suggest a partial shunt of the electric flow to the Müller cells and consequently a reduction of their function.

In conclusion, it seems to us important from a clinical point of view to suggest the recording of the ERG as a reliable and objective test to foresee and possibly prevent a pharmacological overdosage in the treatment of parkinsonism.

REFERENCES

Bloom, F.E., E. Costa & G.C. Salmoiraghi. Anestesia and responsiveness of individual neurons of the caudate nucleus of the cat to acetylcholine norepinephrine and dopamine administered by microelectrophoresis. *J. Pharmacol. Exp. Ther.*, 150: *224* (1965).

Brown, J.H. & M.H. Makman. Stimulation by dopamine of adenylate cyclase in retinal homogenates and of adenosine-3':5'-cyclic monophosphate formation in intact retina. *Proc. Natl. Acad. Sci. U.S.A.*, 69: *539* (1972).

Costa, E. & G.L. Gessa. Non striatal dopaminergic neurons. Advances in Biochemical Psychopharmacology. 16, Raven Press, New York (1977).

Dowling, J.E. & B. Ehinger. Unusual retinal cells in the dolphin eye. *Science*, 181: *747* (1973).

Ehinger, B. & B. Falck. Morphological and pharmacohistochemical characteristics of adrenergic retinal neurons of some mammals. Albrecht von Graefes Arch. Klin. Ophthalmol., 178: *295* (1969).

Ehringer, H. & O. Hornykiewicz. Verteilung von Noradrenalin und Dopamin (3-Hydroxtyramin) im Gehirn des Mensche und ihr Verhalten bei Erkrankungen des extrapyramidalen Systems. Klin. Wschr., 38: *1236* (1960).

Haggendal, J. & T. Malmfors. Identification and cellular localization of the catecholamines in the retina and the choroid of the rabbit. *Acta Phisiol. Scand.*, 64; *58* (1965).

Kebabian, J.W., G.L. Petzold & P. Greengard. *Proc. Natl. Acad. Sci. U.S.A.*, 69: *21145* (1972).

Kramer, S.G. Dopamine: a retinal neurotransmitter. Retinal uptake, storage and light stimulated release of +H3-dopamine *in vivo. Invest. Ophthalmol.* 10: *438* (1971).

Kramer, S.G., A.M. Potts & Y. Mangnall. Dopamine: a retinal neurotransmitter. II. Autoradiographic localization of H3-dopamine in the retina. *Invest. Ophthalmol.*, 10: *617* (1971).

Laties, A.M. & D. Jacobowitz. Histochemical studies of monoamine-containing cells in the monkey retina. *J. Histochem. Cytochem.*, 14: *823* (1966).

Makman, M.H., J.H. Brown & R.K. Mishra. Cyclic AMP in retina and caudate nucleus: influence of dopamine and other agents. *Adv. Cyclic Nucleotide Res.*, 5: *661* (1975).

Miller, R.F. & J.E. Dowling. A relationship between Muller cells slow potential and ERG b-wave. VIII Symposium ISCERG, Pisa (1970).

Nichols, C., D. Jacobowitz & M. Hottenstein. The influence of light and dark on the catecholamine content of the retina and choroid. *Invest. Ophthalmol.*, 6: *642* (1967).

Spano, P.F., S. Govoni, M. Hofmann, K. Kumakura & M. Trabucchi. Physiological and pharmacological influences on dopaminergic receptors in the retina. Advances in Biochemical Psychopharmacology, Costa e Gessa editori, Raven Press, New York, 16: *307* (1977).

Starr, M.S. The effects of various amino acids, dopamine and some convulsants on the electroretinogram of the rabbit. *Exp. Eye Res.*, 21: *79* (1975).

Trabucchi, M., S. Govoni, G.C. Tonon & P.F. Spano. *J. Pharm. Pharmacol.*, 28: *244* (1976).

Author's address:
Istituto di clinica Oculistica
della Università di Pisa
Pisa
Italy

Docum. Ophthal. Proc. Series, Vol. 23

COMPUTER ASSISTED EVALUATION OF CLINICALLY APPLIED VEP IN SOME OPHTHALMOLOGICAL AND NEUROLOGICAL DISEASES*

J. RÖVER, G. SCHAUBELE AND M. HÜTTEL

(*Freiburg, F.R.G.*)

ABSTRACT

Taking 600 VEPs, we determined the latencies of the most frequent peaks and fed them into a microcomputer for further processing. The diagnosis that were confirmed by computer-assisted tomography, neurosurgery, and follow-up, were compared with the evaluations based on earlier results. We found that in spite of specifically different findings in inflammatory, compressive, or vascular diseases, in the VEP trace, the latency of only the first major, positive peak (P4) did not adequately reflect these differences. Including further peaks and their super-position, a more specific differential diagnostic evaluation can be attained.

In clinical application, we found that flash VEP had a lower sensitivity to disturbances in the visual system than had pattern reversal VEP.

Consequently we exclusively used pattern reversal VEP to compile our recordings.

The first three peaks of VEP-recordings with pattern-reversal reflect surprisingly little response to the patients attention or to optic or acoustic stimuli presented in addition. As we have shown in a previous publication, these factors mainly influence P 224 in amplitude and latency. So it seemed reasonable to take the parameters of the first three deflections as a basis for our evaluation.

In 1972 Halliday and co-workers pointed out that nearly all VEPs carried out on patients suffering from multiple sclerosis show considerable increases in latencies of the first major positive peak (P 126), when recorded stimulating both eyes.

Hennerici recalled in 1977, when stimulating the right and the left eye of a patient separately, that a high discrepancy between the latencies in the VEP components is a very probable indication of multiple sclerosis – even when the absolute latencies were within normal range. It has been shown, that the P 126 latency was prolonged in cases of acute glaucoma without major damage to the optic nerve (Bartl 1978), and a reduced amplitude, combined with a moderately prolonged latency was discovered in cases of tumour compressions of the optic nerve (Halliday *et al.* 1976).

We realize that in all tests, especially those performed on patients, the amplitude could only reliably be evaluated when comparing the VEP taken

* Supported by the Deutsche Forschungsgemeinschaft, SFB 7O.

from both eyes. The amplitudes depend on the position of the electrodes on the scalp, their relative position to the occipital lobe, and, to a lesser degree, on the surface conductivity of the electrodes. Therefore the amplitudes, even with normal persons, show a variation up to 50%, whereas the latencies of the first three peaks vary little under constant stimulation.

When evaluating VEP traces considerable difficulty arises from the fact that any lesion of the visual system, all the way from the optical apparatus to the visual cortex, will cause a reduction of amplitude and in numerous cases a prolonged latency of the VEP deflections. We therefore tried to find parameters in the VEP curve to separate these disturbances from each other.

We limited our evaluation to the latencies because – as we have just discussed – they were the only reliable parameters and because they also indicate destructions of the wave form as we can see by comparing them with the normative template.

The correlation of the VEP and clinical diagnosis was established by clinical data compiled from six months to two years after the VEP recordings were made. We formed nine groups from this data: normals; multiple sclerosis; optic neuritis; diffuse cerebral atrophy; intracranial tumours; retinal diseases; glaucoma; diffuse cerebral atrophy; optic nerve atrophy; inflammatory cerebral diseases and optic nerve compression. We grouped the patients into these categories by clinical parameters, including computer assisted tomography, neurosurgery, neurologic examinations, and the clinical course. We compiled all findings in our microcomputer and then compared the final clinical diagnosis with the preliminary evaluation of the VEP.

The VEPs were elicited by monocularly stimulating each eye with an alternating checkerboard pattern, as we described in our previous papers. The outer edge of the screen was visible under an angle of 17°, whereas each square appeared under a visual angle of 0.5°. The dark squares had a luminance of 0,02 cd/m², the bright ones of 7 cd/m². Alternating frequency was 0,5 Hz; 128 stimulus responses were averaged.

Figure 1 shows a standard VEP-recording of a normal test person, indicating the deflections that we used for our evaluation.

Figure 2 shows a histogram of the latencies of those deflections plotted from control subjects. We see that P 126 has the smallest deviation, closely followed by N 94. N 17O is far less restricted in its latencies and P 224 has the widest variability of all.

Figure 3 depicts only P 126 in various diseases. The clinical diagnosis: multiple sclerosis and optic neuritis showed significantly longer latencies. But those patients in whom the diagnosis 'brain atrophy' could be confirmed by computer assisted tomography, had latencies of P 126 that were very similar to those suffering from optic neuritis. All other categories did not give specific VEP-pictures when only using P 126 as a criteria but showed a considerable overlapping of the latencies of P 126.

Using the latencies of all four deflections to differentiate our VEP evaluation, we see in Fig. 4 that the standard error of the traces from patients with optic neuritis is considerably smaller than of M.S., whereas both show a linearly-prolonged latency in all deflections.

Intracranial tumours can hardly be separated by these criteria from brain

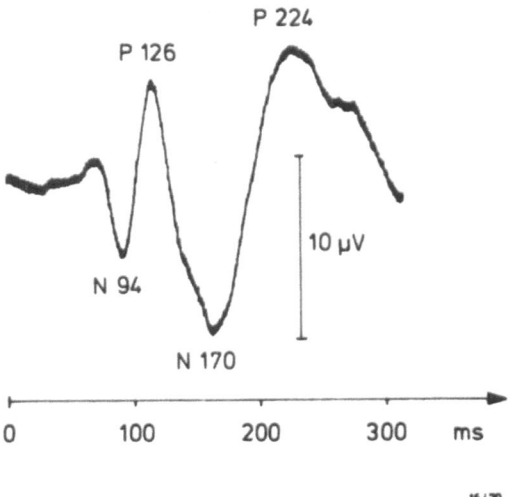

16/79

Fig. 1. Standard VEP-trace, evaluated deflections with their standard latency indicated.

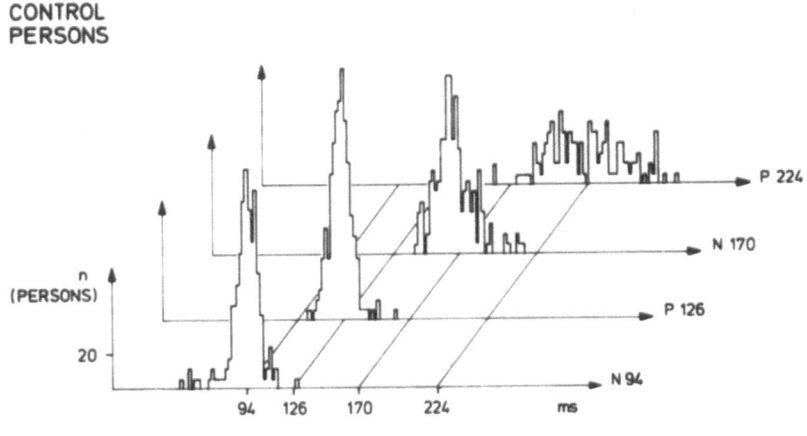

CONTROL
PERSONS

17/79

Fig. 2. Histogram of the latencies of peaks as indicated in Fig. 1, taken from 190 control subjects.

atrophy; both show a linearly prolonged latency in all deflections. Whereas in optic nerve atrophy, the standard error, as an expression of the variation of different peak latencies, is highly augmented, the deflections show a moderate delay when compared to normal VEPs. Orbital tumours seem to have little effect on the latencies or on the variation of the peak.

Furthermore, all those cases were added, where no deflection in the appropriate time range could be detected. A bar on top of each column indicates for

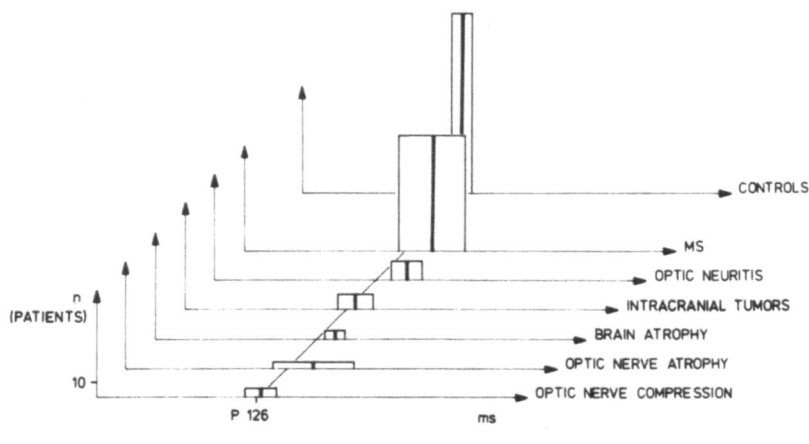

CONTROLS
MS
OPTIC NEURITIS
INTRACRANIAL TUMORS
BRAIN ATROPHY
OPTIC NERVE ATROPHY
OPTIC NERVE COMPRESSION

n
(PATIENTS)

10

P 126   ms

Fig. 3. Mean latencies of P 126 (central bar) and standard deviation (surrounding rectangle) in clinically diagnosed diseases, that occurred most frequently.

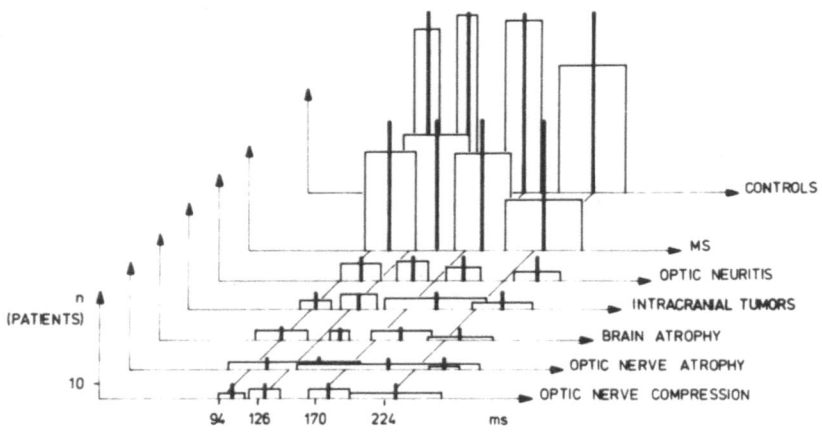

CONTROLS
MS
OPTIC NEURITIS
INTRACRANIAL TUMORS
BRAIN ATROPHY
OPTIC NERVE ATROPHY
OPTIC NERVE COMPRESSION

n
(PATIENTS)

10

94   126   170   224   ms

Fig. 4. Histograms of the latencies of all four evaluated deflections in the same mode as in Fig. 3. Note the wide overlapping of the standard deviation in 'optic nerve atrophy'. The central bars, surmounting the line indicating the standard deviation, represent those cases, where no deflection in the appropriate time range could be found.

each deflection the number of peaks that were not detectible. This 'non-detectibility' of peaks is indicative of the destruction of the recording.

When excluding the least reliable peak, P 224, we realize that the heaviest destructions take place in patients with intracranial tumours and orbital tumours, followed by patients with optic nerve atrophy. Most frequently, the first deflection, N 94, shows the most considerable destruction, whereas P 126

130

is nearly visible. In optic neuritis, the amount of misformed curves is quite high. A number of our patients had a visual acuity of less than 0.3 preventing us from obtaining clear graphs.

On the basis of the table in Fig. 5, where all our parameters are listed, we may discuss one more point: when checking all our MS patients, we found only 10% that had a significant difference in latency for P 126 when stimulating the right and the left eye separately. Quite opposite to this finding, 64% of all cases diagnosed clinically as optic neuritis, showed a significant difference in latencies for P 126. We therefore had the impression that, especially when one of both latencies falls within the normal range, a difference in latencies is not a reliable criteria to support the diagnosis multiple sclerosis.

VEP FINDINGS [%]

CLINICAL DIAGNOSIS	PROLONGED LATENCIES						PEAK DESTRUCTION						Σ [n]
	N 94 xx	x	P 126 xx	x	N 170 xx	x	N 94 xx	x	P 126 xx	x	N 170 xx	x	
M S	24	14	45	10	17	13	9	11	1	5	12	9	132
OPTIC NEURITIS	8	48	16	64	8	40	16	8	8	12	24	16	25
INTRACRANIAL TUMORS	12	18	25	31	37	0	37	12	12	0	24	6	16
BRAIN ATROPHY	16	33	67	16	16	25	0	8	0	8	0	8	12
OPTIC NERVE ATROPHY	15	15	15	30	0	7	15	15	15	15	30	23	13
OPTIC NERVE COMPRESSION	12	0	26	6	26	6	26	26	0	18	0	18	16
RETINAL DISTURBANCES	0	9	36	0	0	9	36	0	0	9	18	9	11
GLAUCOMA	18	9	18	27	9	36	9	27	27	0	27	0	11
NO DIAGNOSIS POSSIBLE	18	8	27	8	16	5	0	24	0	25	0	24	74
NORMALS	3	1	3	2	6	5	6	3	0	1	1	2	153
CONTROLS	0	2	0	8	4	2	0	0	0	0	0	0	37

x x = BINOCULAR
x = MONOCULAR

22/79

Fig. 5. Table of all diseases covered in our study, giving the VEP changes. Monocular and binocular affection separated.

All these parameters considering, we reran our evaluation of VEP tracings that were compiled in our micro-computer: the clinically proved diagnosis and the re-evaluated VEP was compared to see how often we hit correctly. Retinal disturbances and glaucoma cannot be separated from the remaining diseases by VEP, brain atrophy and optic nerve atrophy had a poor correlation with our VEP evaluation, mainly because we are, up to now, suffering from a lack of meaningful understanding of the VEP alterations.

A large number of MS-patients were classified by the VEP evaluation as 'normal,' thus indicating that the reliability of our VEP in these cases only touched 63%. Surprisingly few errors occurred in those patients, who were classified as normal by clinical parameters. However, within this group, 6%

had a bilateral prolongation of peak latencies and were consequently classified as M.S. Possibly these patients will develop M.S. in future.

Great care is required not to classify any patient as a case of multiple sclerosis merely on the basis of a typical VEP-recording: very recently we found that even a bilateral myopia of higher degree can cause prolonged latencies in the VEP recording.

REFERENCES

Bartl, G. Das Elektroretinogramm und das evozierte Sehrinden-potential bei normalen und an Glaukom erkrankten Augen *Albrecht v. Graefes Arch. klin. exp. Ophthal.* 207: *243–269* (1978).

Halliday, A. M., Mcdonald, W. I. & J. Mushin. Visual evoked response in the diagnosis of multiple sclerosis. *British Medical Journal,* iv: *661–664* (1973).

Halliday, A. M. Visually evoked responses in optic nerve disease *Trans. ophthal. Soc. U.K.* 96: *372–376* (1976).

Hennerici, M., Wenzel, D. & H.-J. Freund. The comparison of small-size rectangle and checkerboard stimulation for the evaluation of delayes visual evoked responses in patients suspected of multiple sclerosis. *Brain* 100: 1, *119–136* (1977).

Author's address:
Department of Opthalmology
University of Freiburg
F.R.G.

Docum. Ophthal. Proc. Series, Vol. 23

ERG VARIATIONS
IN MYOTONIC DYSTROPHY (STEINERT'S)

G. CAVALLACCI, C. MARCONCINI AND M. PEROSSINI

(*Pisa, Italy*)

ABSTRACT

The authors have studied the behaviour of the ERG b-wave in patients affected by Steinert's disease. The ERG alterations confirm the existence of the retinal dystrophy in contrast with the minimal or no ophthalmoscopics findings. The authors are persuaded that Steinert's disease is an abiotrophy and they agree with Roses & Appel (1975) who have suggested that the fundamental defect in Steinert's myotonia is of membrane origin and considered it like a diffuse membrane disorder due probably to an inborn error.

Ophthalmologists have long been familiar with lenticular opacities in myotonic dystrophy. Indeed, they have been the first to make the diagnosis since lenticular changes are rather typical and yet precise and may occur early in the disease. Except for the ptosis of the upper lids, the myotonic cataract has been the only ocular sign that ophthalmologists have regularly associated with the disease. More or less sporadic findings have indicated that the ocular involvement in myotonic disease is much more extensive than had previously been reported. The results lead one to suspect that a systematic study of the patients' eyes would yield information which would not only be of ophthalmologic interest but of more importance and would lead to a better understanding of the nature of the disease. Therefore, we have taken the opportunity of making a thorough investigation of patients with myotonic dystrophy available to us through the Institutes of Ophthalmology and Neurology in the Pisa University. The purpose of this study was to observe changes in the ERG of myotonic patients.

MATERIAL AND METHOD

In our present work, we have studied 18 patients aged from 10 to 60 years old. All had well established myotonic dystrophy and all were examined with the same routine laboratory procedures. The ERG was recorded in full dark adaptation after 30 min. and the technique used was that of normal routine in our ERG laboratory: a Burian–Allen electrode served as the active electrode, the indifferent one being placed on the forehead. Leads were taken to a condenser-coupled amplifier of 1 sec. time-constant. The oscilloscope (Tektronix 502 A) was synchronized with the light stimulus by means of a photodiode. A gas discharge lamp of 1 joule instantaneous energy provided the stimulus (2500 lux) and was placed at 30 cm. from the patient's cornea. Tracings were photographed on Polaroid film.

RESULTS

The reported results are in Fig. 1 where can be seen a large decrease of the b-wave (103 ± 34 μV, mean value). Statistical treatment of the results (Student t) showed a highly significant difference. (p $\leqslant 0.01$). No modifications of the a-wave.

ERG b-wave in myotonic patients		
Number of subjects	Mean age	Mean of b-wave scotopic
18	50.2	103 ± 34 μV

Fig. 1.

All patients had prolonged scotopic implicit time (75.42 ± 9 msec., mean value). In photopic conditions the patients' implicit time was similar to that measured in 20 healthy subjects (45 ± 3.5 msec., mean value) (Fig. 2).

Implicit time in healthy and myotonic subjects			
	Number of Subjects	Mean Age	Mean implicit time of scotopic b-wave (msec)
Healthy Subjects	20	45.3	45 ± 3.5
Myotonics Subjects	18	50.2	75.42 ± 9

Fig. 2.

The measure of implicit time was taken from the onset of stimulation until the peak of the b-wave (Fig. 3).

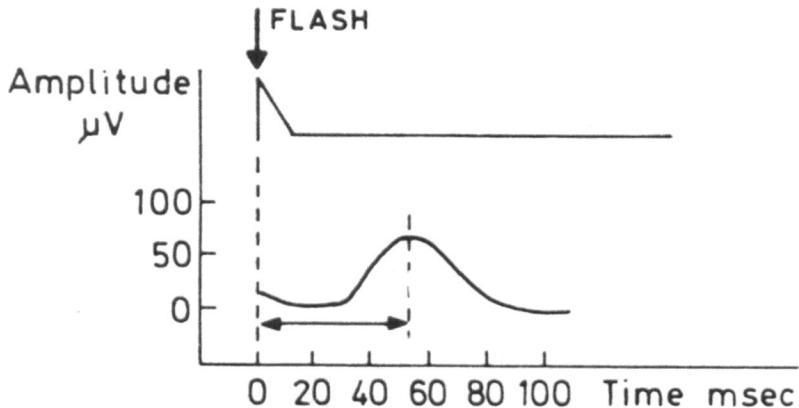

Fig. 3. By Stanescu & Michiels (1975).

DISCUSSION

In contrast with minimal changes or normal ophthalmoscopy in all our patients, the same patients showed a highly significant decrease on the b-wave amplitude of the ERG.

What is the basic defect in Steinert's dystrophy?

Burian & Burns (1967) agreed that this disease is an abiotrophy as Franceschetti *et al.* (1963) had suggested. Recently Roses *et al.* (1973) have suggested that the fundamental defect in Steinert's disease is of membrane origin and considered it like a diffuse membrane disorder with manifestation in many tissues.

The idea of the widespread presence of metabolic alterations in cell membranes are supported by the controlled scanning electron microscopic studies of erythrocytes and abnormalities of endogenous membrane protein-kinesis system in myotonic patients (Roses *et al.*, 1973). Roses & Appel (1975) demonstrated in red cells of myotonic patients the existence of abnormal Ca ions that stimulated K^+ efflux. The same authors considered that many membranes may be affected and that Steinert's disease is due probably to an inborn metabolic error or membrane origin. This could explain the involvement of the eye. Alterations in amplitude and implicit time of the ERG b-wave can be explained by generalized malfunction of cones and rods (Stanescu & Michiels 1975, 1977). Primarily the rod system is implicated: this hypothesis explains the delayed scotopic implicit time and the abnormal dark adaptation curves found by Burian & Burns (1966), (Fig. 4).

Therefore, in conclusion, if in Steinert's dystrophy we also observe minimal or no ophthalmoscopic modifications, the ERG alterations shows the existence of the retinal dystrophy in this disease.

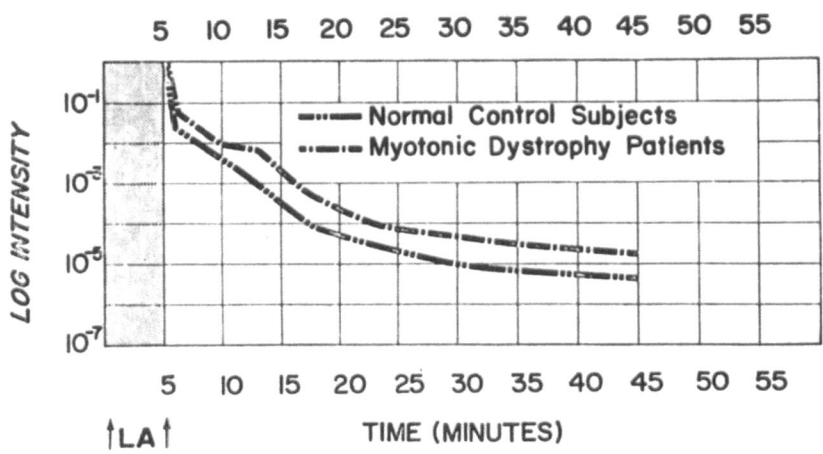

Fig. 4. By Burian & Burns (1966).

REFERENCES

Burian, H.M. & Ch. Burns. Ocular changes in myotonic dystrophy. *Amer. J. Ophthal.* 63: 22 (1967).

Roses, A.D., S.H. Appel, D.A. Butterfield & D.B. Chesnut. Membrane alterations in myotonic muscular dystrophy. New developments in electromyography and clinical neurophysiology. (Desmedt, J. E. Tome I) Karger–Basel, (1973).

Roses, A.D. & S.H. Appel. (1975): quoted in addendum in Roses *et al.* (1973).

Stanescu, B. & J. Michiels. Temporal aspects of electroretinography in patients with myotonic dystrophy. *Amer. J. Ophthal.* 80: 2 (1975).

Stanescu, B. & J. Michiels. Retinal degenerations, electroretinographic aspects in patients with myotonic dystrophy. *Docum. Ophthal. Proc.* 13: 257 (1977).

Authors' address:
Clinica Oculistica
Università di Pisa
56100 Pisa
Italy

ERG IN SOME INBORN ERRORS OF METABOLISM

A. BOHÁR
(Budapest, Hungary)

ABSTRACT

Among the inborn errors of metabolism the clinical and electrophysiologic data of the Tay–Sachs disease, Niemann–Pick disease, Lowe's syndrome and familiar hyperlipoproteinemia are presented. Most remarkable is the unusual disorder of the eyeground associated with an extinct ERG in the case of the hyperlipoproteinemic blind boy.

Among the inborn errors of metabolism two typical forms of sphyngolipidosis were observed within a short time. First the Tay–Sachs disease was identified with the aid of the characteristic fundus picture in a 20-month old girl. The macroscopic, light and electron microscopic, and the biochemical data of the autopsy material of the brain, retina, liver and spleen have confirmed the clinical diagnosis. The biochemical examinations have demonstrated accumulation of gangliosides G_{M2} in the liver and spleen.

Two months prior to death, an ERG examination was carried out. At that time the fundus picture was not characteristic. The cause of blindness was thought to be the atrophy of the optic nerve developing rapidly on both eyegrounds. The retinogram of the 18-month old girl could not yet be considered fully developed as to her age, being rather subnormal; the components, however, were maintained (Fig. 1). As the storage of gangliosides takes place within the gangliar cell layer, the retinogram does not show significant alteration at the time of the development of a characteristic macular change (Straub and Schmidt, 1969).

In the second case the electron microscopy of liver biopsy and sternal puncture disclosed the type of storage disease the 11-month old girl suffered

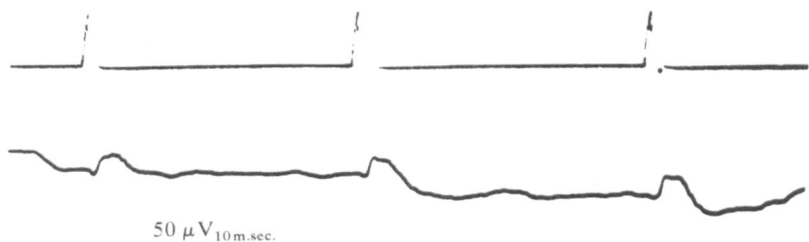

$50\ \mu V_{10 m.sec.}$

Fig. 1. Subnormal ERG of an 18-month old girl affected with the Tay–Sachs disease. Dark adaptation: 10 minutes. Time constant: 0.3. Stimulus intensity: 1.0 Wsec. Local anesthesia.

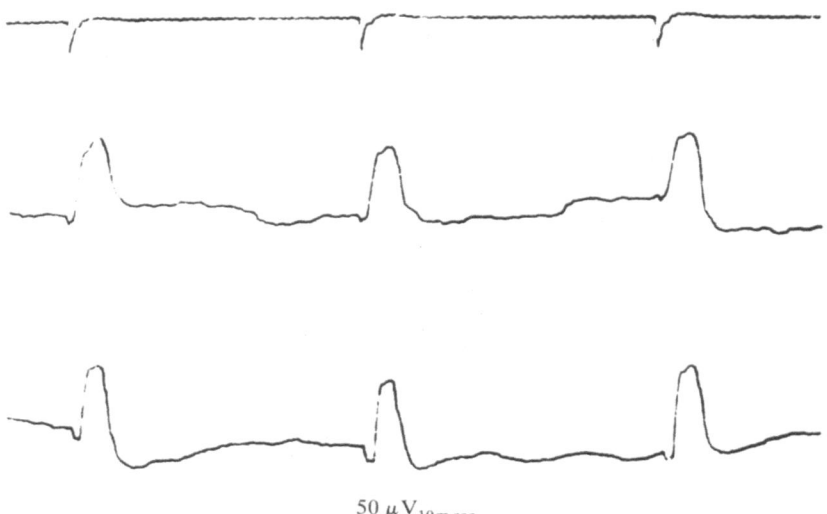

$$50 \, \mu V_{10 \, m.sec.}$$

Fig. 2. Normal ERG of an 11-month old girl affected with the Niemann–Pick disease. Dark adaptation: 10 minutes. Time constant: 0.3. Stimulus intensity: 1.0 Wsec. Local anesthesia.

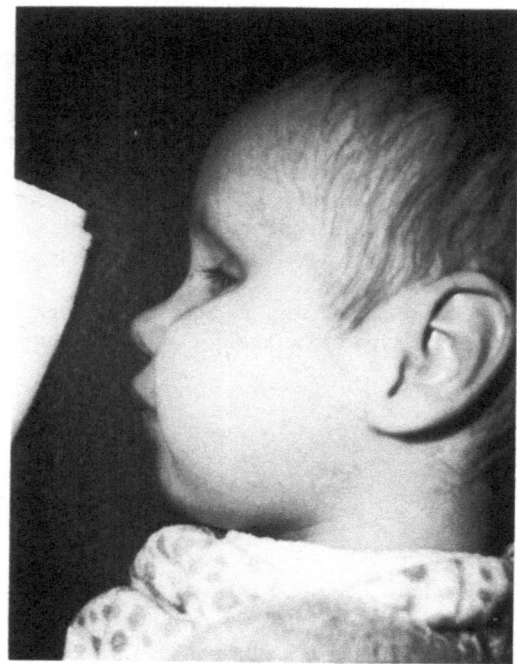

Fig. 3. Characteristic shape of the head, atonic extremities of a child with a Lowe's syndrome. Oculodigital phenomenon.

from. The sphyngomyelin accumulation developing as a result of sphyngomyelinase enzyme lack, is characteristic of the Niemann–Pick disease. Family history: her parents and brother are healthy, her birth weight was 3000 g. According to the mother the abdomen of the newborn was larger. Liver biopsy findings: on the basis of the electron microscopy the accumulated substance corresponds to lipids accumulating in the Niemann–Pick disease. Sternal puncture: within the cytoplasm of the swollen reticular cell numerous cytosomes of various size, resembling the electron microscopic picture of cytosomes of the liver. At the time of the ERG examination the greyish-white macular change was developing and had surrounded the cherry-red area on the eyeground. The retinograms obtained (Fig. 2), were according to age and did not show any pathologic alterations in conformity to most of the data contained in the relevant publications (François, 1976).

Among the inborn errors of metabolism the Lowe's syndrome of a two-year old boy is worth mentioning. A horizontal and vertical nystagmus, proteinuria, a remarkable muscular hypotension and a cataract were first observed at the age of 7 weeks. Intrauterine infection was suspected because of hepatosplenomegaly, but the examinations did not confirm this. The proteinuria (tubular), congenital cataract, muscular hypotension, amino-aciduria and nystagmus correspond to the Lowe's syndrome (Fig. 3). The genetic examinations did not show any alteration and the result obtained in a chromosome examination was normal. The ERG examination was carried out prior to the removal of the cataract and with the objective of a surgical prognosis. In spite of the reassuring ERG finding (Fig. 4) a successful removal of the cataract was not followed by an improved vision, although disorders could not be observed on the eye-ground. According to the data contained in publications, the operative results from the Lowe's oculocerebrorenal syndrome associated with aminoacidopathia cannot be deemed satisfactory (Auricchio, 1976).

The fourth case to be presented is an extraordinary manifestation of familar hyperlipoproteinemia. The blind child, aged 3 years, and of normal physical and mental development, has been observed since its age of 6 months. The

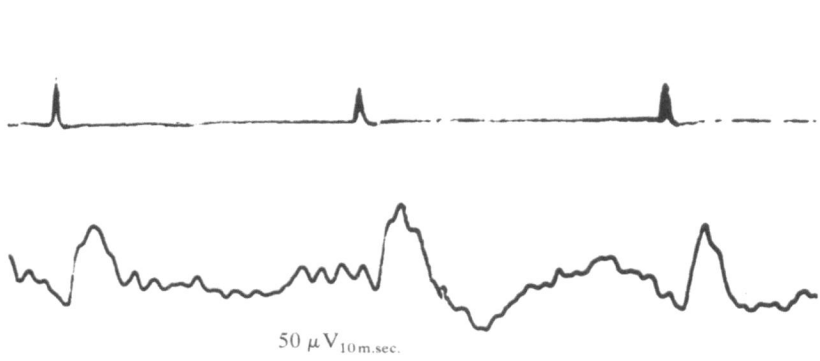

$50 \mu V_{10 m.sec.}$

Fig. 4. Normal ERG of a 2-year old boy with a Lowe's syndrome. Dark adaptation: 10 minutes. Time constant: 0.3. Stimulus intensity: 1.0 Wsec. Local anesthesia.

Table 1. Serum-lipoprotein data of the family.

	Cholest.	TG.	HDL-Cholest. mg/100ml	LDL-Cholest.	HDL-TG	LDL -TG
Our patient	353 <u>336</u>	93 90	<u>29</u>	<u>235</u>	—	—
Mother	358 <u>328</u>	74 104	<u>32</u>	<u>266</u>	35	55
Father	183	65	48	86	—	—
Sister	183	100	—	—	—	—

**Lipoprotein elektrophoreses data of our patient and his mother:
hyperlipoproteinaemia of II/a type**

laboratory data of the mother of an entirely healthy phenotype are essentially identical with those of the child. According to the laboratory data presented in the table, the dominant hereditary clinical picture corresponds to the hyperlipoproteinemia of type II/a (Fredrickson *et al.* 1978). The yellowish, slightly protuberant area of unusual appearance of the eyeground of the boy is most likely due to cholesterol accumulation (Fig. 5). The density of finely granulated

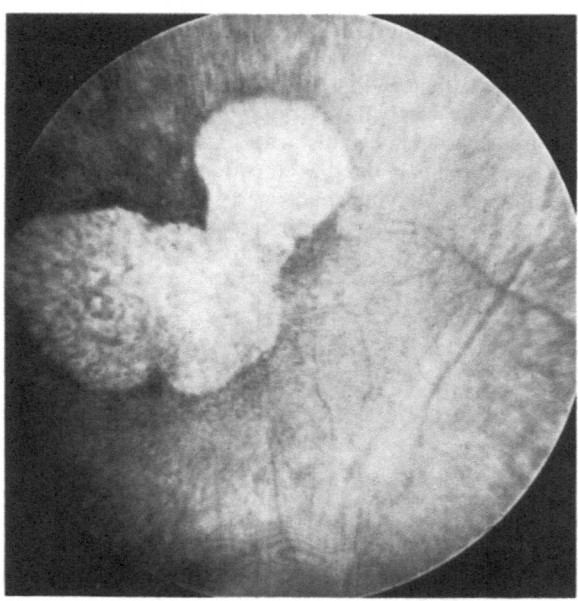

Fig. 5. Picture of the eyeground of a 6-month old blind boy with familiar hyperlipoproteinemia. Atrophic papilla. Yellowish-grey, slightly protuberant area with intensely pigmented margin on the posterior pole.

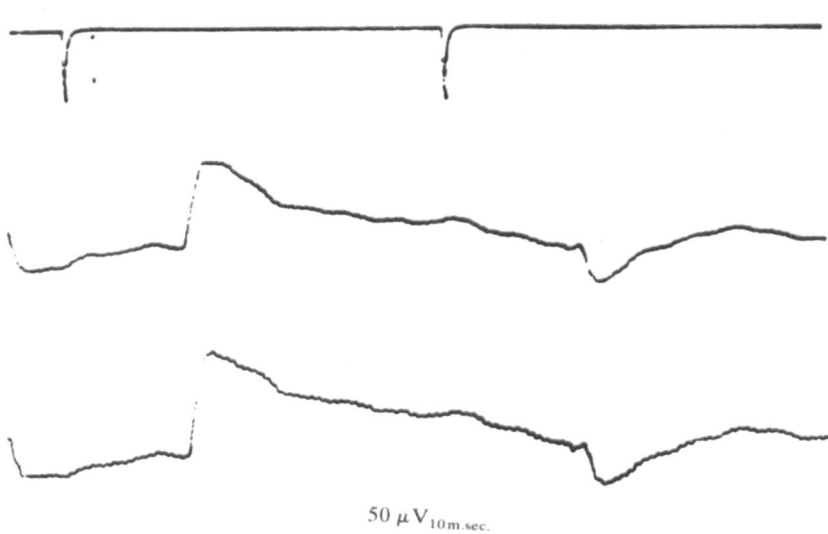

$50 \mu V_{10\,m.sec.}$

Fig. 6. Extinct ERG of a 6 months old boy with hyperlipoproteinemia. Dark adaptation: 10 minutes. Time constant: 0.3. Stimulus intensity: 1.0 Wsec. The ERG was taken without general anesthesia.

pigmentation is most pronounced around the sharply defined yellow area and grows gradually thinner. The retinal change is associated with a yellowish-grey optic papilla of indistinguishable contours, and with narrowed vessels. The ERG is extinct (Fig. 6). As far as we know, no comparable disorder of the eyeground of hyperbetalipoproteinemia has been published so far.

REFERENCES

Auricchio, G. Ocular manifestations of aminoacidopathies, in: XXIIe Concilium Ophthalmologicum Paris 1974. Ed. Masson. Vol. I, pp. 541–581 (1976).

Copenhaver, R.M. & G. Goodman. The electroretinogram in infantile, late infantile and juvenile amaurotic family idicoy. *Arch. Ophthal., Chicago,* 63: *559–566* (1960).

Fredrickson D.S., J.L. Goldstein & N.S. Brown. The familial hyperlipoproteinaemias, in: The Metabolic basis of inherited diseases. Ed. Stanbury, Wyngaarden and Fredrickson, New York, pp. 604–656 (1978).

François, J. Ocular manifestations of inborn errors of carbohydrate and lipid metabolism, in: XXIIe Concilium Ophthalmologicum Paris 1974. Ed. Masson. Vol. I, pp. 541–581 (1976).

Haut, J. & Z. Joannides. A propos de 55 cas de syndrome de Lowe. *Arch. Ophthal., Paris,* 26: *21–28* (1966).

Moreau, P.G. & P. Pichon. L'ophtalmologiste face à une hyperlipidémie. Conduite à tenir. *Arch. Ophthal., Paris,* 32: *53–56* (1972).

Pampiglione G., G. Privett & A. Harden. Neurophysiological studies in 20 children with Tay–Sachs disease. *Electroenceph. Clin. Neurophysiol.* 35: *414* (1973).

Pedriel, G., M. Fontaine, J.J. Aron, J. Cheveleraud & M. Leblanc. Electroretinogram and evoked occipital potentials in blindness cases in children, in: Wirth, A. ed. Proc. VIII. Symp. ISCERG, Pisa, pp. 78–82 (1970).

Straub, W. & B. Schmidt. Le diagnostic des dégénerescences tapetorétiniennes chez l'enfant. *Bull. Soc. Franç. Ophtal.* 82: *5–11* (1969).

Vinger, P.F. & B.A. Sachs. Ocular manifestations of hyperlipoproteinaemia. *Amer. J. Ophthal.* 70: *563–573* (1970).

Author's address:
Dr. Anna Bohár,
II. Szemklinika
Semmelweis Orvostudomanyi Egyetem
Maria ut 39
H-1085 Budapest
Hungary

Docum. Opthal. Proc. Series, Vol. 23

CLINICAL AND ELECTROOCULOGRAPHIC FINDINGS IN CASES OF REGULAR HAEMODIALYSIS

WINFRIED MÜLLER AND H. THIELER

(*Erfurt, G.D.R.*)

ABSTRACT

18 patients from a dialysis programme were called upon for a more accurate electrodiagnostic examination. The clinical ophthalmological results obtained with these and their satisfactory visual functions must be considered good. The electrodiagnostic findings result from the reduction in the overall course of the EOG. The authors take this as an expression of uraemic retinopathy analogous similarly as this is the case with the well known nephrogenic encephalopathy.

Eighteen patients from our dialysis programme were called upon for a more accurate electrodiagnostic examination. As shown in Table 1, the patients concerned were 8 women and 10 men at an average of 34.2 years. As a rule, they had to undergo a highly effective short-time dialysis 3 times a week (the time for the dialysis was 3.5 hours, the high effectiveness was obtained by connecting two filters in parallel).

The period of treatment was about 2 years on the average. In 3 cases the time of treatment was more than 7 years which must be considered a remarkable incident. In the case of 3 of our patients the haemodialysis treatment became necessary despite the kidney transplant effected, in the case of three other patients both kidneys were removed. The clinical diagnoses were: Chronic glomerulonephritis (13), peracute glomerulonephritis (2), chronic pyelonephritis (1), nephrocirrhosis (1), polycystic renal disease (1). All the patients concerned were socially fully rehabilitated. The biochemical data were marked by a general increase in creatinine and bound urea nitrogen (BUN). In the case of potassium and magnesium there was no general increase (see Table 2).

The opthalmological findings were quite good. As shown in Table 3 the visual acuity was from 0.8 to 1.0. There were no colour deficiencies. Impaired

Table 1. General data of kidney patients.

number of patients:	18 (8♀, 10♂)	
age:	34.2 years	(oldest pat. 48 y.) (youngest pat. 18 y.)
dialysis history:	$2^{3/4}$ years	(shortest dur. 5 mon.) (longest dur. 7 3/4 y.)
frequency of dialysis:	3 × weekly = 11 patients 2 × weekly = 7 patients	

143

Table 2. Biochemical values of 18 kidney patients.

	average		
BUN	80.5 mg%	min. value max.value normal value	59 mg % 110 mg % 40 mg %
Creatinine	12.8mg%	min. value max. value normal value	6.9 mg% 17.0 mg% 1.2 - 1.3 mg%
Potassium	5.11 mval	min. value max. value norm. value	3.2 mval 6.2 mval 4.5 - 5.5 mval
Magnesium	3.2 mval	min. value max. value normal value	2.0 mval 4.9 mval 1.3-2.2 mval

vision in immediate adaptation could be proved in one patient only. Cornea and conjunctiva calcinosis was discovered 16 times. The latter findings were dependent on a great number of factors which are not interrelated with the basic disease, but with the methods applied to the dialysis, especially with the composition of the water used in the dialysis. In the case of this small number of patients it also becomes apparent that we could give proof of beginning cataracts in 5 cases which, there is no doubt, must be ascribed to the special way in which we applied the methods of the dialysis treatment. The ophthalmoscopical findings were astonishingly good in all patients. Vascular changes in most cases were only trifling and comparatively inconspicuous. We discovered twice changes of the disc, the picture of a typical retinopathia angiospastica could not be given proof of. Due to these unobjectionable clinical, ophthalmological findings we had good reason to assume that in the electrodiagnostic examination there were hardly noticeable results to be obtained.

Table 3. Ophthalmological findings relative to 18 kidney patients.

Ophthalmological findings (18 pat.)

visus	: 0.8 - 1.0
calcinosis (cornea conj.)	: 16 pat.
cataracta incipiens	: 4 pat.
vascular changes	: 16 pat.
colour	: normal
dark adaptation	: 1 x subnormal

Table 4. Mean values of characteristic EOG data of kidney patients in comparison with those of a control group.

right eye	control-group	haemo-dialysis patients	t-value	signifi-cance
	μV	μV	–	–
0- value	485	358	4. 107	+
dark-trough	333	202	6. 139	+
light - peak	733	569	4. 467	+

We examined the EOG without any special preadaptation. By that we obtained the non-influenced initial value important for the assessment (zero point for the EOG). After a dark phase of 12 minutes a light phase of 12 minutes followed (800 lux). In the evaluation the overall course of each EOG was being assessed. In addition to such an assessment an average EOG of the patient group was established that was compared mathematically and statistically with the average EOG of a control group, of special importance for us being the EOG starting point, the dark trough and the light peak. We have neglected the Arden quotient. Table 4 and Fig. 1 show the results obtained

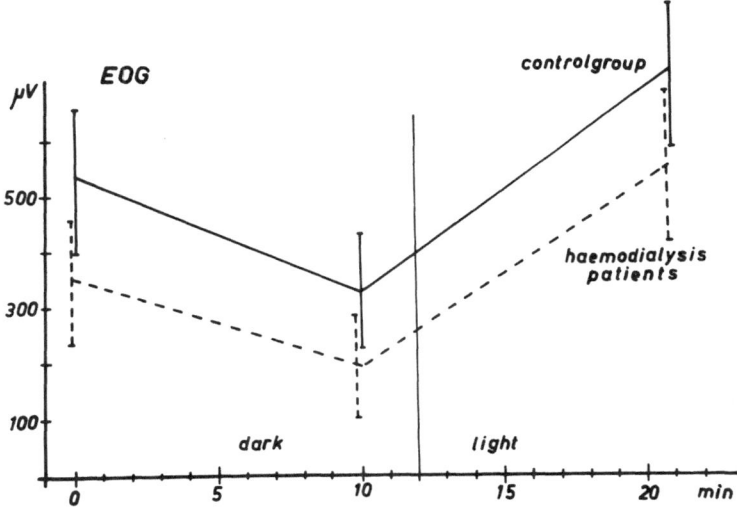

Fig. 1. The average EOG curve of kidney patients is clearly reduced as against that of a control group.

with the comparison of the two average EOGs. The EOG of patients treated with the chronic intermittent haemodialysis was significantly reduced in the overall course, that is to say it was subnormal. We could not give unambiguous proof of a time difference between the dark trough and light peak as compared to the standard group.

The examination of the individual electrooculograms revealed: Only 3 patients have shown an electrooculogram that was in agreement with standard, twice we discovered superelevated potential curves, 13 times we noticed subnormality, two patients were showing a pronounced subnormality. There was not even one case in which an EOG of the flat type could be made out.

Figure 2, for example, shows the electrooculogram of patient No. 14 (surplus EOG) and the EOG of patient No. 18 with subnormality. The indicated data related to blood chemistry and haemodialysis history show that there is no direct relationship between the different EOG curves and the corresponding parameters.

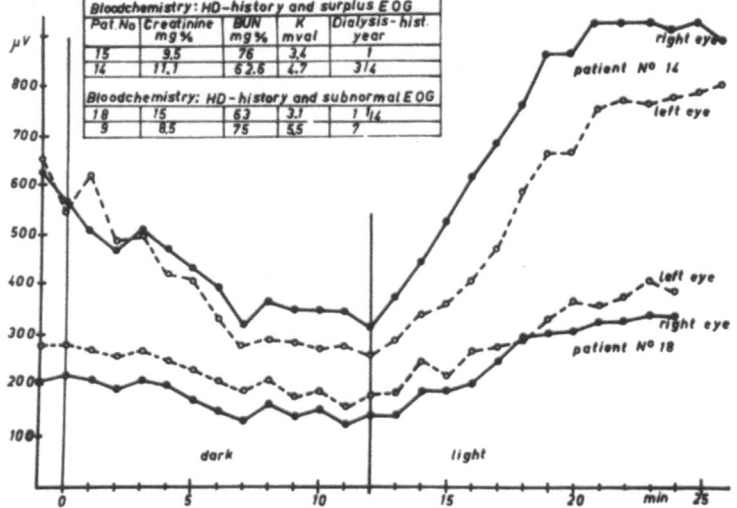

Fig. 2. The biochemical data of two patients with a subnormal EOG and two patients with superelevated potential reactions show no clear differences.

From the data indicated one cannot arrive at the conclusion that there is a superelevated potential curve or subnormality. The apparently distinct change of the EOG in those patients who undergo a chronic intermittent haemodialysis treatment, mainly consists in the reduction in the overall course of the EOG, points to a considerable electrophysiological disorder in the retinal area, and can only be explained as an expression of uraemic retinopathy analogously to the well known uraemic or nephrogenic encephalopathy. Such a uraemic retinopathy – that shows, as do our other studies in this volume and that can be proved by means of the ERG – keeps out of the reach of general, clinical and ophthalmological examinations, since ophthalmological findings are visible only to a limited degree.

REFERENCES

Höhne, W. Zur Auswertung des Elektrookulogramms. *Albrecht v. Graefes Arch. klin. exp. Ophthal.* 192: 36–47 (1974).

Thieler, H., U. Schmidt, M. Marx, N. Otto & N. Jung. 1977. Ein chronisches Dialyse-Programm unter fast ausschließlichem Einsatz hocheffektiver Kurzzeitdialyse. 2. Donau-Symposium für Nephrologie 26–28.9. 1977. Budapest. Verlag C. Bindernagel. Friedberg/Hessen. 1978.

Author's address:
Prof. Dr. med. habil. Winfried Müller
Augenklinik Med. Akademie Erfurt
DDR-506 Erfurt
Nordhäuser Str. 74
German Democratic Republic

ERG ON PATIENTS WITH CHRONIC NEPHROPATHY

A. FARKAS

(*Budapest, Hungary*)

ABSTRACT

The amplitude of b-wave was measured in 20 patients suffering from chronic glomerulonephritis, but without eye disease. Significantly low values ($p < 0.01$) were observed in those who fell ill below the age of 35 years. It was not possible to demonstrate a correlation between the amplitudes of the b-wave and the laboratory values studied. Hypertension could be excluded as a casual factor. Most likely some toxic damage of neural elements must be held responsible for the development of subnormal b-waves. It may be assumed that in younger patients these elements are more sensitive to toxic damage associated with renal disturbance.

Similarly to the action potentials in other structures of living organisms, the retinogram has a membrane potential character (Adams and Hagins, 1960) and thus depends on the ion transport through the cell membrane. Therefore it seems to be obvious to consider the characteristics of the retinogram as influenced by the actual ionic conditions. As early as in 1949 Hodgkin and Katz pointed out the relationship between the action potential and the sodium concentration of the surrounding fluid. However examinations in this field–especially in humans–must be considered complex due to several factors. Therefore it is easy to understand why most of the publications report on "in vitro" experiments carried out with isolated retinal preparations (Sillman *et al.*, 1969; Winkler, 1973).

After giving a glycocorticoid injection Wirth and Tota (1968) have observed an increased amplitude in the ERG of cats. After aldosteron injection administered to rats the b-wave showed a rise of 45 per cent. In healthy human eyes Zimmerman *et al.* (1973) noted significantly increased a- and b-waves during the treatment with prednisolon. The cause of increased ERG amplitudes in these cases most likely is due to the fact that the corticosteroids are changing the sodium-potassium balance by exerting an influence on the distal renal tubules.

One of the reasons why the examination of ions which influence the retinogram recorded in living persons must be considered difficult may be explained by the fact that the values of serum electrolytes determined clinically are not necessarily equal to the ionic composition of the interstitial and intracellular fluid, playing a decisive role in the ion exchange.

Although there are quite a few uncertainties in the above examinations, careful estimation of the ERG data may give valuable information for the assessment of the patient's condition suffering from chronic renal disease.

We studied the retinogram of 20 patients suffering from chronic glomerulonephritis, by giving special regard to the amplitude of the b-waves. The age of the patients ranged from 16 to 55 years, the time that had passed since establishing the diagnosis was between 2 and 10 years. They had no eye disease, the visual acuity was good. One third of the patients (6 persons) had normal blood pressure, two thirds (14 persons) had hypertension of a moderate degree. The eyeground was intact in about half of the cases, the remaining half had hypertonic vascular manifestations of various degrees, distinct retinopathy, however, was not observed. In the urine of the patients, proteinuria of various degrees and in general, decreased specific weight was found. As far as the electrolytes are concerned, pathologic values of the sodium concentration were not observed, whereas five patients showed a moderately increased serum potassium level. The values of BUN (blood urea nitrogen) and serum creatinin were pathologically increased in about half of the cases.

The retinographic examinations were carried out according to the method of Karpe, the amplification and registration with a 4-channel EMG encephalograph. An EMG photostimulator was used. The amplitude of b-wave registered under photopic conditions was measured. [Its normal value being between 150 and 300 μV under our laboratory conditions.]

Figures 1 and 2 show the results obtained. It may be noticed, that in "younger" patients (on the average 18.2 years) the amplitude of the b-wave is distinctly subnormal, whereas in "older" ones (39 years on the average, at the beginning of the illness) the amplitude of the b-wave is within normal limits.

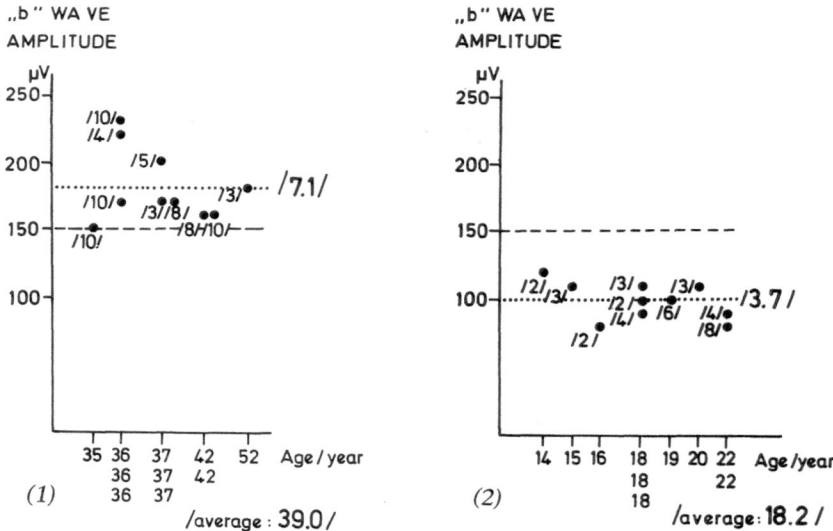

Fig. 1 and 2. Correlation between the b-wave amplitude and the patient's age at the time of diagnosis. The small Arabic numbers show the duration of the disease. The difference of b-wave amplitudes between "younger" and "older" groups is highly significant (p < 0.01).

The difference between the amplitudes of b-waves of the two groups is highly significant (p < 0.01).

It was neither possible to correlate the above tendency of the b-wave amplitudes with the seriousness of the illness nor with the laboratory values.

One retinogram is demonstrated from each group. Figure 3 shows the subnormal retinogram of a patient aged 18 years. In Figure 4 the retinogram was taken from a patient aged 42 years; the b-wave amplitude is normal.

We were cautious not to overestimate the results obtained in examinations carried out in a comparatively low number of cases. However, the consistent incidence of subnormal b-waves in youth is hardly accidental. In the case of our patients we consider that the damaging effect caused by hypertension may be excluded. Among the authors dealing with the retinogram of hypertensive patients Henkes (1954) noted that the b-waves were normal or supernormal. In the case of moderate hypertensive vascular alterations Karpe (1945) and Schmöger (1955) reported normal values.

In our cases most likely some toxic damage to particularly sensitive structures must be held responsible for the ERG pattern. The younger the patients with chronic renal failure clearer becomes the ERG change. Thus it may be assumed that the sensitivity of the cells will be reduced after some years.

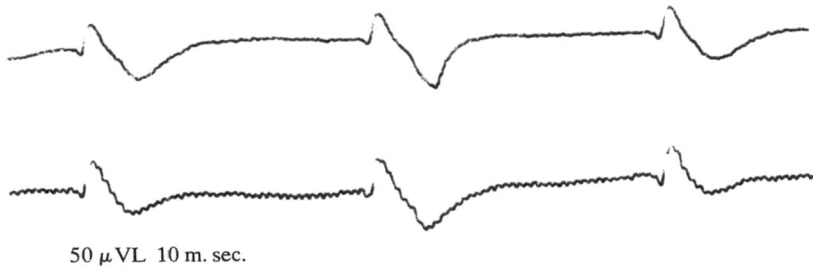

50 μVL 10 m. sec.

Fig. 3. subnormal retinogram of an 18-year old patient.

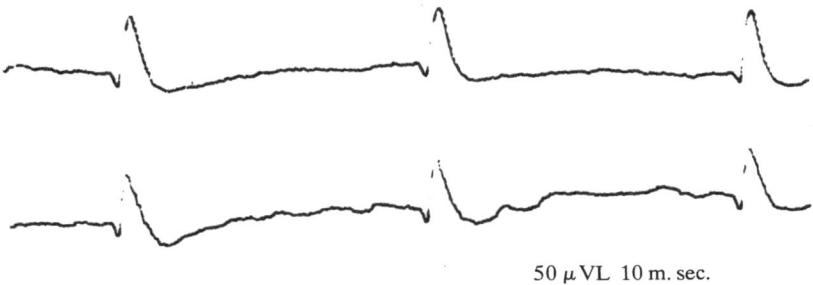

50 μVL 10 m. sec.

Fig. 4. Normal retinogram of a patient aged 42 years. After dark adaption of 10 minutes. Time constant: 0.03 sec. Intensity of light: 1.0 Ws

151

REFERENCES

Adams, R.G. & W.A. Hagins. The ionic composition of squid photoreceptors. *Biol. Bull.* 119: *300–301*, (1960).

Henkes, H.E. Electroretinogram in circulatory disturbances of the retina IV. Electroretinogram in cases of retinal and choroidal hypertension and arteriosclerosis. *Arch. Ophthal.* 52: *30–41*, (1954).

Henkes, H.E., J.P. van der Kam- & A.J.S. Westhoff, Electroretinographic studies in arterial hypertension. Effect of reduction in blood pressure on electrical responses of human retina. *Arch. Ophthal.* 52: *221–233*, (1954).

Hodgkin, A.L. & B. Katz. The effect of sodium ions on the electrical activity of the giant axon of the squid. *J. Physiol.* 108: *37–77*, (1949).

Karpe, G. The basis of clinical electroretinography. *Acta ophthal. (KBh.), Suppl. 24* (1945).

Schmöger, E. & W. Thieme Das klinische Elektroretinogramm. *Dtsch. Gesd. wes. 10: 1159–1164*, (1955).

Sillman, A.J., H. Ito & T. Tomita Studies on the mass receptor potential of the isolated frog retina II. On the basis of the ionic mechanism. *Vision Res.* 9: *1443–1450*, (1969).

Winkler, B. S. Dependence of fast components of the electroretinogram of the isolated rat retina on the ionic environment. *Vision Res.* 13: *457–463*, (1973).

Wirth, A. & G. Tota Electroretinogram and adrenal cortical function. Advances in electrophysiology and pathology of the visual system. Sixth ISCERG Symposium 1967. Ed. by E. Schmöger. Thieme Leipzig. 347–350. 1968.

Zimmerman, T.J., W.W. Dawson & C.R. Fitzgerald Electroretinographic changes in normal eyes during administration of prednisone (Part I.) *Ann. Ophthal.* 5: *757-765*, 1973.

Author's address:
Dr. Agnes Farkas
Second Department of Ophthalmology
Semmelweis Medical University
Maria ut 39
H-1035 Budapest
Hungary

LOGISTIC FUNCTION IN THE ANALYSIS OF THE ERG IN DIALYSED PATIENTS

J. SVĚRÁK, J. PEREGRIN, D. HEJCMANOVÁ, J. ERBEN
AND J. GROH
(*Hradec Králové, Czechoslavakia*)

ABSTRACT

The ERG intensity-response function of the b-wave in 32 patients undergoing regular hemodialysis treatment was evaluated using a logistic equation. Statistically significant lowering of the retinal sensitivity (M-parameter of the logistic function) has been observed. 37.5% of the patients displayed the subnormal values of the b-waves (A), lower slope (S) and significant lower retinal sensitivity (M). The immediate effect of a single dialysis manifests itself in about 30 per cent of the patients by a transient, statistically significant lowering of the retinal sensitivity.

There is an increasing amount of evidence suggesting that the ERG of patients undergoing the regular hemodialysis treatment is pathologically changed (1, 3, 5). Our previous experience (4) showed that a depressed retinal activity in these patients manifested itself by the depression of the ERG intensity-response curves. The aim of the present study is a detailed quantitative analysis of the ERG intensity-response function.

METHODS

Thirty two patients (aged 36 years on average), undergoing a regular hemodialysis treatment (143 dialyses on average), were studied. All were suffering from the chronic terminal renal insufficiency on the basis of the chronic glomerulonephritis or interstitial nephritis. The patients were compensated using 14 to 18 hours of dialysis weekly by means of two coil kidneys of $1 \, m^2$ dialysis cuprophane or nephrophane area.

The ERG examination (2) covers the registration of 11 ERG curves in the intensity range of 5 log units using 11 intensity levels in steps of 0.5 log units. The maximum intensity of the xenon discharge tube is 70 Ws. Under these conditions the amplitudes of the ERG b- and a-waves display a sigmoidal shape (Fig. 1.). Mathematically, these curves can be well described by a logistic function (Fig. 2). In a reparametrised form this equation is helpful for the description of the retinal functions.

The logistic equation was computed using s digital computer ODRA 1204. The programme allowed the estimation of the principal parameters and their standard deviations, and a statistical comparison of different groups of patients.

153

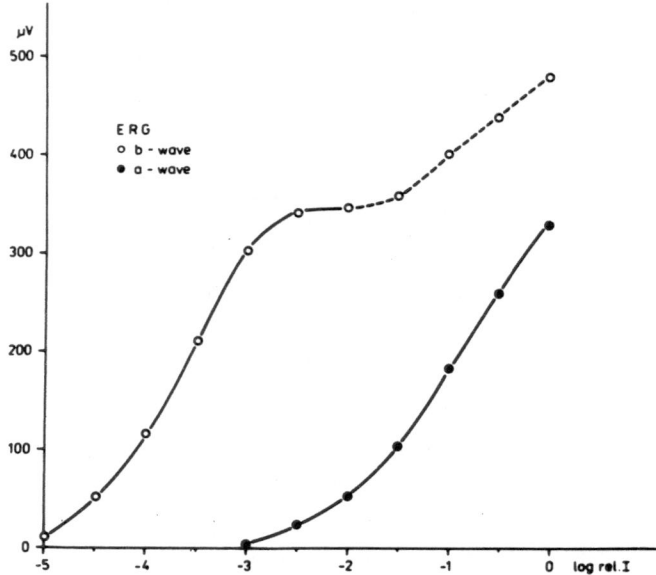

Fig. 1. ERG I–R curves.

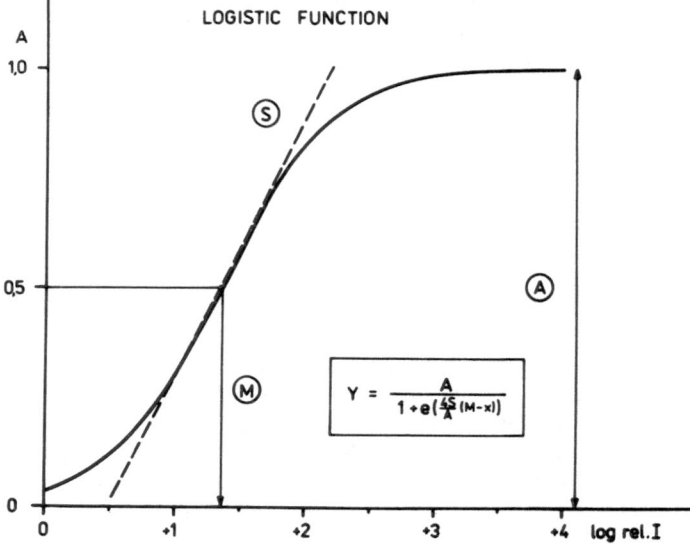

Fig. 2. A: The maximal value of the b-wave potential. M: The photo-stimulation intensity at 50 per cent of the maximal amplitude. S: The slope of the curve at the inflexion point.

RESULTS

The mean values of the intensity-dependent b-wave amplitudes in groups of 50 controls and in 32 dialysed patients are presented in Fig. 3. The values of all three evaluated parameters (M, S, A) in the patient-group are distinctly lower (Fig. 4). Statistically significant is the lowering of the retinal sensitivity only. An analysis of the individual intensity-response curves showed, that lower values are present in 12 patients (37.5%).

The immediate effect of a single dialysis on the ERG in a group of 14 patients (Fig. 5) gives evidence about the statistically significant lowering of the sensitivity (M) and nonsignificant lowering of the amplitude (A) and the slope of the curve (S).

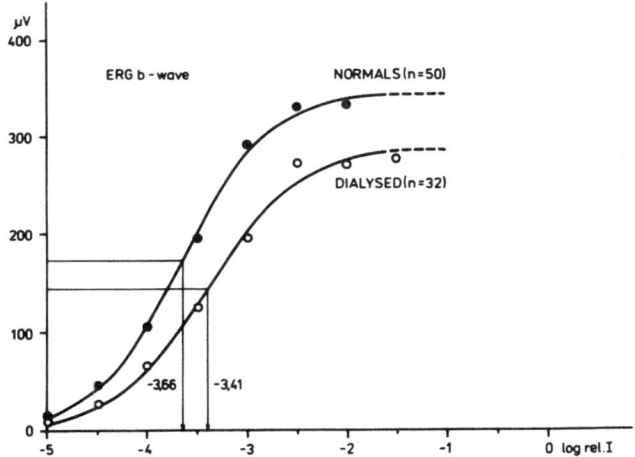

Fig. 3. Intensity-reaction changes expressed by logistic function.

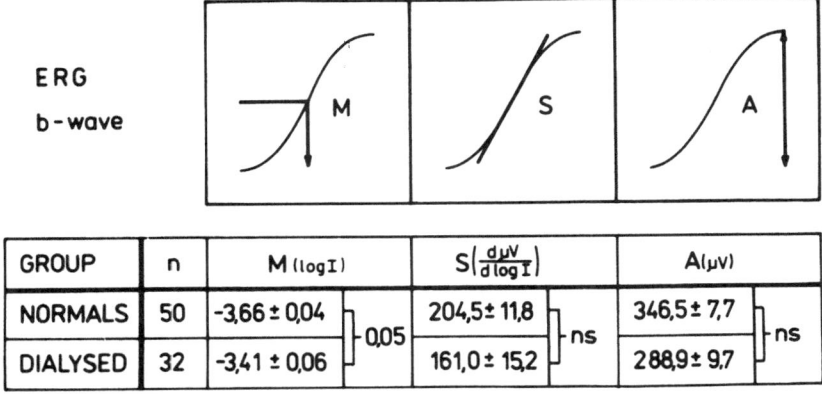

GROUP	n	M (logI)		$S\left(\frac{d\mu V}{d\log I}\right)$		A(μv)	
NORMALS	50	-3,66 ± 0,04	0,05	204,5 ± 11,8	ns	346,5 ± 7,7	ns
DIALYSED	32	-3,41 ± 0,06		161,0 ± 15,2		288,9 ± 9,7	

Fig. 4. Statistical evaluation of the M-, S- and A-parameters.

GROUP	n	$M_{(\log I)}$		$S\left(\frac{d\,\mu V}{d\log I}\right)$		$A_{(\mu V)}$	
PRE-DIAL.	14	−3,41 ± 0,03	} 0,05	181,12 ± 10,8	} ns	292,7 ± 5,5	} ns
POST -	14	−3,28± 0,03	} 0,01	165,18± 7,3	} 0,01	278,3 ± 4,4	} 0,01
POST -	5	−3,01 ± 0,05	} 0,01	119,35± 9,3	} 0,01	196,4 ± 6,4	} 0,01
POST -	9	−3,35± 0,02		195,6 ± 8,1		324,7 ± 4,5	

Fig. 5. Statistical evaluation of the pre- and post-dialysis values of the M-, S- and A-parameters.

In 5 out of the 14 patients examined before and after the dialysis, great subjective discomfort (headache, nausea) has been stated. If the group was divided according to the subjective feelings, it could be shown, that the subgroup with subjective discomfort displays a statistically significant lowering of all parameters of the logistic equation after the dialysis in comparison to the rest of the group. These 9 patients did not differ in the postdialysis values from the predialysis b-wave potentials.

The ERG findings in the entire group of 32 patients were correlated with the values of BUN, Vitamin A, residual glomerular filtration rate and some ions. No significant correlation between the abnormaly ERG findings and these characteristics has been found.

DISCUSSION

The analysis of the results of the ERG examination using a logistic equation confirms previous findings of the subnormal ERG b-wave in dialysed patients (1, 3). Moreover the analysis allows a more detailed classification of the subnormality of the ERG responses.

Using this method it could be shown, that 37.5% of the dialysed patients display subnormal values of the ERG b-wave, lower slope and statistically significant lower retinal sensitivity. The effect of a single dialysis manifests itself in about 30 per cent of the examined patients by the transient alteration of the retinal activity.

The correlation between the ERG findings and several characteristics of the physical status of the patients was found to be non-significant. Further work is needed in this area.

REFERENCES

1. Mihara, A. The studies on the eyes of the subjects of renal disease with the treatment by the hemodialysis and the peritoneal dialysis. Report II. The correlation between the EOG and ERG. *Acta Soc. Ophthal. Jap.* 77: *1116–1123* (1973).

2. Peregrin, J. & Svěrák, J. Die elektroretinographischen Intensitäts-Reaktionskurven. I. Physiologische Grundlagen. Advances in electrophysiology and pathology of the visual system. Proc. VIth ISCERG Symp. Erfurt 1967, 355–361. Thieme Verlag Leipzig 1968, edit. E. Schmöger 1968.
3. Perossini, M. & G. Tota. Electroretinographic findings in chronic uraemics treated with periodic haemodialysis. *Docum. Ophthal., Proc. Series,* 15: *257–263* (1978).
4. Svěrák, J., J. Peregrin, J. Groh, J. Erben J. & D. Hejcmanová Změny elektrické aktivity sítnice při chronické intermetentní dialyze Čs. oftal., 35: *332–338* (1979).
5. Zimmermann, T.J., W.W. Dawson & J.R. Cade. Electroretinographic changes: pre- and postrenal dialysis. *Ann. Ophthal.* (Chic.). 5: *769–772* (1973).

Author's address:
Dept. of Ophthalmology
University Hospital
500 36 Hradec Králové
Czechoslovakia

157

CHRONIC HAEMODIALYSIS AND ERG

WINFRIED MÜLLER, E. HAASE, R. NIEDLICH, J. GAUSS
AND N. JUNG

(*Erfurt, G.D.R.*)

ABSTRACT

Eighteen kidney patients showing a comparatively good compensation and satisfactorily clinical ophthalmological results were examined. The results showed: (1) Photopic ERG was normal in all cases. (2) In comparison with a control group scotopic ERG showed a statistically significant reduction in amplitudes of a- and b-waves in about two thirds of the cases. Two eyes showed superelevated potential reactions. (3) No peak time differences as to the normal values were found. (4) Dynamic ERG showed distinct reductions in amplitudes in nearly all of the cases. (5) There was no correlation between biochemical data, length of dialysis history and ERG. (6) The authors consider the failure of the scotopic system as an expression of uraemic retinopathy.

INTRODUCTION

If one examines the mass of ERG literature, information on the ERG in cases of patients undergoing a chronic intermittent haemodialysis in renal diseases is given comparatively seldom, even when taking diseases such as the Senior Looken syndrome and Alport syndrome into consideration. B. Dyszynska-Rosciszewska and coworkers (1975), J. Pneck (1976), D. Huck and coworkers (1976), R. Severin (1975), Goldberg and coworkers (1973), H. Hatano and coworkers (1976) a.o. reported on the problematical nature recently. The sub-normality of the ERG seems to be the substantial ERG result obtained with all patients affected with a renal failure, given that the Senior Looken syndrome, coming along with an extinguished ERG, is ignored.

The photopic, scotopic and dynamic ERG in 18 patients from our dialysis programme was recorded just before the dialysis treatment.

The Photopic ERG

Recording was effected after 10 minutes adaptation in a bright room. The potentials were recorded by an amplifier and an oscilloscope; subsequently they were measured. The average curves, standard deviations and a mathematical and statistical comparison were determined for one control group (F- and t-test).

The amplitudes and peak times of the a- and b-waves of the photopic ERG of our dialysis patients showed no statistically significant difference in comparison to that of a control group.

Recording was effected after dark adaptation of 20 minutes. The amplitudes and peak times of the a- and b-waves were measured. After estimation of the average curves and standard deviation the mathematical and statistical determination was effected. The t-test resulted in a significant diminution of the

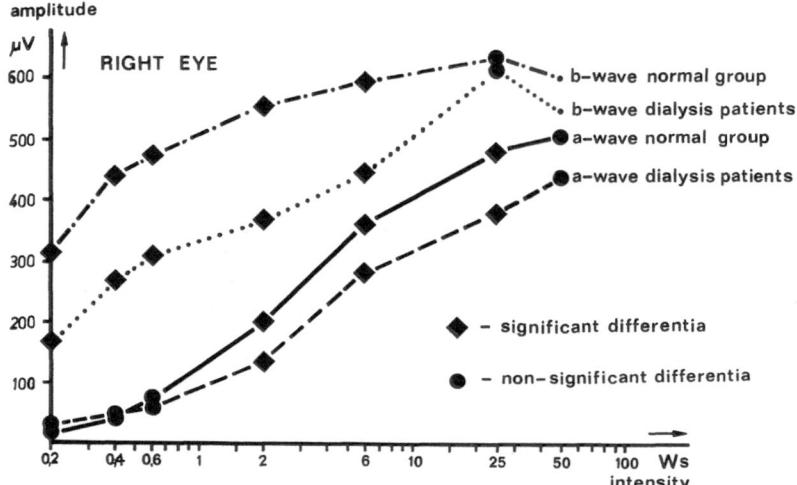

Fig. 1. Average ERG of the standard group and average ERG of the dialysis patient. Right eye

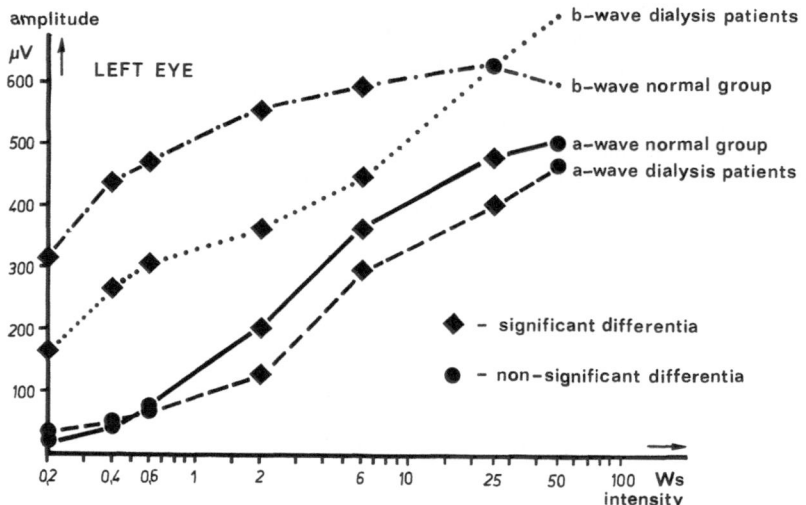

Fig. 2. Average ERG of the standard group and average ERG of the dialysis patient. Left eye

amplitudes of the scotopic ERG from those of a control group whose eyes and kidneys are perfectly sound. These variations apply to both the a-wave and the b-wave. Figures 1 and 2 show the average ERG of the standard group and the average ERG of the dialysis patient. Marking the deviation was dispensed with.

The areas of the differences determined mathematically and statistically were marked by crosses, and those areas in which no significant diminution could be proved were marked by a circle. The reduced curve of the retinal electric answers in dialysis patients becomes clearly discernible.

If the individual cases were analysed the result in such incidents must be regarded more differentiated (Table 1). In the case of 10 eyes the a-wave and the b-wave acted according to standard. In the case of 11 eyes only the b-wave was reduced, in the case of 13 eyes we found the reduction of a and b. Two eyes showed potentials distinctly superelevated.

Table 1. Individual ERG results

waves	diagnosis	eyes
a and b	normal	10
a and b	reduced	13
only b	reduced	11
a and b	elevated	2

The peak time of the a- and b-wave showed no distinct variation compared with the control group. All in all, however, the reduction in the retinal potentials must be taken – in the case of two thirds of the investigated eyes – as an expression of a uraemic retinopathy that is not discernible clinically and ophthalmoscopically, but that will become perfectly clear electroretinographically. We always pay special attention to the electroretinogram whose electric answers are always in the area of superelevated curves, unfortunately indicated as "supernormal" by other authors.

Figures 3 and 4 show the superelevated potential curve of the a- and b-wave of our patient No. 16 who has been treated with a chronic intermittent haemodialysis for two years and nine months. The illustrative figure also shows the data found in the laboratory. The creatinine and urea levels are increased. In this case there is no difference with the other dialysis patients. It should be noticed, however, that the patient concerned is the only one who shows a markedly reduced potassium value; perhaps this has something to do with it. Whereas the b-wave is considerably increased in all stimulus intensities, an a-wave increase can be proved only from 6.0 Ws forward. The electrooculogram shows no relevant curve, in other words: there is no superelevated potential reaction.

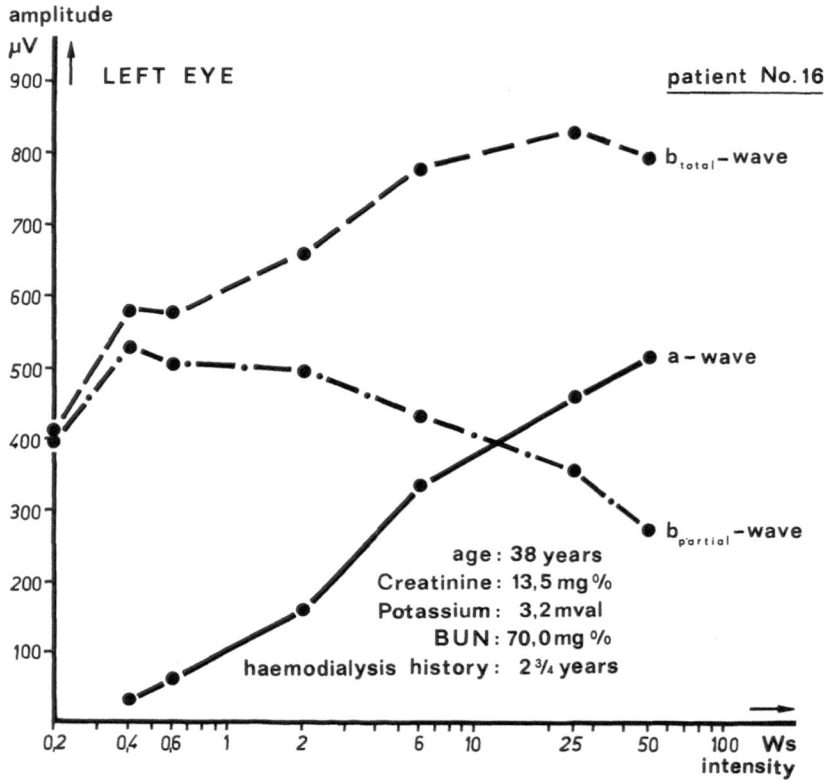

Fig. 3. Superelevated potential curve and the data found in the laboratory. The potassium value is markedly reduced. Left eye

The Dynamic ERG

After 10 minutes light adaptation, ERG recording takes place for a period of 20 minutes under scotopic conditions at a stimulus intensity of 2.0 Ws. Recording is effected by a common EEG amplifier and oscilloscope. The amplitudes of the a- and b-waves were measured.

Behaviour of b-wave amplitudes: Of 18 patients only 2 showed a curve that was in agreement with that of a control group. 16 patients showed a distinct subnormality, in 3 of them the subnormality being more pronounced (Figs. 5 and 6). There was no direct relationship with the biochemical data as to urea, creatinine, potassium and with the time of the dialysis treatment.

Behaviour of the a-wave amplitudes: The a-waves of 15 patients were within the lower standard range, only in the case of 3 patients did the subnormality of the a-waves become distinctly discernible. These were the same patients whose b-waves were so much reduced.

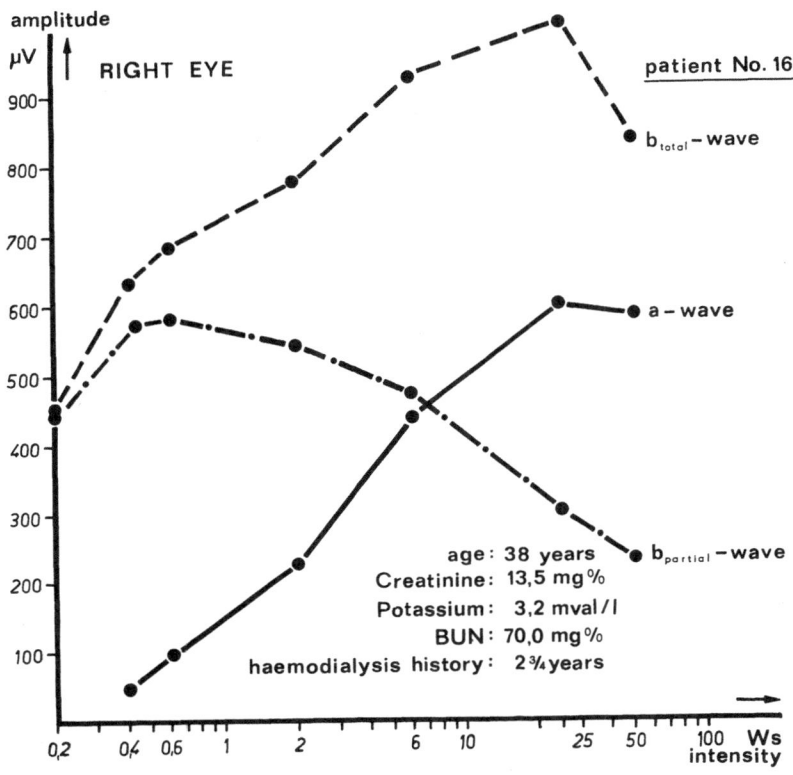

amplitude

μV | RIGHT EYE   patient No. 16

900 —

800 —   • b_{total} – wave

700 —

600 —   • a – wave

500 —

400 —

300 —

age: 38 years
Creatinine: 13,5 mg%
Potassium: 3,2 mval/l   • $b_{partial}$ – wave
BUN: 70,0 mg%
haemodialysis history: 2¾ years

100 —

0,2 0,4 0,6 1   2   6   10   25 50   100 Ws
                                              intensity

Fig. 4. Superelevated potential curve and the data found in the laboratory. The potassium value is markedly reduced. Right eye.

The time curve of the dynamic ERG showed that there also was a remarkable difference between the standard group and that of dialysis patients. While the increase in the b-wave of the control group was largely completed after 10 minutes, the dialysis group completed their wave increase in the dynamic ERG not earlier than after 15 minutes. The dynamic ERG reveals, same as the scotopic ERG, a considerable change as an expression of uraemic retinopathy.

Summarizing we can state: In our 18 kidney patients with a comparatively good compensation of the pathological process and satisfactorily clinical ophthalmological results we were able to prove;

1. The photopic ERG was normal in all incidents.
2. The average ERG recorded under scotopic conditions showed a statistically significant reduction in the amplitudes of the a- and b-waves as compared to the control group. Of 36 eyes only 10 showed a response of the a-wave and b-wave according to standard. 2 eyes showed superelevated potential reactions, 24 showed differently strongly reduced ERGs.

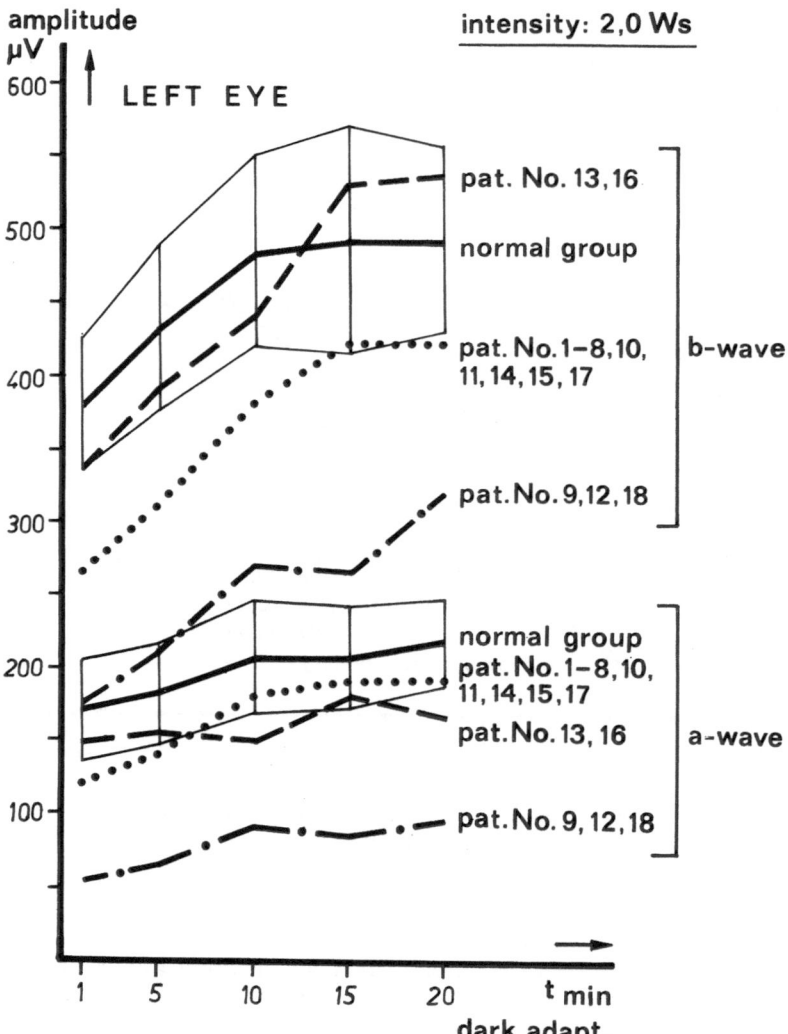

Fig. 5. Behaviour of the dynamic ERG. Left eye

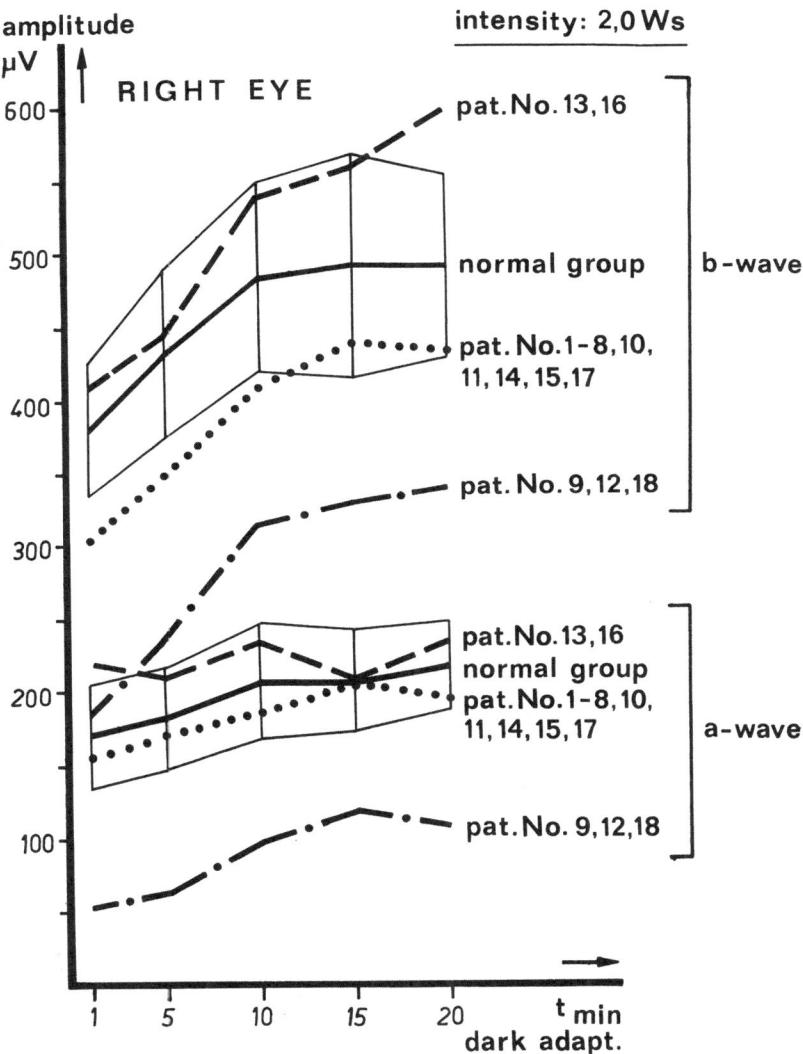

Fig. 6. Behaviour of the dynamic ERG. Right eye

165

3. Proof could not be given of a secured peak time difference between the group of these patients, suffering from a kidney disease, and the control group.
4. The dynamic ERG likewise shows a distinct reduction in the amplitudes. Only in the cases of 2 patients a standard behaviour could be noted. The a-waves were less concerned in the reduction. The time curve of the ERG in the cases of patients who had not to undergo a haemodialysis treatment was likewise changed as compared to standard. The increase in the b-waves in dialysis patients was completed not earlier than after 15 minutes, that of the control group already after 10 minutes.
5. There was no direct relationship with the biochemical data, the length of the dialysis history and the electrodiagnostic changes.
6. We take the failure of the scotopic system as an expression of uraemic retinopathy.

REFERENCES

Dyszynska-Rosciszewska, B. *et al.* Some observations on the status of visual system in patients with transplanted kidneys. *Klin. Ocna* 45/8: *921–926* (1975).
Goldberg, M. *et al.* Retinal infarction during haemodialysis. *Lancet* 2 (7881): *667* (1974).
Hatano, H. *et al.* Research on chronic renal failure patients, under an artificial dialysis treatment. *Folia Ophthal. Jap.* 27/11: *1086–1091* (1976).
Huck, D., H. Meythaler & R. Rix. Alport-Syndrom mit Hornhautbeteiligung und Veränderungen des ERG. *Klin. Mbl. Augenhk.* 168: *553–556* (1976).
Severin, M. Augenveränderungen bei juveniler Nephronophthise. *Klin. Mbl. Augenhk.* 166: *674–686* (1975).

Author's address:
Prof. Dr. med. habil. W. Müller
Augenklinik der
Medizinischen Akademie Erfurt
Nordhäuser Str. 74
DDR–506 Erfurt
German Democratic Republic

ELECTRORETINOGRAPHIC STUDIES IN PATIENTS AFTER RENAL TRANSPLANTATION

EWA DRÓBECKA-BRYDAK
AND ALICJA MOSZCZYŃSKA-KOWALSKA
(*Warsaw, Poland*)

ABSTRACT

Seventy two patients, aged from 14 to 52 years, were examined. The study describes scotopic ERG changes at different periods after renal transplantation. A relationship was found between the type of the ERG curve and the changes in the eye due to hypertension including arteriosclerosis and choroidal sclerosis. In spite of normal function of the transplanted kidneys, in the majority of the patients, abnormal ERGs have been found. Other observations are indispensable to find out whether the retinal dysfunction is progressive.

The development of transplantation techniques in recent years has led to an increasing number of publications estimating the state of the eye in patients after renal transplantation. Since 1968 periodic complex ocular examinations have been carried out in the Eye Clinic of Warsaw on haemodialised patients affected with renal insufficiency and on patients after renal transplantation. The purpose of this study was the electroretinographic examination of the retinal function on post renal transplant patients in relation to the arterial blood pressure, observation period after transplantation and changes of the eye fundus.

MATERIAL AND METHODS

Seventy two patients (17 women, 55 men) aged from 14 to 52 years had been examined. The age groups were as follows; below 20 years – nine patients, from 21 to 30 years twenty seven, from 31 to 40 years twenty-three, from 41 to 52 twelve. Renal transplantation was carried out on these patients due to the fact that they were suffering from chronic renal insufficiency resulting from glomerulonephritis or pyelonephritis.

Before the transplantation was carried out the disease lasted: up to 5 years in 26 patients, from 6 to 10 years in twenty-three patients, from 11 to 15 years in eight patients, over 15 years in twelve patients, not defined in 3 patients. In 33 out of these patients the arterial diastolic blood pressure exceeded 110 mmHg.

All patients received immunosuppressive therapy after the transplantation (Prednisone, Azathioprine or Cyclophosphamide. Hypotensive agents were administered to 35 patients. All patients were subjected to complex ocular examinations including visual acuity, slit lamp examination and ophthalmoscopy. ERG recordings were performed using an electroretiongraphor Alvar.

167

The first ocular examinations were carried out with 53 patients within a time of from 1 to 2 months following transplantation, with 12 patients from 3 to 6 months, with all the remaining cases up to 5 years. Thirty patients were subjected to a single examination, in the remaining patients such examination was carried out repeatedly.

The observation periods after transplantation were as follows: up to 6 months in 37 patients, 7 to 12 months in 13 patients, 1 to 2 years in 12 patients, 3 to 5 years in 7 patients and over 5 years in 3 patients.

RESULTS

The initial examination carried out with 72 patients (144 eyes) revealed a reduced visual acuity in 35 eyes. This was due to macular degeneration in the course of hypertension (22 eyes), posterior subcapsular cataract (9 eyes), or to preceding amblyopia (4 eyes). Control examinations revealed a slight reduction in the visual acuity in 10 eyes resulting from progressive lens opacification, and considerable diminution in 3 eyes due to cytomegalic virus (CMV) retinitis.

Vascular changes of the eye fundus were estimated according to the Keith–Wagener classification. During the first examination the eye fundus was normal in 6 cases, angiopathia hypertonica retinae I° or I/II° was diagnosed in 37 patients, angiopathia hypertonica arteriosclerotica in 29 patients.

Vascular changes in the eye fundus in relation to the duration of the disease before transplantation are shown in Table 1.

Apart from vascular changes related to hypertension the retina was very thin in some patients with a clearly visible choroid. The retinal periphery was pale with pigmentation, and mascular degenerative changes could be seen.

Table 2 shows central and peripheral retinal changes in relation to the duration of the disease.

Control examinations of the eye fundus have not shown any regression of vascular and degenerative changes.

Types of ERG recordings during the first examination are shown in Table 3.

The ERG performed on 42 patients from 6 months to 5 years, following the first examination, has not shown any significant differences. Evolution of the ERG changes was observed in 2 patients with CMV retinitis, 6 years and 6 months after transplantation. In one of these patients a 5 year follow-up

Table 1

Duration of the disease in years	Number of patients	Normal fundus	Hypertensive changes	
			I° and I/II°	II°
$\frac{1}{2}$–5	24	3	14	7
6–10	25	2	11	12
10	20	1	9	10
unknown	3	—	3	—

Table 2

Duration of the disease in years	Macula		Periphery	
	Normal	Pathological	Normal	Pathological
$\frac{1}{2}$–5	8	16	3	21
6–10	10	15	10	15
10	10	10	10	10
unknown	—	3	—	—

Table 3

Period after trans-plantation	Type of record				Remaining
	Supernormal	Normal	Subnormal	Negative	
1–2 months		27	67	5	7
3–6 months	2	8	5	2	
6–12 months		—	6	—	
1–3 years		6	—	2	

examination has shown an ERG with a high amplitude of the a-wave, and the b-wave must be considered negative +. One year ago the incidence of viral infection the ERG record changed to negative −. Residual ERG was obtained at the time of typical diffuse changes in one eye, and was subnormal when incipient changes in the second eye appeared.

In the second patient with unilateral CMV retinitis and partial retinal detachment the ERG was not recordable. In previous examinations the b-wave was bilaterally slightly diminished. In 8 patients the ERG was recorded before and after transplantation. A slight improvement in the ERG recordings was detected in only 3 patients; in the remaining cases the type of recording remained unchanged.

DISCUSSION

Many authors link the incidence of ocular complications in renal transplant patients with long-term administration of immunosuppresive therapy (Hovland (1967), de Venecia (1971), Porter (1972), Astle (1974), Murray (1977), Pavlin (1977), Pfefferman (1977)).

These complications include: increase in the intraoccular pressure, posterior subcapsular cataract and CMV retinitis. Periodic ocular examinations carried out in our Clinic confirmed the presence of those complications. A posterior subcapsular cataract was observed in 5 patients, CMV retinitis with a typical clinical course in 2 cases. The present study analyses scotopic ERG changes in patients at different periods following renal transplantation.

A relationship between the type of ERG recording and changes in the eye fundus due to hypertension with arteriosclerosis and choroidal sclerosis was found.

A normal ERG was obtained in patients with an unchanged eye fundus as well as in those affected with angiopathia hypertonica I° or I/II°. Apart from retinal vacular changes no other alterations have been found. Subnormal and negative ERG were detected in patients with evident sclerosis of the arteries and incipient peripheral alteration often manifested as increased pigmentation. In patients who survived the malignant phase of hypertension and exhibited diffuse and irreversible degenerative changes with abundant pigmentation in the central and peripheral retina, residual ERG was obtained.

As other authors have described in patients with retinal vascular changes resulting from hypertension and arteriosclerosis associated with advanced changes in the eye fundus, the ERG may be subnormal (François 1954, Henkes 1954). Summarizing it should be stressed that in spite of normal function of the transplanted kidneys, in the majority of the patients, abnormal ERG have been found.

Further observations are needed to detect whether the retinal dysfunction is progressive.

REFERENCES

Astle, J. & P. Ellis. Ocular complication in renal transplant patients. *Ann. Ophtal.* 6: *1269–1273* (1974).

François, J. & A. De Rouck. L'électrorétinographie dans la rétinopathie diabétique et dans la rétinopathie hypertensive. *Acta Ophtal.* 32: *391–404* (1954).

Henkes, H. Electroretinogram in cases of retinal and choroidal hypertension and arteriosclerosis. A.M.A. *Arch. Opht.* 52: *30–41* (1954).

Hovland, K. & P. Ellis. Ocular changes in renal transplant patients. *Amer. J. Ophtal.* 63: *283–289* (1967).

Murray, H.W., D.L. Know, R.W. Green & R.M. Susel. Cytomegalovirus retinitis in adults. *Amer. J. of Med.* 63: *574–584* (1977).

Pavlin C.R., G.A. De Veber, G.T. Cook & L.D. Crisholm. Ocular complications in renal transplant recipients. *Can. Med. Assoc.* J. 117: *360–362* (1977).

Pfefferman, R., G.M. Gombos & S.L. Koutz. Ocular complication after renal transplantation *Ann. Ophtal.* 9: *467–473* (1977).

Porter, R. A.L. Crombie, P.S. Gardner & R.P. Uldall. Incidence of ocular complications in patients undergoing renal transplantation. *Brit. Med. J.* 3: *133–136* (1972).

De Venecia, G., Rhein, G.Z.M., Pratt, M.V. Cytomegalic inclusion retinitis in an adult. *Arch. Ophtal.* 86: *44–57.* (1971).

Author's address:
Dr. Ewa Drobecka
Ophthalmic Clinic of the Medical Academy
Warsaw
Poland

INVESTIGATION BY MEANS OF VECP IN PATIENTS WITH CHRONIC NEPHROPATHY

WINFRIED MÜLLER, E. HAASE, J. GAUSS AND N. JUNG

(*Erfurt, G.D.R.*)

ABSTRACT

The authors investigated VECP in 18 patients who had to undergo a highly effective short-time dialysis just before the dialysis. Results: VECP showed a prolonged peak-time; changes in amplitudes could not be proved. There were neither direct relations to pathological biochemical data, nor were there any to the length of the dialysis history.

INTRODUCTION

There are a number of authors dealing with the condition of the EEG in patients suffering from renal failure and who undergo a chronic intermittent dialysis treatment. The investigators found pathological EEGs as a sign of nephrogenic encephalopathy or uraemic encephalopathy. Mann and coworkers (1977) emphasized that these EEG changes consist of a generalized shifting of basic activities and even more of a sudden appearance of short-time EEG changes in the basic activities due to different frequencies, amplitudes and steepness. Spehr et al. (1977) with the majority of their patients described a moderate uraemic encephalopathy. In general, the EEG abnormality consisted of diffuse or slightly paroxysmal slowing. There were no statistically significant relations between visually assessed EEG qualities and the lengths of the haemodialysis history, or the general clinical state before and after the haemodialysis. They found also no significant correlation between creatinine and visually assessed EEG abnormality. The computerized EEG showed that EEG slowing was largely connected with the creatinine level, and EEG acceleration with hyperkalaemia, which in most cases was accompanied by a high urea level. Hamel and coworkers, too, described the increased slow wave activity in EEG as a well-known correlate of advancing renal failure. A disorganization of the background activities was found by K. Hazafi et al. (1977).

Kiley and Hines (1965), Bourne et al. (1975) have reported the same findings.

There is only little information on the conditions of VECP in cases of renal failure.

Hyman and Kooi (1969) investigated 7 patients and found that the latencies of the VECPs (5 components of the responses) were increased, that is to say slowed.

Hamel and coworkers (1978) studied 129 patients over a period of 4 years. Data were collected from 49 patients who did not undergo any dialysis treatment with varying degrees of renal failure, and 36 patients who did undergo a dialysis treatment when entering the programme. Data were recorded from 20 patients with kidney transplantations. The basic overall findings are those that the VECP latencies increase as a patient's clinical condition deteriorates and normalizes as the condition improves.

However the data collected offer compelling evidence that this retinocortical measure is directly influenced by uraemic toxicity. They found a significant interrelationship between latency and creatinine, calcium, potassium measures. It is also important that they described large intersubject differences for VECP latencies but small subject variability. Thus large intersubject differences tend to mask within subject differences and may be the reason for producing an insignificant correlational analyses result. Lewis, Dustman and Beck (1978) studied 8 patients who were being maintained on chronic haemodialysis and 3 patients who had received successfully kidney transplants. It could be seen that the means derived from the VECP of haemodialysis patients were all of longer latency than those derived from the responses of the control group. These differences reached statistical significance for 8 of the 13 waves analysed. In most instances, evoked potential amplitudes of haemodialysis patients were larger than those of the control group. The prolonged latencies and increased amplitudes, found in the response of haemodialysis patients, did not appear to be related to the related time on dialysis.

Note: In other brain diseases, a combination of increased amplitude and prolonged latency is found rather infrequently. A correlational analysis revealed no consistent relationship between blood chemistries and evoked potential characteristics (*e.g.* creatinine, BUN).

METHODS

We investigated the VECP behaviour in 18 patients who had to undergo a highly effective short-time dialysis just before the dialysis. Stimulation was effected in a monocular way. The hemisphere of a diameter of 1.5 m, developed by us for electroperimetry, was used as stimulation device. The macular area and an area that was 10° temporal of the foveola were stimulated. The flash discharge energy was 0.2 joules, the flash exit aperture was of a diameter of 8 mm which corresponds to a determined retinal area of below 1 degree. Stimulation was in cycles of 1 Hz, 50 stimuli per stimulus point. The surrounding brightness of the hemisphere was approximately 10 lux. The output of the results obtained was plotted as analogue-mean value curve, the maxima and minima were being printed additionally in terms of digital values.

The visually assessed EEG showed slight or moderate abnormalities, severely abnormal EEGs were not found (Endler *et al.* 1978). In regard of these facts the evaluation of the VECP was more complex. The visual recognisability and the visual correlation of the potentials were lowered. Table 1 shows the data collected from 18 patients, that is to say the peak time of N_2 in bipolar and unipolar recording. The normative data are also shown (n = 52 age-matched persons). The renal patients show a significantly longer peak time of N_2 in comparison with the data of the control group (Fig. 1).

172

Table 1. Peak times of N_2 in 18 kidney patients and the control group.

Mean peaktime and amplitude values from 18 dialysis patients

	bipolar				central			
	10° nasal peaktime N₂ ms	s ms	amplitude μV	s μV	peaktime ms	s ms	amplitude μV	s μV
r. e.	118	19	3.3	2.6	118	21	5.1	2.5
l. e.	118	19	3.2	2.4	119	21	5.6	4.2
	unipolar							
r. e.	124	18	5.6	1.4	119	15	5.6	4.5
l. e.	123	14	4.2	3.8	123	13	4.5	4.5
				Normal group				
			bipolar	103	12	5.2	4.3	
			unipolar	105	12	6.7	6.2	

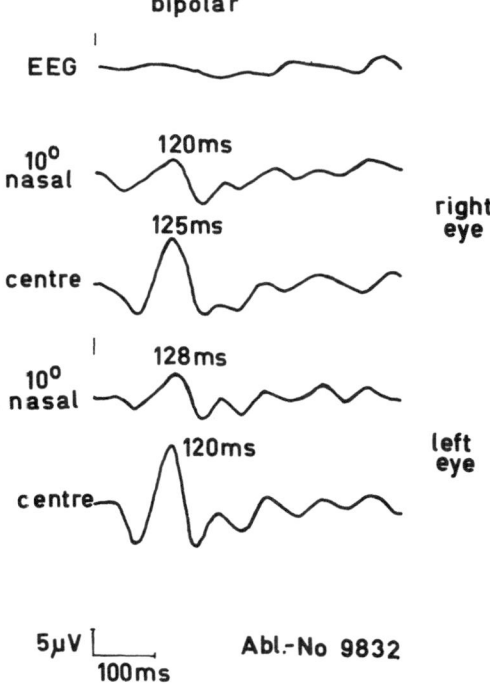

bipolar

EEG

10° nasal — 120ms — right eye

centre — 125ms

10° nasal — 128ms — left eye

centre — 120ms

5µV 100ms   Abl.-No 9832

Fig. 1. Example of a mean value response of a patient, peak time prolongation becoming clearly discernible.

173

These findings are in agreement with other investigators (Hyman and Kooi, Hamel et al., Lewis et al.). Lewis and coworkers described an increase in the amplitude in the most cases of renal failure. In our investigation this could not be stated. N_2-amplitudes were like the amplitudes of the control group. There was also no direct connection between the blood chemistries and the peak time. The level of bound urea nitrogen (BUN) and the level of creatinine were increased in all patients, and the level of potassium in most of them (Table 2).

Table 2. Laboratory data regarding our 18 patients.

Blood chemisty of our 18 dialysis patient

			normal:
Creatinine	12.28 mg%	17 max 6.9 min	1.2 − 1.3 mg%
Urea	80.5 mg%	110 max 59 min	40 mg%
Potassium K	5.11 mval	6.2 max 3.2 min	4.5 − 5.5 mval

But it was not possible to find out that a very high level of one of them was correlated with an especially longer peak time. Like the other investigators we also found that the prolonged peak time, found in the responses of haemodialysis patients, did not appear to be related to the related time on dialysis (see Table 3).

The dialysis treatment over a period of 7 years and even longer must be considered important, but none of the three patients showed any remarkable prolongation of the peak time. This is explicable. In these cases the severity of the disease and the necessity of dialysis treatment must be in relationship one with another, which must be considered well balanced. Efficient balancing and

Table 3. Peak times of N_2 in patients who had to undergo a chronic intermittent haemodialysis treatment.

Patients with a dialysis history of more than 7 years

pat.No		bipolar				unipolar			
		10° nasal peak(ms)	ampl.(μV)	central peak(ms)	ampl(μV)	10° nasal peak(ms)	ampl.(μV)	central peak(ms)	ampl.(μV)
1	r. e.	96	7.2	92	6.2	108	4.0	108	3.3
	l. e.	100	2.2	96	3.1	108	4.1	100	3.9
9	r. e.	116	1.1	108	15.1	120	2.8	128	8.4
	l. e.	'0	0	116	15.6	116	3.6	132	7.9
13	r. e.	88	1.0	92	4.8	116	1.3	108	10.5
	l. e.	104	1.6	92	2.7	124	1.5	120	6.5

a long survival are expressed by the electrophysiological data, which must be considered optimum to a certain extent.

Summarizing we can say:
(1) The VECP of haemodialysis patients shows a prolonged peak time
(2) Changes in the amplitude could not be proved
(3) In all cases BUN, creatinine and potassium were increased.
There was no direct relation of these data with a ,prolonged peak time.
(4) The VECP did not show any connection with the length of the dialysis history.

REFERENCES

Bourne, J.R., J.W. Ward, P.E. Teschan, M. Musso, H.B. Johnston Jr. & H.E. Ginn. Quantitative assessment of the EEG in renal disease. *Electroencephal. clin. Neurophysiol.* 39: *377–388* (1975).

Endler, S., E. Müller, M. Marx & H. Thieler. Vergleichende EEG-Untersuchungen bei Patienten vor und nach konventioneller Dialyse sowie hoch-effektiver Kurzzeitdialyse. Dt. Gesundheitswesen (1979) (im Druck).

Hamel, B., J.R. Bourne, J.W. Ward & P. Teschan. Visually evoked cortical potentials in renal failure: Transient potentials. *Electroenceph. clin. Neurophysiol.* 44: *606–626* (1978).

Hazafi, K., L. Györi & L. Grofman. Neuropsychiatric and EEG examinations in patients on intermittent hemodialysis. 2. Donau-Symposium für Nephrologie 26.-28.9.1977, Budapest. Verlag C. Bindernagel, Friedberg/Hessen 1978, S. 406, (1977).

Hyman, P.R. & K.A. Kooi. Visually evoked cortical responses in renal insufficiency. *Univ. Mich. Med. Center J.* 35: *177–179* (1969).

Kiley J. & O. Hines. Electroencephalographic evaluation of uraemia. *Arch. intern. Med.* 116: *67–73* (1965).

Lewis, E.G., R.E. Dustman & E.C. Beck. Visual and somatosensory evoked potential characteristics of patients undergoing hemodialysis and kidney transplantation. *Electroenceph. clin. Neurophysiol.* 44: *223–231* (1978).

Spehr, W., H. Satorius, K. Berglund, B. Hjorth, C. Kablitz, U. Plog, P.H. Wiedemann & K. Zapf. EEG and haemodialysis. *Electroenceph. clin. Neurophysiol.* 43: *787–797* (1977).

Author's address:
Prof. Dr. med. habil. W. Müller
Augenklinik der Medizinischen
Akademie Erfurt
Nordhäuser Str. 74
DDR-506 Erfurt
German Democratic Republic

PART TWO

VISUAL ELECTROPHYSIOLOGY
AND LOCALIZED STIMULATION

Docum. Ophthal. Proc. Series, Vol. 23

LOCALIZATION OF DISTAL RETINAL ACTIVITY WITH THE TRANSRETINAL ERG

Development of a rapid procedure

ANNE B. FULTON, KAREN A. MANNING AND RONALD M. HANSEN

(*Boston, U.S.A.*)

ABSTRACT

A wide range of normal human scotopic ERG responses obtained in background adaptation are compactly represented by Rushton H_2 curves; (1) sensitivity and (2) scaling of response size are two separable adaptive properties of both a- and b-waves (Vision Research *18*, 1978). A similar H_2 analysis of ERG responses from developing rat retina in background adaptation was done to determine age related changes in a- and b-wave sensitivity and scaling. Correlations of developing ERG to maturing distal retina suggest anatomical sites in photoreceptors and outer plexiform layer which influence sensitivity and scaling of ERG responses. Furthermore, ERG studies of background adaptation in a strain of mutant mouse (pcd) having progressive retinal degeneration which begins in the photoreceptor inner segments have revealed sensitivity and scaling changes which are clearly distinguishable from normal. We have now devised an abbreviated procedure which allows rapid assessment of sensitivity and scaling of human ERG responses in conditions of background adaptation ranging from dark to those which saturate the psychophysical increment threshold. In human retinal diseases localization of the site of early degeneration in rods may become possible through this technique.

Localization of retinal sites generating ERG voltages and currents has been based largely on studies employing microelectrodes or manipulation of the retinal circulation (*e.g.* Granit, 1962; Arden and Brown, 1965; Brown, 1968; Penn and Hagins, 1969; Miller and Dowling, 1970; Newman, 1969). Recent ERG experiments have suggested another means of localizing distal retinal activities in the intact eye.

In the laboratory, the human scotopic ERG recorded via a contact lens electrode (in a manner similar to that used clinically) under various conditions of background adaptation has generated the stimulus/response curves shown in Fig. 1. For each background condition, b-wave amplitude is related hyperbolically to stimulating flash. The smooth curves drawn through the experimental points are called H_2 curves (Alpern, Rushton and Torii, 1970). These curves plot the relationship $V/V_{max} = I/(I+\sigma)$ on log-log coordinates. I is the flash intensity, V a measure of the response, σ a constant (semisaturation) and V_{max} the saturating value of V. The position of an H_2 curve is defined by a unique *apex point*, the intersection of the horizontal and oblique asymptotes to the curve. (Fulton and Rushton, 1978a; Hemila, 1977). The single *apex point* defines the entire H_2 curve. The abscissa of the *apex point* meets the curve 0.3

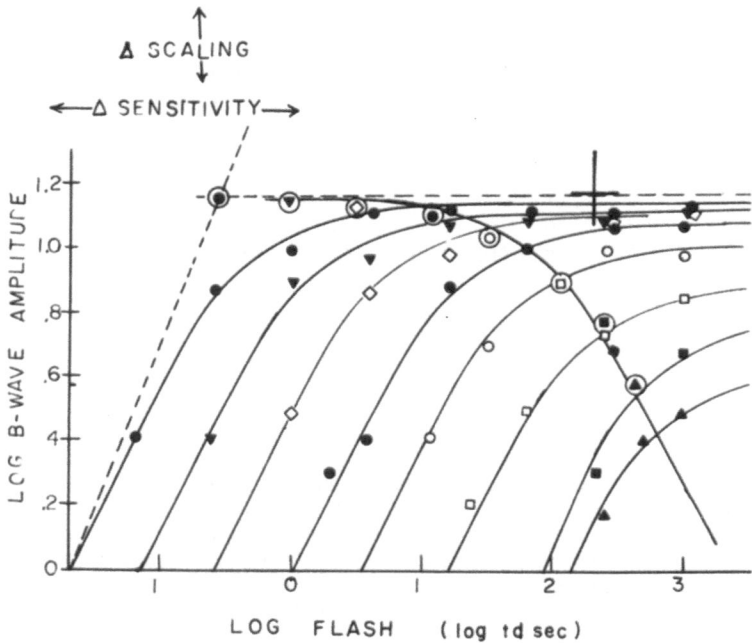

Fig. 1. The effects of steady red backgrounds (Jena-Schott RG-2; $\lambda > 630$ nm) on the ERG elicited by 50 msec white flashes. *Log b-wave amplitude* is plotted as a function of *log flash* in log td-sec for 8 different background conditions. Symbols for backgrounds are: ● no background; ▼ −0.4 log td; ◇ +0.2 log td; ● +0.8 log td; ○ +1.4 log td; □ +0.2 log td; ■ +2.9 log td; ▲ +3.2 log td. Each point is the average of at least 20 stimulations. Interstimulus intervals (ISI) were chosen to maintain a stable adaptation level; in this experiment ISI's ranged from 5 to 20 sec.

log units below the *apex point*; thus the abscissa represents the stimulating flash that produces a half maximal (semisaturated) response. The ordinate of the *apex point* represents the maximum response size. Therefore, the vertical variation of *apex points* indicates a change in maximum response size; the vertical shift of *apex points* will be referred to as scaling. A horizontal shift of *apex points* indicates a change in sensitivity of the response.

The circled points are the *apex points* that were obtained for the dark adapted eye and then in conditions of background adaptation ranging from very dim to those bright enough to saturate the psychophysical increment threshold function. Thresholds of the b-waves, or the log σ values, fit a Weber-Fechner function, having a slope of +1.0 in its linear portion.

The locus of *apex points* is a left facing H_2 curve with its apex point at the large +. The abscissa of the large + is the Log I value that semisaturates the a-wave H_2 curve obtained from the dark adapted eye. The sensitivity of the

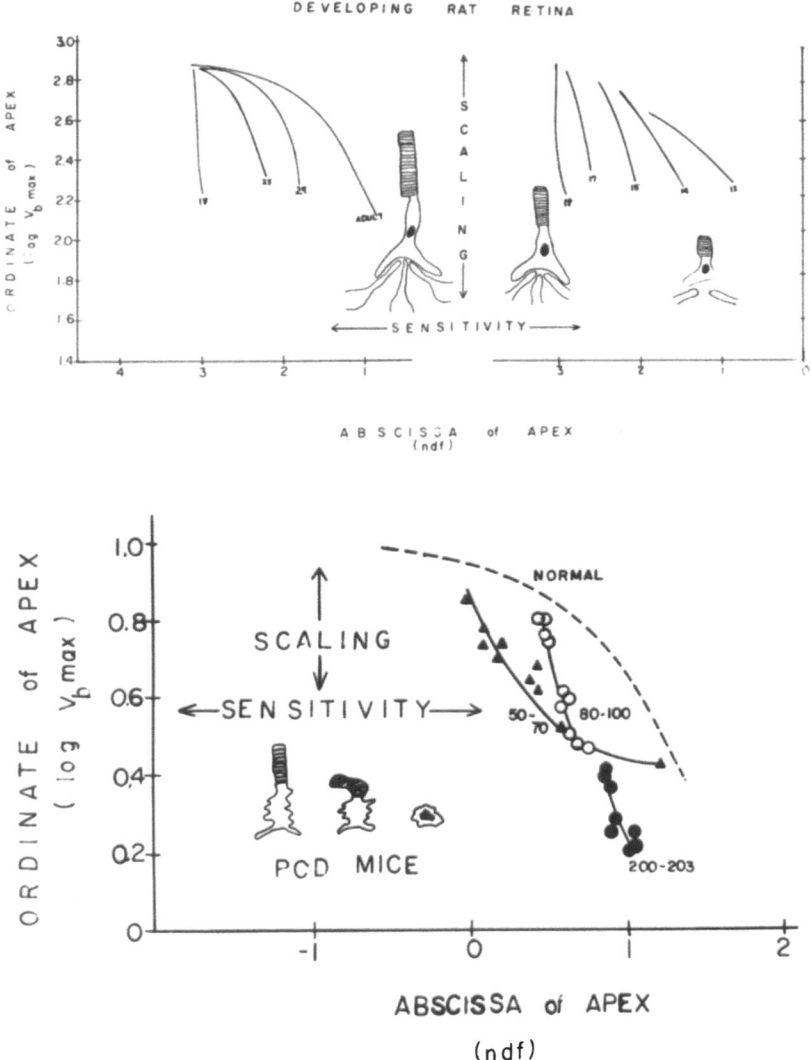

Fig. 2. A. Age related changes in background adaptation measured in the developing rat retina. Stimulus-response relations were measured in the dark, and with different backgrounds at ages 13 days through adult. Figure 2 plots *ordinate of apex*, that is, log maximum b-wave amplitude, as a function of the *abscissa of apex*, the flash producing a half-maximum response. The lines are smooth curves drawn through the loci of *apex points* for that age group. Also shown are schematic drawings of photoreceptor maturation during that period. B. Age related changes in background adaptation with mutant (PCD) mice. Once again, only the apex points are plotted. Loci of apex points for 3 age groups (▲ 50–70 days; ○ 80–100 days; ● 200–203 days), and normal adult mice (dashed line). These curves show changes in scaling and sensitivity which parallel the schematically illustrated retinal degeneration. Other features are the same as in *A*.

a-wave is not much changed by backgrounds; the slope of the Weber-Fechner function is about +0.4. The vertical variation of the *apex points* (scaling) is about the same for a- and b-waves. The left facing H_2 curve has also been found to describe the locus of b-wave *apex points* for mudpuppies and normal adult rats and mice.

To date two examples have been found in which the loci of *apex points* are not left facing H_2 curves. One is in the developing retina of rats. The ERG can be recorded in the post natal period when the retina is still developing. The b-wave is present when outer segments are short and outer plexiform connections are not yet mature. Then outer segments grow longer, the outer plexiform connections become mature and finally the receptor cell itself becomes mature. The curves in Fig. 2 show the progressive change in loci of the b-wave *apex points* at various ages from age 13 days to adult. The range of scaling (total vertical variation of the curves) becomes the same as measured in adults by age 18 days. For dark adapted eyes, b-wave sensitivity is equal to adult sensitivity, by age 18 days (see also Dowling and Sidman, 1962). However, changes in sensitivity (horizontal variation of the loci of *apex points*) caused by backgrounds become adult only after the receptor cell itself becomes mature. This is consistent with the results of microelectrode studies which show that the receptor response has an increment threshold relationship with a slope of + 1.0 in its linear portion.

The other example is the mutant mouse, purkinje cell degeneration (gene symbol pcd/pcd) (Mullen and LaVail, 1975; Mullen, Eicher, and Sidman, 1976). These animals have a gradual, progressive degeneration of photoreceptor cells which starts in the inner segments (Blanks, Mullen and LaVail, 1978). For these animals the loci of b-wave *apex points* show less change in sensitivity in the presence backgrounds than normal litter mates. (Fig. 2B). When large amounts of outer segment material have also degenerated, the range of scaling also decreases.

Thus studies on animal eyes suggest changes in scaling and sensitivity of b-wave responses obtained under various conditions of background adaptation can be linked to different sites in the photoreceptor cell and its neural connections. A procedure to determine scaling and sensitivity for patients retinas might also have value in localizing retinal abnormalities. However, families of curves such as shown in Fig. 1 take 3 to 4 hours to collect. Therefore, we set out to develop an abbreviated procedure to determine scaling and sensitivity which would be more suitable in a clinical setting.

METHODS

The two channel stimulator used is similar to that previously described by Fulton and Rushton (1978b). One beam was used to deliver 50 msec blue flashes and the second, steady red backgrounds. Subjects had their pupils dilated with Tropicamide 1% and dark adapted 30 minutes before the test session. A bipolar Burian-Allen contact lens electrode was next placed on the anesthetized eye. Responses were amplified (dc coupled; OHz–3KHz) and summed with a signal averager. B-wave amplitudes were later measured from the records obtained.

Experiment 1. Normative Data. Stimulus/response curves were collected from the dark adapted eye and then under the six levels of background adaptation indicated in Fig. 3. Stimuli were presented every 5 sec, and incremented in 0.3 log unit steps from -1.2 log td sec to 3.0 log td sec. Twenty or 40 responses to each stimulus intensity were collected to generate a full H_2 curve for each condition of adaptation. Twenty complete families of curves were collected. The average of the *apex points* obtained in these twenty runs are shown in Fig. 3. It took two to three hours to complete such as run -- too long for clinical use.

Experiment 2. Rapid procedure. Instead of collecting full H_2 curves, a method to determine quickly the locus of b-wave *apex points* has been developed.

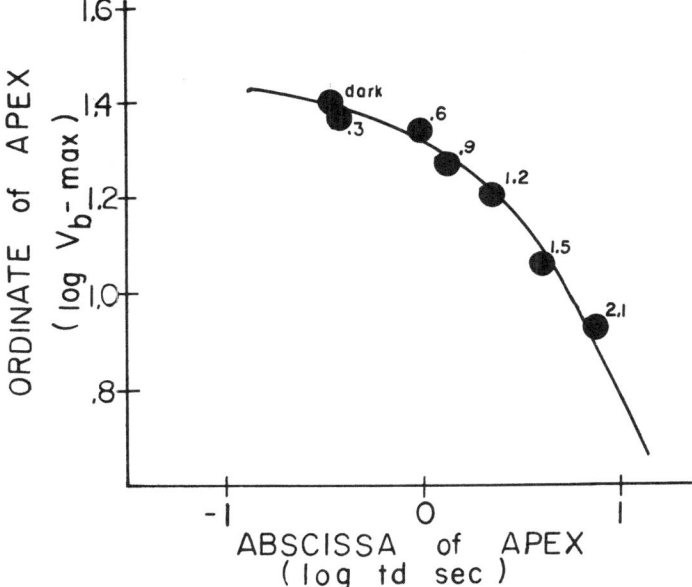

Fig. 3. Summary of the effects of red backgrounds (Jena-Schott RG-2; $\lambda > 630$ nm) on ERG responses elicited by 50 msec blue (Ilford 621) flashes. A Burian-Allen contact lens electrode was used to record ERG's from 3 dark adapted subjects when there was no background (dark) or at backgrounds of .3; .6; .9, 1.2; 1.5, or 2.1 log td. Twenty or 40 responses were summed at each flash intensity. Flash intensity was increased in 0.3 log unit steps from -2.1 log td sec to $+1.8$ log td sec. The *apex point* of the best fitting H_2 curve through the data was then determined. Each subject participated in 20 such runs. Figure 3 plots the average *apex points* obtained with this procedure. The *ordinate of apex*, the log maximum b-wave amplitude, is plotted as a function of *abscissa of apex*, the flash that produces a half-maximum response. The smooth curve through the points is a left-facing H_2 curve.

Based on the normative data obtained in Experiment 1, for each adaptation condition, the flash intensity *expected* to produce a half maximal (semisaturated) response was selected. The response to the estimated semisaturating flash would serve as a check that the estimated semisaturating flash was, indeed, about half the maximum response. A flash intense enough to saturate the response was then put on and this maximum response recorded. In each background condition the log of the maximum response gave the ordinate of the *apex point* and the pre-determined semisaturating flash, the abscissa of that *apex point*. The backgrounds are the same as used in Experiment 1.

RESULTS

An example of *apex points* obtained with the rapid procedure is shown in Fig. 4. For each adaptation condition the ordinate of the filled circles represents the experimentally measured log maximum b-wave response. The abscissa is the

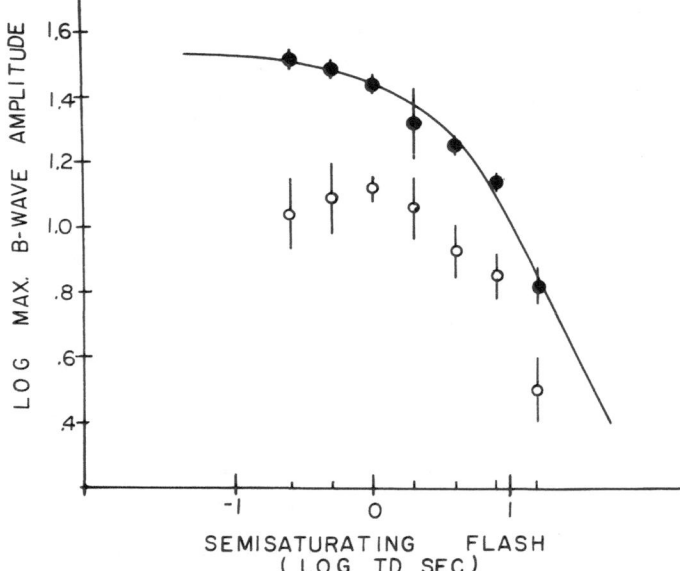

Fig. 4. Results of the rapid procedure. Log b-wave amplitude is plotted as a function of semisaturating flash in log td sec. The filled circles (●) represent the measured log maximum b-wave amplitude at the *expected* log semisaturating flash for each background used. The smooth curve drawn through the points is a left facing H_2 curve. The open circles (O) plot the measured log b-wave response to the semisaturating flash; these points confirm that the *expected* semisaturating flash produced, within experimental error, a half maximal response. Each point is the mean of 7 runs consisting of 4 stimulating flashes per point with the same subject. Error bars show ±2 standard errors of the mean.

log stimulating flash which, based on Experiment 1, was estimated to be the stimulus that would produce a half maximum response. The open circles are the responses to the estimated semisaturating flash which were measured during the course of the rapid procedure. Within experimental error the measured half amplitude responses are equal to the predicted half amplitude responses.

The smooth curve drawn through the experimentally determined *apex points* is a left-facing H_2 curve. The average test time required to determine the locus of b-wave apices by the rapid procedure has been about 10 minutes.

DISCUSSION

These results have demonstrated that the *apex points* of H_2 curves can be used to describe compactly the effects of various levels of background adaptation on scotopic b-wave sensitivity and maximum response size. In the normal adult retina, the *apex points* have a characteristic locus. Specifically, the points fall on a left-facing H_2 curve as shown in Figs. 1, 3 and 4. This relation may change during development of the retina and during the course of retinal degeneration as suggested by the results presented in Fig. 2.

Correlation of scaling and sensitivity changes with morphological characteristics of the animal retinas suggests anatomical sites in the photoreceptor cell and its outer plexiform connections which influence the *apex point* loci. A procedure to determine *apex points* in patients might help to localize the primary site of abnormalities early in the course of a variety of retinal degenerations which affect adaptation. Thus, the development of a procedure for rapid assessment of the locus of *apex points* described in the second experiment may be useful because it can be easily incorporated in clinical electroretinographic testing.

REFERENCES

Alpern, M., Rushton, W.A.H. & S. Torii. The size of Rod Signals. *J. Physiol.*, Lond. 206: *193–208* (1970).

Arden, G.B. & K.T. Brown. Some properties of components of the cat electroretinogram revealed by local recording under oil. *J. Physiol.* 176: *429–461* (1965).

Blanks, J.C., Mullen, R.J. & M.M. LaVail. Ultrastructural Study of Slow Photoreceptor Degeneration in PCD, a Cerebellar Mutant Mouse. *Invest. Opth. Visual Sci.* 18 (Suppl.) *158* (1978).

Brown, K.T. The electroretinogram: its components and their origins. *Vision Res.* 8: *633–677* (1968).

Dowling, J.E. & H. Ripps. Visual Adaptation in the Retina of the Skate. *J. Gen. Physiol.* 56: *491–520* (1970).

Dowling, J.E. & R.L. Sidman. Inherited Retinal Dystrophy in the Rat. *J. Cell Biol.* 14: *73–109* (1962).

Fulton, A.B., Graves, A.L. J.L. Craft. Development of ERG Signals in Light Adaptation. *Invest. Ophth. Visual Sci.* (Suppl.) 17: *218* (1978).

Fulton, A.B. & W.A.H. Rushton. Rod ERG of the Mudpuppy: Effect of Dim Red Backgrounds. *Vision Res.* 18: *785–792* (1978a).

Fulton, A.B. & W.A.H. Rushton. The Human Rod ERG: Correlation with Psychophysical Responses in Light and Dark Adaptation. *Vision Res.* 18: *793–800* (1978b).

Granit., R. Reviewed in *The Eye*, Vol. 2, pp 575–691 (edited by Davson, H.). Academic Press, New York. (1962).

Hemila, S. Background adaptation in the Rods of the Frog's Retina. *J. Physiol.* 265: *721–741* (1977).

Miller, R.F. & Dowling, J.E. Intracellular responses of the Muller (glial) cells of mudpuppy retina: Their relation to b-wave of the electroretinogram. *J. Neurophysiol.* 33, 323–341 (1970).

Mullen, R.J., Eicher, E.M. & Sidman, R.L. Purkinje cell degeneration, a new neurological mutation in the mouse. *Proc. Nat. Acad. Sci. U.S.A.* 73: *208–212* (1976).

Mullen, R.J. & LaVail, M.M. Two new types of retinal degeneration in cerebellar mutant mice. *Nature* 258: *528–530* (1975).

Newman, E.A. B-wave Currents in the Frog Retina. *Vision Res.* 19: *227–234* (1979).

Penn, R.D. & Hagins, W.A. Signal transmission along retinal rods and the origins of the electroretinographic a-wave. *Nature*, Lond. 223: *201–205* (1969).

Author's address:
Department of Ophthalmology
Children's Hospital Medical Center
300 Longwood Avenue
Boston, MA 02115
U.S.A.

Docum. Ophthal. Proc. Series, Vol. 23

ERG BY LOCALISED SINUSOIDAL STIMULATION

P.A. GROUNAUER, VO VAN TOI AND CH. HUBER

(*Lausanne, Zürich, Switzerland*)

ABSTRACT

Five normal subjects were tested with our stimulator. A new relation between ERG and stimulus field size is demonstrated. Pathological conditions were also tested and confirm the possibility of eliciting an ERG from the posterior pole.

INTRODUCTION AND METHOD

Many authors have used sinusoidal stimulation and shown the relations between ERG and luminance, modulation or frequency. Shortly we present the relation between ERG and stimulus field size from one degree to sixty degrees. Based on our previous psychophysical results we have chosen five hertz and hundred percent modulation, to have a maximum retinal response.

We use the visual stimulator commercially available, about which technical information has been published. This instrument, the Papillometer, gives a sinusoidal stimulus waveform, white light, luminance from 40 to 56 nits. Two hundred stimulations are averaged in a Pantops 500. On the screen of the cathode ray tube a square wave takes the place of the sinusoidal waveform. This mark allows us to localise accurately stimulus extrema.

After dilatation with Mydriaticum the cornea is anaesthesied with Novesine. During these preparations and before setting the Henkes lens electrode, the observer is adapted at the light of our laboratory, 12 lux. The inactive electrode is on the homolateral ear, the ground electrode on the forehead. The observer looks through the Maxwellian eye piece. The experiment is monocular, the other eye being covered.

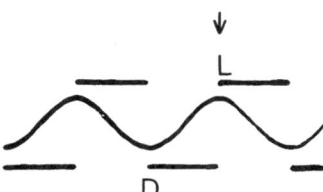

Fig. 1. Sinusoidal stimulus waveform and its square mark. Arrow: maximum of light L. D = darkness.

RESULTS AND DISCUSSION

We have tested 5 normal subjects, among them 2 protans. The ERG of these protans are identical with that of the normal colour vision subjects. Figure 2 shows the ERG of a normal subject elicited by sinusoidal waveform stimulus.

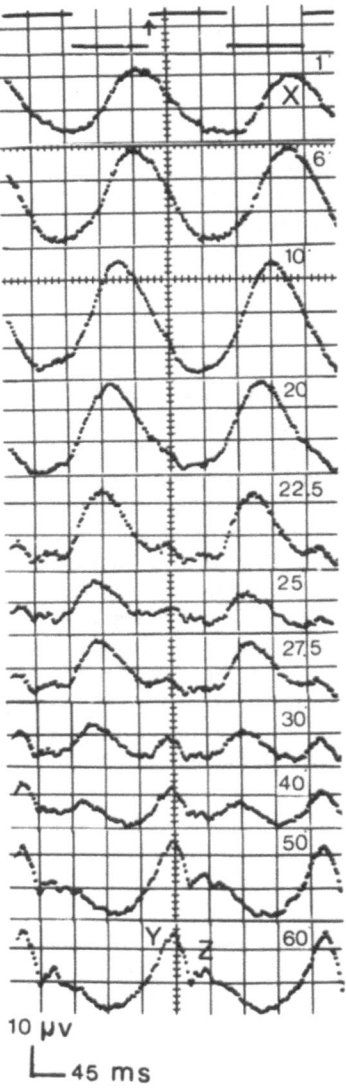

Fig. 2. Normal ERG result. Arrow: maximum of light. Angle of vision: 1° to 60°. Scale: right bottom. X, Y, Z: waves responses.

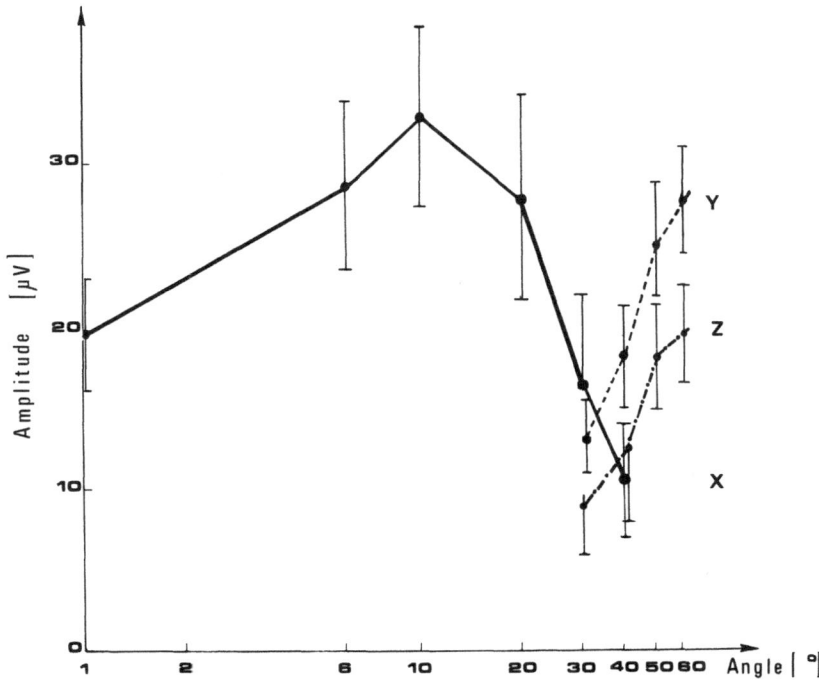

Fig. 3a. Amplitude versus angle of vision, with standard deviation for X, Y, Z.

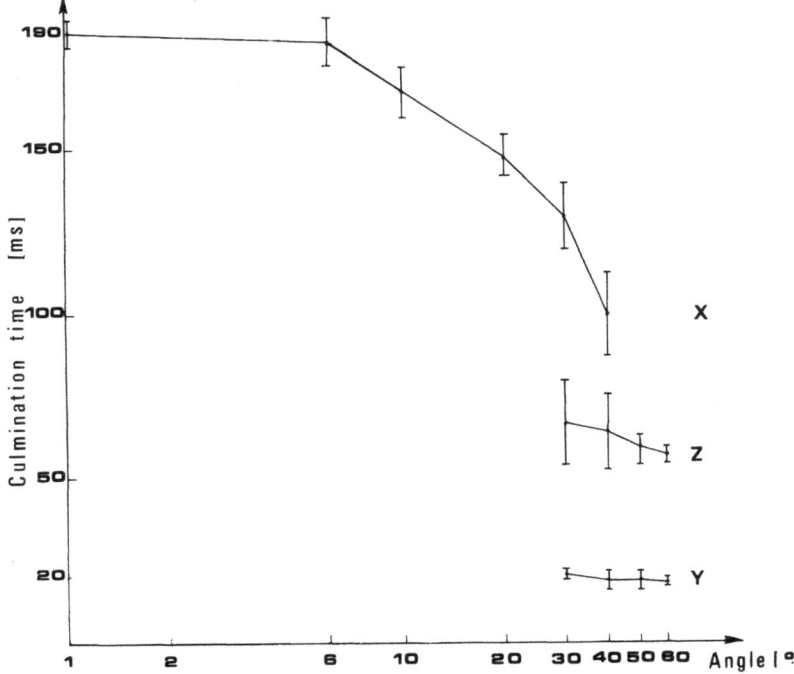

Fig. 3b. Culmination time versus angle of vision with standard deviation for X, Y, Z.

189

The response is linear between 1° and 20°, then non linear. There is a transition zone around 30° field size, the amplitude of the waves being nearly equal.

It is not possible to define and to compare the waves obtained in this work to the wellknown waves a, e, bl, b2, obtained with flash stimulus. So that we call deliberately X, Y, Z, the waves obtained by sinusoidal waveform stimulus. The peak to peak amplitudes of the waves are shown in Fig. 3a. The amplitude of X wave increases until 10° then decreases as the field size increases. Above 40° it is quite difficult to localise this wave because it is submerged. The Y and Z waves appear at 20° and increase continuously when the field size increases.

To determine the culmination time of the waves we consider that the wave which follows immediately the maximum luminance of the stimulus is its response. If this choice should be incorrect the culmination time would have only a constant error and Fig. 3b should be shifted vertically.

Figure 4 shows the ERG of a normal observer when we used a ring form stimulus. The result is non linear but with 1° field size stimulus and lateral fixation the result is linear, but the culmination time is appreciably shorter than that of 1° field size stimulus and central fixation (see Fig. 2.). So that the non linearity is probably due to the lateral inhibition effect.

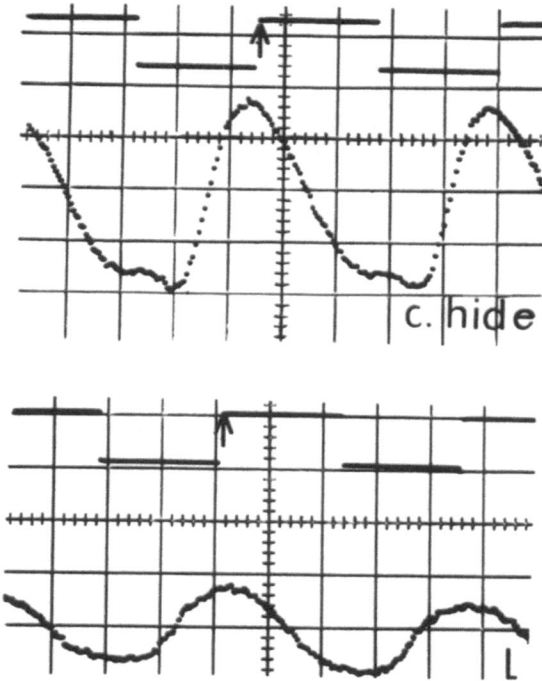

Fig. 4 (above) ERG with a ring form stimulus (c. hide).
(below). ERG with a 1° angle and lateral fixation (L).
Scale see Fig. 2.

A. Troelstra *et al.* used a sinusoidal waveform stimulus, 10° field size, 5 hertz, and found that the ERG is non linear. Their response has a resemblance with our's at 25°. This can be due to the stray light of their optical system.

Figure 5a shows a posterior dystrophy of Stargardt type. The ERG obtained with a flash stimulus is quite normal (Fig. 5b top) whereas the ERG elicited by

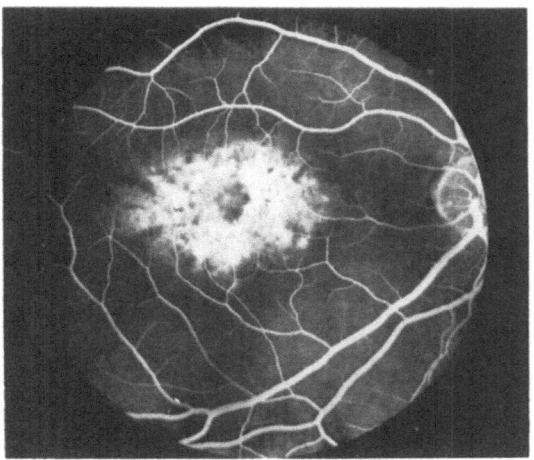

Fig. 5a. Posterior dystrophy of Stargardt type.

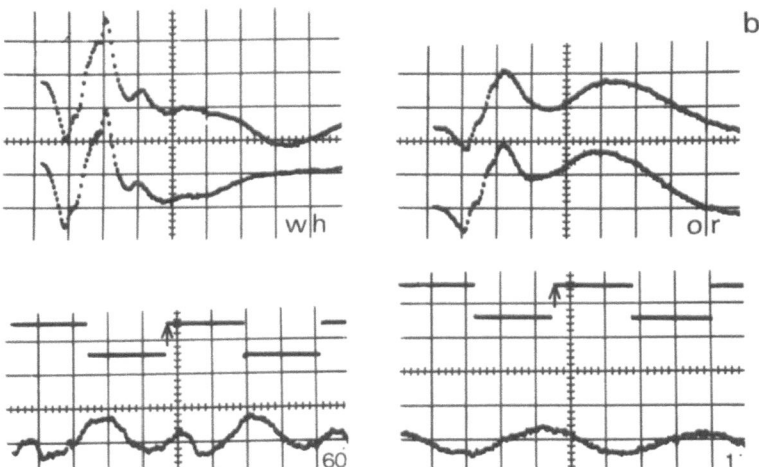

Fig. 5b. Comparison between flash ERG and sinusoidal ERG of case of Fig. 5a. Wh.: white light response. Or.: response with orange light, after dark adaptation. 60°: response with 60° sinusoidal stimulation. 1°: response with 1° degree angle. Compare 60° and 1° results with Fig. 2. Scale top: 40 μV and 25 ms.

sinuoidal 1° and 60° (Fig. 5b bottom), are different to that of the normal observer (Fig. 2). Such differences between flash ERG and sinusoidal ERG were found in other diseases as well retrobulbar neuritis. So we think that ERG elicited by sinusoidal waveform stimulus can be useful in the diagnosis of macular lesions and also in optic nerve diseases.

SUMMARY AND CONCLUSIONS

1. A response can be obtained from the posterior pole.
2. A transition zone of linear and non linear responses is found around 30°.
3. Amplitude of X wave increases until 10° and then decreases, while his culmination time decreases when the field size increases.
4. Amplitude of Y and Z waves increase continuously. Their culmination times are nearly constant when the field size increases.
5. No differences were found between normal colour vision subjects and protan subjects.

REFERENCES

Grounauer, P.A., Vo Van Toi & Streiff E.B.: Vom perzeptiven Flicker zum makulären ERG durch sinusoidale Stimulation. *Klin. Mbl. Augenheilk.* 170: *821–823* (1977).

Grounauer, P.A., Balmer, A., Geinoz, J. & S. Stress: Electrorétinogramme maculaire et tests psychophysiques comparés dans la rétinopathie diabétique avec oedème intrarétinien. Adv. Ophthal. 36, *24–42*, Karger Basel, 1978.

Henkes, H.E. & L.H. Van der Tweel: Flicker. Proc. Symp. Physiol. of flicker and Proc. 2nd ISCERG on Flicker Electroretinography. *Documenta Ophthal.* 18, 1964.

Troelstra, A. & C.A. Garcia: The electrical Response of the Human Eye to sinusoidal light stimulation. *IEEE Trans. Biomed. Engin.* 22, 5, *369–378*, 1975.

Van der Tweel & P. Visser: Electrical responses of the retina to modulated light. *Acta. Fac. med. Univ. Brun.* 4. *185–196*, 1959.

Vo Van Toi. & P.A. Grounauer: The visual stimulator. *Rev. scient. Instrum.* 49, *1403–1406*, 1978.

Author's address:
P.A. Grounauer, M.D.
Clinique Ophtalmologique Universitaire
15 Avenue de France
CH-1004 Lausanne
Switzerland

THE LOCAL ERG WITH LASER AND LIGHT EMITTING DIODES STIMULATION

P. MIERDEL, A.I. BOGOSLOWSKI, A.A. KABAN, E. MARRÉ
AND A.M. SHAMSHINOWA

ABSTRACT

For the purpose of carrying out the stimulation a helium-neon laser (632 nm) and high-efficiency red-light emitting diodes (635 nm, half-width 40 nm) and a blue-green background were used. The ERG was recorded by applying a special silver hook electrode. The stimulus size is 1.5° and adequate for testing the function of the macular region. The LED-stimulator provides a local ERG suitable for clinical evaluation. However, in special investigations, at a background that is more or less intense, a laser will be preferred.

INTRODUCTION

In the last 10 years the electrophysiologists' attention was directed to problems involved in ERG recording of local stimulation of the retina. On the one hand, the role of evoked potentials associated with the retina for the information transmission to the visual centre is not enough known, on the other hand, the pathogenesis of several hereditary congenital and acquired deficiencies localized in the central part of the retina including a therapy of these diseases, according to the pathogenesis, were not sufficiently clear. Different methods of local retinal stimulation exist (Brindley and Westheimer (1965), Aiba *et al.* (1967), Van Lith and Henkes (1968), Nagata and Honda (1970), Bogoslowski *et al.* (1973), Bagolini *et al.* (1973), Brunette (1973), Hirose *et al.* (1977)). The aim of the presented work is to directly compare the stimulation with laser and light emitting diodes (LED) and to seek the physiological interpretation of the recorded local ERG.

METHODS

For the stimulation of a helium-neon laser (632 nm) and high efficiency red LED (635 nm, half-width 40 nm) were used. The stimulus size is 1.5°. The laser light has on the level of the cornea a maximal radiance of about 1.9 μW, the LED produces there a radiance of about 0.008 μW. The experiments were carried out without and with a blue-green background (400–560 nm) in order to avoid the effect of light scattering in the eye and to activate relatively the red primary colour vision mechanism. The stimulus duration varied from 10 to 500 ms. As a rule, 100, 128 or 200 responses were being summed on a digital averager, the stimulus frequency ranges from 0.2 to 1 Hz. The ERG was recorded using a special silver hook electrode attached at the lower lid. All potentials were derivated from healthy normal subjects.

RESULTS

The typical response obtained from the macula region under mesopic conditions consists of a negative component (a-wave with a peak latency of about 30 ms) and of a positive one (b-wave with a peak latency of some 70 ms). Both laser and the LED stimulus excite the same response form (Fig. 1). The time course of the response stimulated with LED is somewhat later, explicable by the lower intensity. But the "b"-wave is prevailing, also in this low intensity range.

During dark adaptation in the first five minutes only a decrease in the b-component to about 3.5 μV could be detected. In this period a second b-component (b_2) occurs which reaches its maximal value of 1.5 μV after 10 minutes and remains significantly smaller than the main component "b" until 30 minutes of dark adaptation. The peak latency of this component is 120 ms in the beginning and later it shifts to shorter values. This behaviour can also be discerned in LED stimulation (Fig. 2). After 2 minutes of new light adaptation the b_2-component completely disappears and the ERG receives its initial form.

Recordings with a blue-green background show no changes in the peak latency, but a decrease in the b-component occurs as a function of the background luminance. Experiments at different stimulus times showed that in a period of 10 and 50 ms no off-effect became discernible. Without background an increase in the laser stimulus radiance produced an increase in the b-component of up to some 0.9 μW. The b-component remained constant for a higher radiance (up to 1.9 μW). The stimulus intervals result in a response to the effect that at intervals of less than 2 s the b-component is diminished.

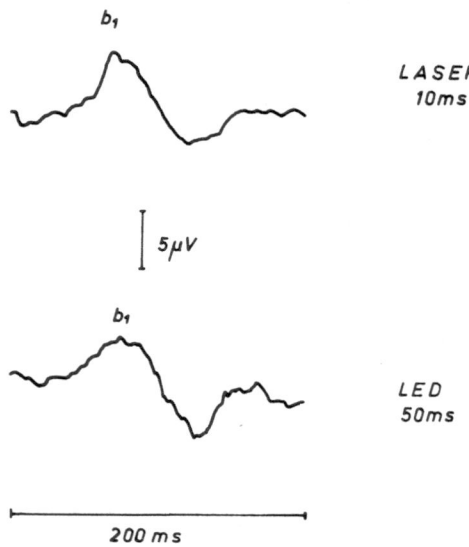

Fig. 1. Local ERG with laser and LED stimulation under mesopic conditions (stimulus 1.5°).

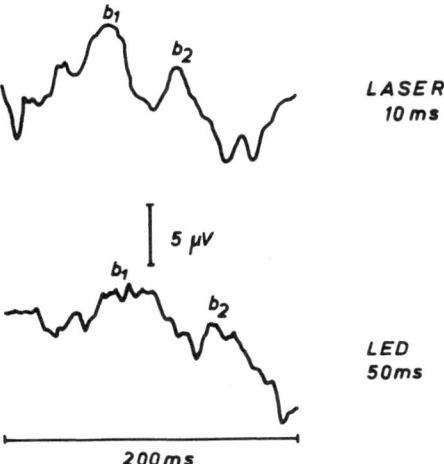

Fig. 2. Local ERG with laser and LED stimulation
after 20 minutes dark adaptation.

DISCUSSION

The high radiance and monochromasy of the laser and the relatively simple
and inexpensive LED stimulator were the reasons to use this source. To
guarantee a clear perception of the stimulus and to avoid any loading of the
cornea the special hook electrode has been used. The recorded response
amplitude is 70 per cent of the response using a corneal electrode.

The mesopic conditions are preferred, because the ERG response is well
recognizable and the used relatively high laser stimulus intensity mainly excites
the cones. Under these conditions the use of a small stimulus size (1.5°) is
employed to test the function of the macular region.

It is clear that the determination of the functional state of the macular region
depends on an exact localization of the stimulus on the retina. A directly
simultaneous observation of the stimulated area is not advisable in normal light
to avoid a retinal loading. The fixation of the patients eye must be checked
prior to the ERG and secured during the recording process by using special
arrangements.

The LED stimulator provides an adequate local ERG for clinical purposes.
However in special investigations, at a background that is more or less intense,
a laser will be preferred.

REFERENCES

Aiba, T.S., U. Alpern & F. Maaseidvaag. The electroretinogram evoked by the excitation of human foveal cones. *J. Physiol.* 189: 43–62 (1967).

Bogoslowski, A.I., A.D. Volcova, L.S. Urmacher, W.K. Shdanow & E.I. Shapiro. Laser-Electroretinogram. *Vest. Ophthal. USSR*, 2: *3–6* (1973).

Brindley, G.S. & G. Westheimer. The spatial properties of the human electroretinogram. *J. Physiol.* 179: *158–537* (1965).

Brunette, J. Standardisable method for separating rod and cone responses in clinical electroretinography. *Amer. J. Ophthalm.* 75/5: *833–845* (1973).

Bagolini, V., V. Barbaro, C. Bosi, M. Neroni & G. Ravalico. Une nouvelle technique pour l'enregistrement de ERG localisés. *Bull. Soc. Ophthal. Fr.* 85: *345–354* (1973).

Hirose, T., Y. Miyake & A. Hara. Simultaneous recording of electroretinogram and visual evoked response. *Arch. Ophthal.* 95: *1205–1208* (1977).

Nagata, M. & Y. Honda. Studies on local electric response of the human retina. *Acta Soc. Ophthal. Jap.* 74: *388–394, 511–528, 582–586, 957–964* (1970).

Van Lith, G.H.M. & H.E. Henkes. The local electric response of the central retinal area. Proc. VI. ISCERG Symp. Erfurt, 1967; Advances in Electrophysiology and Pathology of the Visual System. Leipzig. pp. 163–170, ed. E. Schmöger, 1968.

Author's address:
Dr. rer. nat. Peter Mierdel,
Augenklinik, Medizinische Akademie
Fetscherstr. 74,
DDR-8019 Dresden
German Democratic Republic

196

Docum. Ophthal. Proc. Series, Vol. 23

THE LASER ELECTRORETINOGRAM
AND ITS SIGNIFICANCE IN THE INVESTIGATION OF
THE FUNCTIONAL STATE OF
THE RETINAL MACULAR REGION

A.M. SHAMSHINOWA, A.I. BOGOSLOWSKI, E. MARRÉ
AND P. MIERDEL
(*Moscow, U.S.S.R. and Dresden, G.D.R.*)

ABSTRACT

A laser stimulator and a special silver hook electrode were used to record the local ERG for investigation of the functional state characteristics of the macula. Patients affected with hereditary retinal diseases and diabetic retinopathy were examined. The results show that the laser ERG changes depend on origins and states of macular diseases.

INTRODUCTION

For the diagnosis of diseases of the retina it is very important to know the functioning state of the macula. However, the existing methods of examination have a subjective character and have frequently equal results in different diseases. The registration of biopotentials of the retina with local stimulation is a possible objective method. Some authors (Hedin 1967; Bogoslowski *et al.* 1973; Shapiro 1974; Hirose *et al.* 1977) have shown that the laser light stimulation can be used for adequate local stimulation of the retina.

MATERIAL AND METHOD

In the present work a helium-neon gas laser with a wavelength of 632 nm was used to record the local response of the retina. The stimulus spot was 2–3° at an intensity on the corneal level of $0.5 \cdot 10^{-6}$–$1.15 \cdot 10^{-6}$ W. This corresponds to a stimulated area of the retina of 0.5–0.8 mm^2. Under this condition one neural element of the retina receives $0.02 \cdot 10^9$ light quants.

The laser ERG was recorded by means of a special silver hook electrode placed on the lower eyelid. The indifferent electrode was attached to the ear lobe.

The differences of potentials between these electrodes were amplified by means of an electroencephalograph (Alvar-Electronic). The averaging was carried out with the MOPEV computer 27 (Alvar). The recording equipment was a H 327 · 3 three-channel recorder (USSR). 100 responses were averaged. The analysis time amounts to 200 ms. The fixation was effected by light emitting diodes. The pupil was not dilated.

RESULTS

The described stimulation produces a bioelectrical response consisting of two principal components: a negative a-wave of 1–2 μV with a peak time 30–36 ms

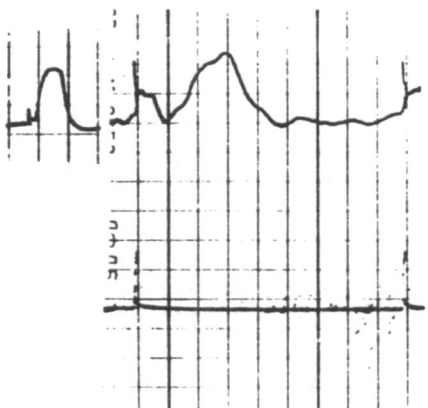

Fig. 1. Normal Laser ERG

and a positive b-wave of 3–6 μV with a peak time of 80–90 ms under mesopic conditions of the adaptation (Fig. 1).

With this method 49 patients with different phases of hereditary dystrophy of the macula (type Stargardt), retinitis pigmentosa and initial state of retinopathy diabetica were examined. Data from 3 patients with retinitis pigmentosa correlate with data by Sandberg *et al.* (1978) and demonstrate that the recorded laser ERG responses are the true local responses of the retina. These patients showed a typical clinical manifestation of the retinitis pigmentosa in the peripheral retina, visual fields were concentrically reduced to 10–15°, visual acuity was either normal 1.0 or no lower than 0.6. The normal clinical ERG did not exist or the micro ERG was recorded, respectively. However the response amplitude of laser ERG amounts to 3 μV with normal peak times, corresponding to normal laser ERG (Fig. 2).

Twenty four patients affected with Stargardt diseases were also examined. Visual acuity was decreased to 0.8–0.1 in dependence on the stage of the

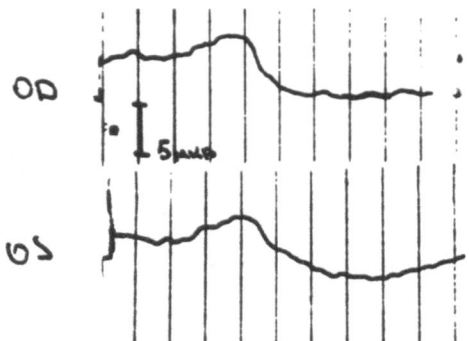

Fig. 2. Laser ERG in the patient M., 35 years, with retinitis pigmentosa. Vis. 0,7; concentrical field defect of about 85°.

198

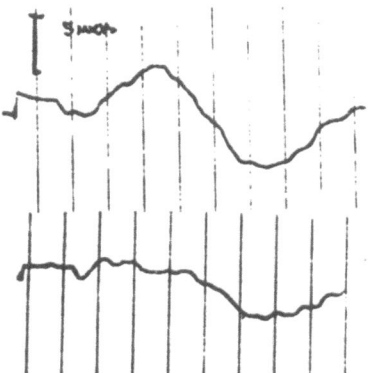

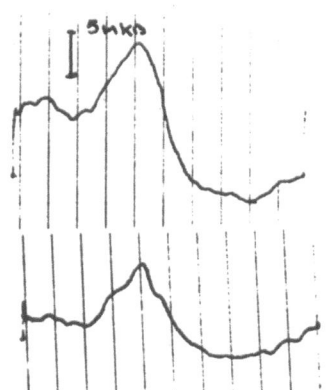

Fig. 3. Laser ERG in the patient E., 24 years, with macular dystrophy type Stargardt. Upper curve: the right eye with initial stage. Vis. 0,5 Laser ERG normal; lower curve: the left eye with a developed stage of the disease. Vis. 0,1, central scotoma 3°, Laser ERG subnormal.

Fig. 4. Laser ERG in the patient C., 40 years, with initial phase of retinopathia diabetica. Vis. 1,0. Upper curve: right eye, ERG supernormal; lower curve: left eye ERG normal.

disease. Some of these had central scotoma of about 3°. The normal clinical ERG and Flicker ERG in white and red light showed normal values.

In the initial stage of Stargardt diseases the laser ERG was normal; while the process is being developing, the local laser ERG is decreasing until it disappears (Fig. 3).

In another 22 patients with early stages of diabetic retinopathy the pathological process in the fundus of eye did not become evident, but microaneurisms were found angiographically only. Visual field, visual acuity and normal clinical ERG of these patients were normal or increased in the amplitude of the a-wave of the ERG. The laser ERG was either normal or increased in amplitude (Fig. 4).

DISCUSSION

We believe that the laser beam is sufficiently adequate to the local stimulation of the retina, as it has a very high radiance and monochromatism. The direct control of the fundus (acc. to Hirose, 1977) and a special background were not being used, in contrast to Aiba (1967); Brindley, Westheimer (1965), because the interaction between the two systems is more complex and the bioelectrical response of the retina is not so large. On the other hand a stimulation at high intensity and in a small size under mesopic conditions enable to register the local response, i.e. that of the macula region, mainly consisting of cones. The previous stimulation of the blind spot made this clear.

The relative low stimulation frequency was used to get the complete transient response of the retina, in contrast to the other authors as van Lith, Henkes (1968); Hirose (1977) and Sandberg et al. (1978).

After 10 minutes of dark adaptation a second b-wave component as described by Brunette (1973 and 1974) has appeared, therefore it was supposed that under the used mesopic conditions the laser ERG of the macula is a bioelectrical response of the photopic system. The used hook electrode allows clear perception of the stimulus and avoids any additional light scattering as this is the case when using the corneal lens. The investigation of hereditary dystrophy of macula showed the correlation between the decreased amplitude of the laser ERG and the development of the disease. The increase in the laser ERG amplitude in patients at an initial phase of diabetic retinopathy might be a result of irritation of the neuro-receptor elements of the macula which possibly must be considered as a function of oxygen insufficiency in tissues.

Thus the laser ERG represents a sensitive indicator for initial functional deficiencies of the macula. First steps in the application of this method for the functional characterisation of the macula region facilitate the detection of initial pathological processes; we hope that it will help us to understand the pathogenesis and differential diagnosis of macular diseases.

REFERENCES

Aiba, T.S., U. Alpern, & F. Maaseidvaag. The electroretinogram evoked by the excitation of human foveal cones. J. Physiol. 189: 43–62 (1967).

Bogoslowsky, A.I., A.D. Volcova, L.S. Urmacher, W.K. Shdanow, & E.I. Shapiro. Laser-Electroretinograma. Vest. Ophthal. USSR 2: 3–6 (1973).

Brindley, G.S. & G. Westheimer. The spatial properties of the human electroretinogram. J. Physiol. 179: 518–537 (1965).

Brunette, J. Standardisable method for separating rod and cone responses in clinical electroretinography. Amer. J. Ophthalmol. 75.5: 833–845 (1973).

Hedin, A. The laser as light source in electroretinography. Acta. Ophthal. 45: 475 (1967).

Hirose, T., Y. Miyake & A. Hara. Simultaneous Recording of Electroretinogram and Visual Evoked Response. Arch. Ophthal. 95: 1205–1208 (1977).

Sandberg, M.A., M.H. Effron & E.L. Berson. Focal cone electroretinograms in dominant retinitis pigmentosa with reduce penetrance. Inv. Ophthal. 17.11: 1095–1110 (1978).

Shapiro, E. I., W.K. Shdanow, A.I. Bogoslowski, L.S. Urmacher & Shamshinowa, A.M. About registration of the Laser ERG (russ), in: Electrophysiology of the visual system in practice of ophthalmology. Moscow (1974).

Van Lith, G.H.M. & H.E. Henkes. The local electric response of the central retinal area. Proc. of the VI.ISCERG Symp. Erfurt. 1967. Advances in Electrophysiology and pathology of the visual system. Leipzig: 163–170 (1968).

Authors' address:
Dr. A.M. Shamshinova
Prof. Dr. A.I. Bogoslovsky
Helmholtz Institute of Ophthalmology
Sadovo-Chernogriasskaya 14/19
Moscow 103064, USSR

Prof. Dr. sc. E. Marré
Dr. P. Mierdel
Augenklinik der Medizinischen Akademie
Fetscherstr. 74, DDR 8019 Dresden,
German Democratic Republic

EARLY POTENTIALS EVOKED BY MACULAR STIMULATION: OPTIC NERVE POTENTIALS?*†

JOHN B. SIEGFRIED

(*Philadelphia, U.S.A.*)

ABSTRACT

Electrical potentials were recorded from the region of the human "temple", and compared with simultaneously recorded ERG and VECP records. The properties of the "temple" recordings are such that they are not explained by volume conduction of ERG or VECP potentials, in these initial experiments.

INTRODUCTION

I have recorded electrical potentials from the skin of the "temple" (caudal to the fronto-zygomatic suture, on a level with the eye) referenced to the ear lobe on the same (ipsilateral) side. These potentials which are triggered by light striking the retina, are very similar in shape and time course to those recorded from the whole, exposed optic nerve in cat (Steinberg, 1966). An initial series of experiments has demonstrated that these potentials are not simply volume conducted electroretinographic (ERG) potentials arising from the inner layers of the retina, nor are they volume conducted evoked cortical potentials (VECP) of the brain.

MATERIAL AND METHODS

Gold skin electrodes (Grass Instrument co.) were affixed to the temple and ear lobe. ground for all experiments was the high center of the fore-head (see Fig. 1). Stimulation was provided by means of a Maxwellian view optical system. For most experiments, a 30 degree visual angle field (3×10^5 Trolands) was centrally fixated by means of incomplete cross-hairs. 20 mS duration flashes were presented at a rate of 2 Hz, except where otherwise noted. Computer summation was employed, and the bandpass of the recording system, which was limited on the high end by the sampling rate of the computer, was 1 Hz to 2500 Hz. In all cases, responses from the temple and from the cortex were elicited to 1000 flash presentations.

* The experiments reported here were performed in my laboratory at the Pennsylvania College of Optometry. Partial funding and some of the clinical patients were generously supplied by Wills Eye Hospital, Philadelphia, Pennsylvania.
† Some of this work was reported at the annual meeting, Association for Research in Vision and Opthalmology, Sarasota, Florida, 1979.

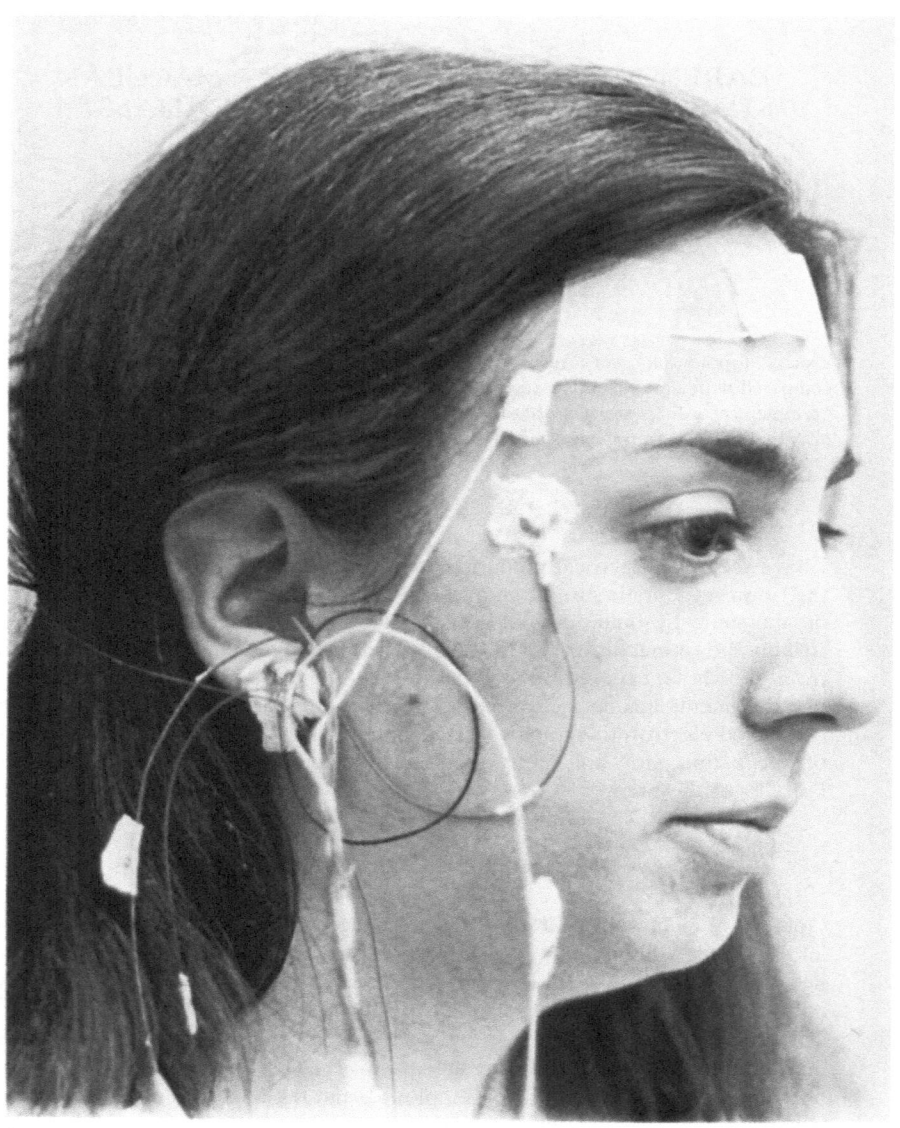

Fig. 1. Electrode configuration for recordings between temple and ear lobe, with ground on the forehead. Electrode leads from temple and ear lobe were input to a differential amplifier (Grass P-15).

RESULTS AND DISCUSSION

In order to demonstrate that the potentials recorded from the temple were not cortical in origin, skin electrodes were affixed to the temple and earlobe of both sides of the head, and recordings obtained for right eye stimulation. Results show (Fig. 2) that repeatable waveforms (each the summed response to 1000 flashes of light) are obtained on the side ipsilateral to the stimulated eye, and that little (subject NC) to no (subject DB) response is obtained on the contralateral side. At the optic chiasm, approximately 50% of the fibers making up the optic nerve cross to the contralateral side, while the others remain on the ipsilateral side. By this anatomical arrangement, the left visual field is projected to the right half of the brain, and the right visual field is projected to the left half of the brain. Thus, stimulation of one eye with a centrally fixed field of light produces neural responses which activate both sides of the brain about equally. If, therefore, the electrical potentials recorded from the temple were of cortical origin, it would be expected that similar responses

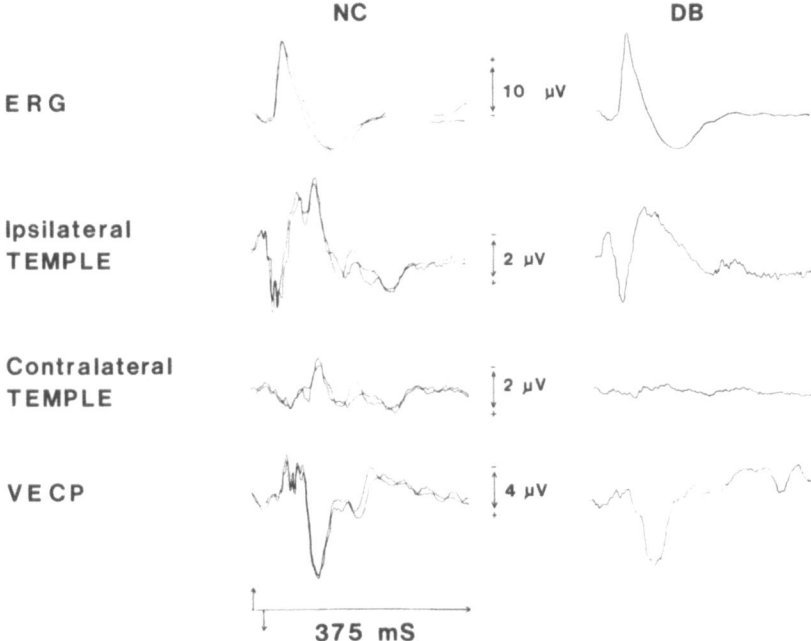

Fig. 2 Recordings from two normal subjects (NC and DB), showing ERG, ipsilateral temple, contralateral temple, and VECP. (Electrode configuration for VECP was 1 cm anterior to occipital protuberance, in the midline, referenced to ipsilateral ear lobe). Each tracing in this and subsequent figures represents the summation of 1,000 flash elicited potentials, except for ERG, where n = 100. For subject NC, two consecutive such summations are superimposed to show consistancy of response. Upward and downward arrows on the time calibration of this and subsequent figures indicate onset and offset of light stimulus, respectively.

would be recorded from *both* left and right temples, following stimulation of *either* eye. That such is not the case, as exhibited in Fig. 2, proves that the potentials are not of cortical (or optic radiation) origin, and in fact must originate anterior to the optic chiasm. In support of this conclusion, it may also be seen in Fig. 2 that implicit times of major peaks are shorter in the temple recordings than in the VECP recordings.

In order to demonstrate that these potentials are not volume conducted ERG potentials, simultaneous recordings were made of the ERG, by means of one platinum electrode in contact with cornea of the eye referenced to an electrode affixed to the cheek on the same side; and of recordings from the temple, with additional simultaneous recordings of VECP included for comparison. In Fig. 2 it can be seen that the major potential recorded from the temple reaches its peak approximately 10–15 mS *prior* to the peak of the ERG b-wave. In Fig. 3, typical results are exhibited for a long duration flash (1.0 S

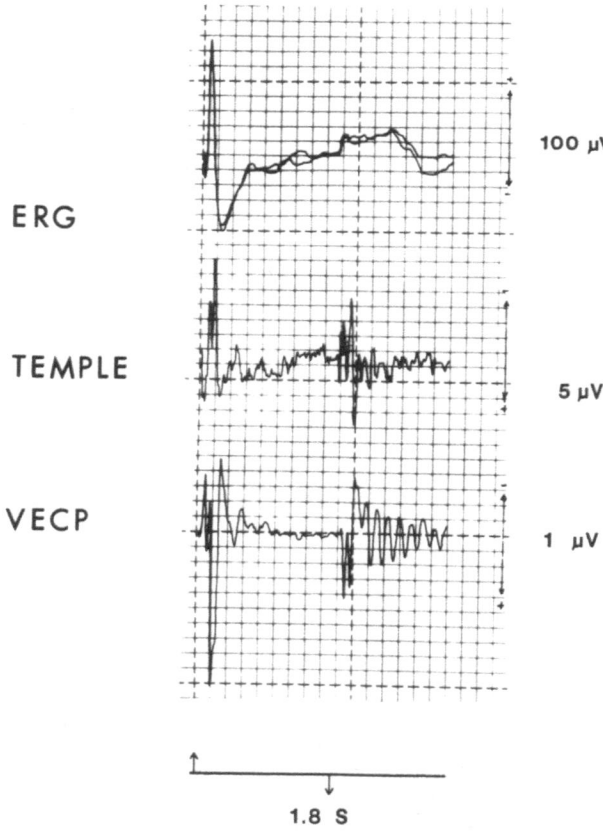

Fig. 3. Recordings from normal subject showing ERG, ipsilateral temple, and VECP. For the ERG, two consecutive summations are superimposed.

204

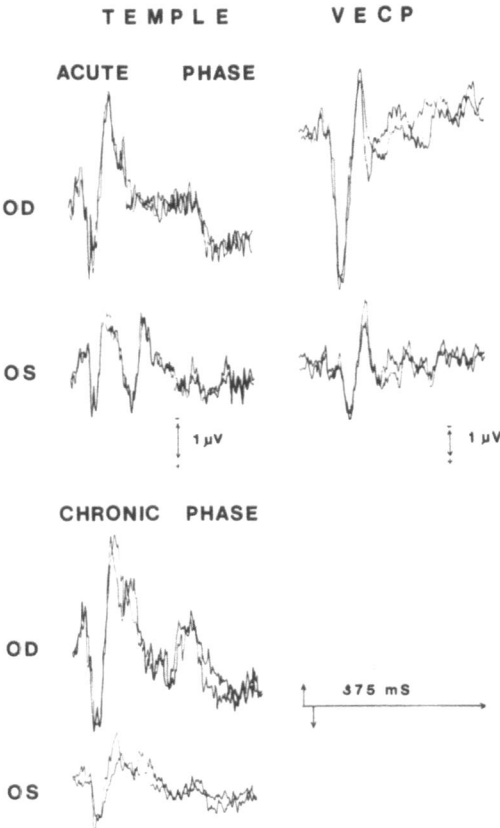

TEMPLE   VECP

ACUTE   PHASE

OD

OS

1 µV   1 µV

CHRONIC   PHASE

OD

375 mS

OS

Fig. 4. Recordings from patient with optic neuritis, on two occasions, showing temple and VECP during acute phase (top) and chronic phase (bottom). All temple recordings are from the side ipsilateral to stimulation. OS was the affected eye.

on, followed by 1.0 S off). A typical, small off-effect is seen in the ERG, however, the recording from the temple exhibits a vigorous off-response, whose amplitude is approximately equal to that of the on-response. In published records of whole optic nerve potentials in rabbit (Bartley & Bishop, 1942), the response of the nerve to light offset is almost as large as the response to light onset. On the other hand, the human ERG is known to exhibit only a very diminutive effect of light offset (Armington, 1974). Thus, it is clear that the relative magnitude of the off-effect in recordings from the ipsilateral temple resembles that of the optic nerve, and not that of the ERG.

Results from the testing of several clinical patients lend further support to the conclusion that the potentials recorded from the temple are not electroretinographic in origin. One patient had unilateral optic neuritis, with papillitis. Optic neuritis is an inflammation of the optic nerve, which results in

205

suddenly reduced visual acuity, afferent pupillary defect, and demyelinization of some optic nerve fibers. Such patients visual perception is altered in a manner which can be partially simulated by the interposition of a neutral density filter before the affected eye. Demyelinization results in a decreased neural conduction velocity, which has been demonstrated to result in delays in the VECP. The observation of papillitis (an abnormality of the optic disc, observable with funduscopic examination) indicates that the partial optic nerve lesion extends anteriorly to the point where ganglion cell axons first exit the back of the eye. Since the ERG is fully developed by retinal structures encountered *prior* to ganglion cells in the neural chain, it is fully normal in the eye of a patient with optic nerve disease. For this patient results of simultaneous recordings from the ipsilateral temple and from the cortex in response to light flash stimulation are exhibited in Fig. 4. "Acute phase" recordings were obtained when visual acuity in the left (affected) eye was 20/400, and visual

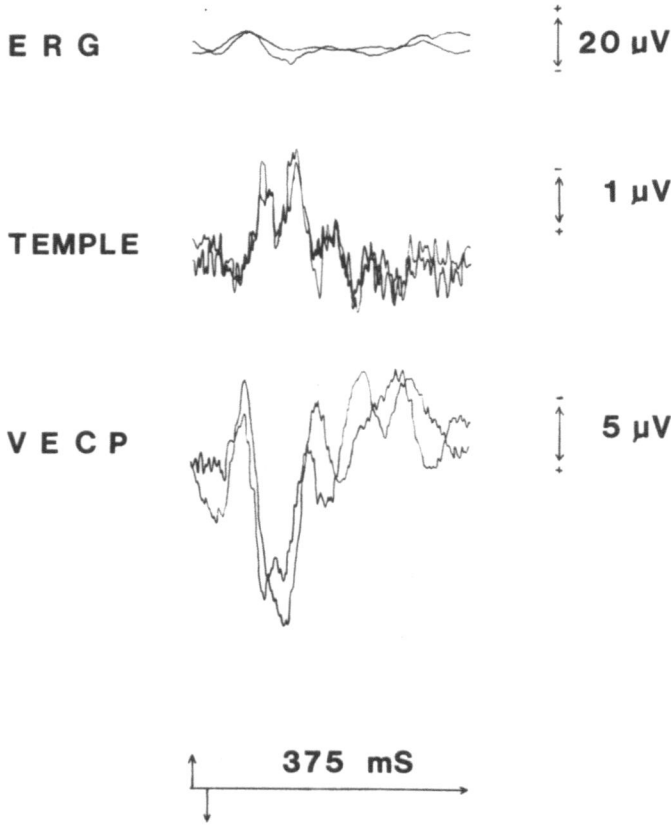

Fig. 5. Recordings from patient with retinitis pigmentosa, showing ERG, ipsilateral temple, and VECP. Two consecutive summations are superimposed in each case.

fields exhibited a partial central scotoma. VECP records exhibit the typical findings in optic neuritis; namely, a reduction in amplitude and increased implicit time for stimulation of the affected eye. The ipsilateral temple recordings, however, exhibit gross asymmetry for stimulation of the two eyes, with the affected eye exhibiting a reduction in amplitude, and a doubling of the response waveform. Since the potentials recorded from the ipsilateral temple are clearly different for the two eyes, their origin cannot be the ERG, since it was the same for both eyes. "Chronic phase" recordings were obtained after an interval of 10 days, with no medication, when visual acuity had returned to 20/25, and no field defects were measurable in the affected eye. The recordings from the ipsilateral temple were still markedly asymmetric in amplitude for the two eyes, but most of the second, delayed response had disappeared.

A second patient had retinitis pigmentosa, a pigmentary degeneration of the retina. This inherited, progressive disease leads to complete blindness eventually, but at an intermediate stage the patient may retain good central visual fields. Characteristically, such patients exhibit a markedly reduced, or extinguished, ERG. However, since the optic nerve is made up of approximately 90% fibers which have their receptive fields in the macular region of the retina, it would be expected to remain vigorous. Similarly, the VECP emphasizes macular input, and is therefore little changed from normal as long as central vision is relatively intact. For this patient, results of simultaneous recordings from the ipsilateral temple, ERG, and VECP in response to light stimulation are exhibited in Fig. 5. The ERG, in this case result of computer summation of 100 flash elicited records, is essentially extinguished, whereas a repeatable response is still present in recordings from the temple and in the VECP.

The results of these initial experiments support the conclusion that the recordings from the temple as performed here reflect activity of the optic nerve.

REFERENCES

Armington, J.C. The electroretinogram. Academic Press, New York. (1974).
Bartley, S.H. and Bishop, G.H. Some features of the optic-nerve discharge in the rabbit and cat. *J. cell. comp. Physiol.* 19: 79–93 (1942).
Steinberg, R.H. Oscillatory activity in the optic tract of cat and light adaptation. *J. Neurophysiol.* 29: 139–156 (1966).

Neuro-visual Sciences Tract
Pennsylvania College of Optometry
1200 West Godfrey Avenue
Philadelphia, Pennsylvania 19141
U.S.A.

MULTISPOT STIMULI REVEAL SPATIAL ORGANIZATION IN THE HUMAN ELECTRORETINOGRAM (ERG)

R. DIEHL AND E. ZRENNER

(*Bad Nauheim and Frankfurt, West Germany*)

ABSTRACT

As shown in the arterially perfused cat eye, multispot patterns, appropriately adjusted to the receptive field properties of cells in the inner nuclear layer, can abolish the b-wave under certain spatial conditions, even though the total number of quanta and the area illuminated are kept constant (Nelson, Zrenner and Gouras, 1979). This raised the hypothesis, that the b-wave reflects an annular or circular surround structure of the spatially organized ERG-generators.

In order to study similar spatial effects in the human ERG, a multispot pattern was constructed, with the size of the individual spots increasing towards the retinal periphery, according to perceptive field estimations in man. The ERG was recorded in response to the flashed pattern. Defocussing the pattern decreased the b-wave about 40%, even though the total number of quanta and the size of the visual field illuminated were kept constant. This effect cannot be explained by the influence of diffuse stray light; control experiments with homogeneous fields, bars and several checkerboard patterns showed only a comparably small effect.

Since only the spatial configuration of the test pattern can be made responsible for the change of the b-wave amplitude, these data support the idea, that the ERG-generators have a spatial organization of the center/surround type. Therefore, under certain conditions of illumination, the influence of this functional structure can be demonstrated also in the human ERG by means of specific patterns, which take into consideration the inhomogeneous distribution of these ERG-generators.

INTRODUCTION

There are only a few reports (Millodot and Riggs, 1970; Sokol and Bloom, 1977), which indicate spatial interaction in the electroretinogram (ERG), recorded by corneal electrodes in response to patterned stimuli. Local ERGs, however, recorded by intraretinal electrodes, suggest that there is spatial interaction between adjacent retinal areas as shown by Motokawa *et al.* (1959) and Arden and Brown (1965). Many retinal neurons show a discrete spatial organization in their receptive field structure; some of them certainly contribute to the ERG. Nelson, Zrenner and Gouras (1979) reported that a multispot pattern can show striking effects also in the ERG of the cat – recorded from the arterially perfused eye-cup preparation – if the receptive field size of cells in the inner nuclear layer, as measured in intracellular recordings, is considered. Their results are shown in Fig. 1. A hexagonally arranged multispot pattern heavily influenced the b-wave, if the diameter of

SPOT DIAM.
(µm)

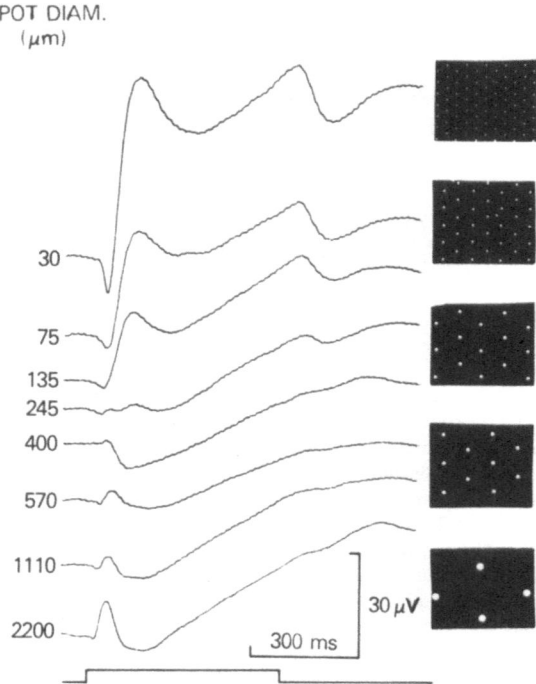

30

75

135

245

400

570

1110

2200

30 µV

300 ms

Fig. 1. Averaged d.c.-ERG recordings in the cat's perfused eyecup preparation in response to hexagonally arranged multispot patterns (right). The spot diameters are indicated beside each trace (left); the area stimulated by each pattern and the total number of quanta impinging on the retinal surface was held constant (from Nelson, Zrenner and Gouras, 1979).

each spot was adjusted to the size of the receptive field center and if the distance between the spots corresponded to the surround of such cells. In such a pattern each spot is surrounded by a dark ring-like area. At certain spatial configurations, with a spot diameter of 245 micrometer, the b-wave could be abolished. A spot diameter of 400 micrometer even reversed the polarity of the b-wave, although the number of quanta and the total area illuminated were kept constant in all stimuli. If the pattern with spot diameter of 245 micrometer was defocussed, which means that all quanta in the pattern were evenly distributed over the retina, the original b-wave returned, clearly indicating spatial organization in the ERG.

In the present study a similar technique was applied in man, in order to examine a spatial function of cells in the inner nuclear layer, contributing to the ERG b-wave.

The hexagonal arrangement of spots was not appropriate for human observers, since the size of their receptive field increases rapidly towards the retinal periphery. Therefore we constructed a pattern, in which the size of the spots and the distance between them increases from the center to the periphery (Fig. 2), corresponding to the change of the perceptive field size in man as reported

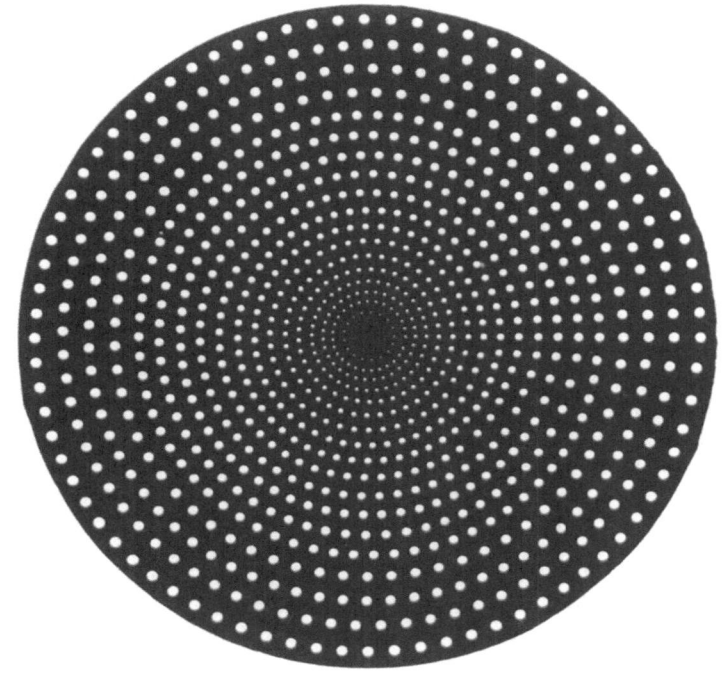

Fig. 2. Circular spot pattern for human observers (example). The size of the spots and the distance between them increases with eccentricity, corresponding to the change of the perceptive field size in man, as reported by Ransom and Spillmann (1978). The relation of spot diameter to distance was kept constant.

by Ransom and Spillman (1978) based on Westheimer's (1965, 1967) technique. We found that defocussing such a pattern with a certain spatial configuration produces a change of the b-wave amplitude between 30% and 40%. This result was not found using other patterns, explaining, why Brindley's (1956) stimulus arrangement did not reveal such spatial effects in the ERG. Thus, the b-wave of the human ERG can be a sensitive indicant of the spatial arrangement of a pattern stimulus.

METHOD

Five healthy students (age 18 to 25) with normal vision served as subjects (3 males, 2 females). They were trained to accommodate to two fixation spots in the center to insure a focussed image of the pattern on the retina.

The concentric spot pattern subtended a visual angle of 85°, presented at a distance of 30 cm. Combined with a red test filter (Schott OG 5) it was flashed every second for 15 ms with an illumination of 9 lm/m^2 on a background of blue light (Schott BG 28) of 0.3 lm/m^2, as measured by a photometric detector,

PIN-10 AP (United Detector Technology Inc.) in the position of the observers eye. The ERG was recorded with a Henkes contact lens electrode and averaged 64 times (Nicolet 1070). Each pattern was presented in a focussed as well as in a totally defocussed state. In the latter case it looked like a homogeneous field.

Control experiments were performed by presenting checkerboard and other differently structured contrast patterns as well as a homogeneous field (see text).

RESULTS

ERG a- and b-waves in response to various focussed (solid line) as well as defocussed patterns (dashed line) are shown in Fig. 3. Usual checkerboard patterns (left) caused a small amplitude decrease of only 11% when focussed. When a circular spot pattern (middle), here with 17 concentric circles, was presented in the focussed state, an average amplitude decrease of 33% was observed, in comparison to the defocussed state, even though the same number of quanta had been delivered. Moreover, control experiments with unstructured homogeneous fields (right) showed that the method of focussing used in these experiments was not responsible for the amplitude decrease, observed with the circular multispot pattern. In fact focussing even increased the amplitude because of a slight increase in aperture. No difference was found in the average peak latency between focussed and defocussed stimuli. When focussed, the concentrical spot pattern showed the maximum effect compared to all other patterns used, which were stripes, checkerboard patterns and other randomly structured patterns. The probability of error (P) that the responses of these two experimental conditions statistically belong to the same group is less than 1%.

Having found the pattern structure which gave a reliable effect, the next step was to improve this effect by varying the magnification of the circular spot pattern (Fig. 4). This variation keeps constant the relation of spot diameter to distance between the spots as well as the total number of quanta delivered on the retina.

The optimum effect of nearly 40% (in the middle) was obtained by a pattern consisting of 13 concentric circles, while coarser (left) or finer patterns (right) show a smaller effect between 32% and 34%. This means that there is a favoured spatial configuration. The 3 records shown are only representatives of 10 different magnifications used, the amplitude decrease of which has values in between these examples.

The probability of error (P) that the response obtained with 13 circles belongs to the same group as the responses obtained with 10 and 21 circles is less than 1%. Obviously a particular pattern magnification favours a maximal decrease of the b-wave amplitude.

DISCUSSION

Since the work of Spekreijse (1966), White (1969), Armington, Corwin and Marsetta (1971) and Regan (1972) it is known that the visually evoked cortical

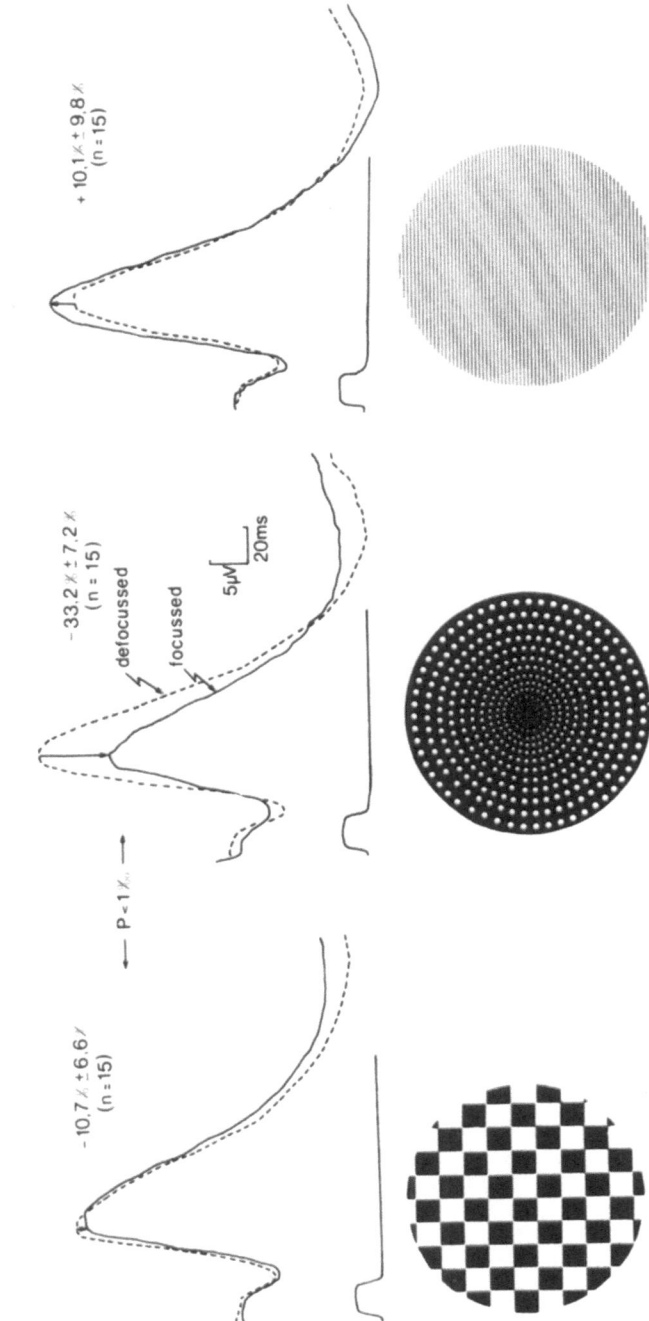

Fig. 3. ERG a- and b-waves in response to various focussed (solid line) as well as defocussed patterns (dashed line). The lowermost record indicates the flash duration. The patterns shown below are schematic examples. Responses to a checkerboard pattern (50′ check size) on the left, to a circular concentrical spot pattern in the middle and to an unstructured homogeneous field on the right side. The average decrease of b-wave amplitude (15 experiments) and the standard deviation is denoted (in percent) besides each pair of records. The probability of error (P) between checkerboard and circular spot pattern is indicated in between the records.

213

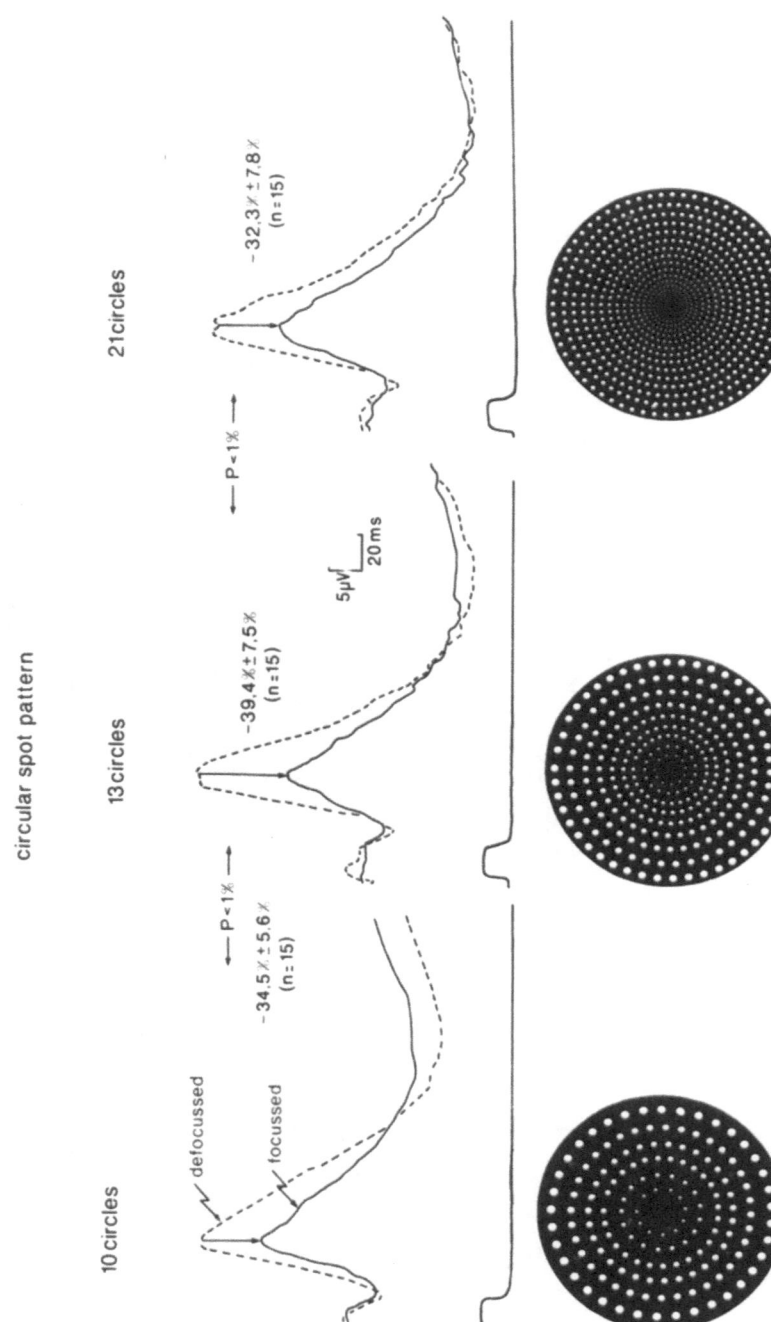

Fig. 4. Same as Fig. 3 for circular concentrical spot patterns of various magnifications (10, 13 and 21 circles).

potential reveals a spatial sensitivity. This was shown by Barber and Galloway (1976) also for a dartboard like pattern, which takes into account differences between the central and peripheral retina in the spatial domain. Our data support the idea, that the human ERG is sensitive to the spatial arrangement of the stimulus pattern and therefore possibly reflects lateral interactions in the inner nuclear layer of the retina.

The model in the cat of Nelson, Zrenner and Gouras (1979) suggests that the b-wave originates mainly from the annular or circular surround structure of cells in the inner nuclear layer: When the surround area of these cells is kept in dark while the center is illuminated, the b-wave is minimized or abolished. A similar effect was achieved by our circular spot pattern in man. A polarity reversal and a total b-wave suppression could not be obtained in man. Obviously, the saccades and the influence of the optic media which could be avoided in the cat's enucleated and perfused eyecup preparation prevented a stabilized and in all parts focussed image in human observers. Furthermore, to obtain the optimum effect a coarser pattern had to be used than predicted by the perceptive field size data on which the original pattern was based. This suggests that the retinal receptive field sizes might be more extended than the cortical perceptive field sizes. Therefore in some cells whose center was illuminated by a spot, the surround might not have been totally kept in dark, still generating a small amount of b-wave potentials. Nevertheless an obvious spatial effect could be demonstrated with patterns, which take into consideration the perceptive or, in certain magnifications, possibly the receptive field size in the human visual system.

It should be noted that the contrast of the focussed pattern was higher than 3 logarithmic units; since the test flash was only about 1 logarithmic unit above the b-wave threshold the straylight in the dark areas of the pattern was kept well below b-wave threshold and could not contribute to this response. The straylight deliberately produced by defocusing was equal in all spot patterns, because the relation of spot size to spot distance was not varied. Also the luminance and the area were kept constant (± 0.1 log units); therefore the influence of changes in the area luminance relation, caused by defocussing, could not vary among the different patterns presented.

Since the only variable was the spatial arrangement of photons in the various patterns, we have to assume, that the decrease in b-wave amplitude (found to be different for each pattern) reveals spatial sensitivity of the human ERG.

ACKNOWLEDGEMENT

We are grateful to Prof. E. Dodt and Dr. R. Nelson for helpful discussions and Mrs. E. Wulfken for technical assistance.

REFERENCES

Arden, G.B. & K.T. Brown. Some properties of components of the cat electroretinogram revealed by local recording under oil. *J. Physiol.* 176: *429–461* (1965).

Armington, J.C., T.R. Corwin & R. Marsetta. Simultaneously recorded retinal and cortical responses to patterned stimuli. *J. Opt. Soc. Amer.* 61: *1514–1521* (1971).

Barber, C. & N.R. Galloway. A pattern stimulus for optimal response from the retina. *Doc. Ophthal. Proc. Ser.* 10: *77–86* (1976).

Brindley, G.S. The effect on the frog's electroretinogram of varying the amount of retina illuminated. *J. Physiol.* 134: *353–359* (1956).

Millodot, M. & L.A. Riggs. Refraction determined electrophysiologically. *Arch. Ophthal.* 84: *272–278* (1970).

Motokawa, K., T. Oikawa, K. Tasaki & T. Ogawa. The spatial distribution of electric responses to focal illumination of the carp's retina. *Tohoku J. Exp. Med.* 70: *151–164* (1959).

Nelson, R., E. Zrenner & P. Gouras. Patterned stimuli reveal spatial organization in the electroretinogram 16th ISCEV Symposium. Morioka, Japan, pp. 161–169 (1979).

Ransom, A. & L. Spillmann. Estimates of perceptive field size at various eccentricities using the Westheimer paradigm, and a test of its decrement counterpart. Poster presented at the Experimental Psychology Meeting, Marburg, West Germany (1978).

Regan, D. Evoked potentials in psychology, sensory physiology and clinical medicine. Chapman and Hall, London (1972).

Sokol, S. & B. Bloom. Macular ERG's elicited by checkerboard pattern stimuli. *Doc. Ophthal. Proc. Ser.* 13: *299–305* (1977).

Spekreijse, H. Analysis of E.E.G. responses in man, evoked by sine wave modulated light. Academisch Proefschrift, Universiteit van Amsterdam (1966).

Westheimer, G. Spatial interaction in the human retina during scotopic vision. *J. Physiol.* 181: *881–894* (1965).

Westheimer, G. Spatial interaction in human cone vision. *J. Physiol.* 192: *309–315* (1967).

White, C.T. Evoked cortical responses and patterned stimuli. *Am. Psychologist* 24: *211–214* (1969).

Authors' address:
R. Diehl
Max-Planck-Institute for Brain Research
Frankfurt a. Main
F.R.G.

E. Zrenner
Max-Planck-Institute for Physiological and Clinical Research
D-6350 Bad Nauheim
Parkstr. 1, and
University Eye Clinic
Frankfurt a. Main
F.R.G.

HUMAN FAST RETINAL POTENTIALS STUDIED WITH PATTERN REVERSAL STIMULI

MATTHIAS J. KORTH AND VIKTOR REIMANN

(*Erlangen, F.R.G.*)

ABSTRACT

High-frequency wavelets of the human ERG obtained with alternating stimulus patterns were observed predominantly on the ascending slope of the b-wave. With increasing stimulus intensity, the peak latency of the b-wave decreased at a higher rate than that of the fast components and the number of the wavelets decreased. The spectral sensitivity of the wavelets obtained with a checkerboard pattern was purely photopic at all adaptation levels. When the spatial frequency of alternating square wave stripe and checkerboard patterns was varied between 0.3 and 8 c/deg, typical changes in the behaviour of the fast components could be observed. Around a spatial frequency of 3 c/deg, two wavelets showed increased amplitude values. Above 1 c/deg, up to five wavelets and below 1 c/deg, only three wavelets were observed. Most of the fast components evoked with a checkerboard pattern were of smaller amplitude and, when plotted as a function of the spatial frequency of the fundamental Fourier component of the checkerboard pattern, showed a behaviour similar to that of the wavelets obtained with the stripe pattern.

INTRODUCTION

The contribution of the scotopic and the photopic system to the generation of human ERG wavelets has been investigated by several authors. Based on observations using single flashes of white light the fast ERG components were ascribed either to cone or an interaction of rod and cone function (*e.g.*, De Molfetta *et al.*, 1968; Jacobson *et al.*, 1967; Algvere and Westbeck, 1972; Wachtmeister, 1972, 1973; Auerbach, 1964). Spectral sensitivity studies of the wavelets are also in disagreement. Functions were obtained suggesting either scotopic or photopic or a mixture of both activities (Adams and Dawson, 1971; Fujimura *et al.*, 1972; Kojima and Zrenner, 1978; Stodtmeister, 1972, 1973a, b; Wachtmeister, 1974).

In the present experiments the human ERG wavelets were examined using the method of pattern reversal (Johnson *et al.*, 1966). This stimulus procedure allows an excellent control over the level of the eye's adaptation and, since stray light does not contribute to the response, is suitable for studying spectral sensitivity of the ERG. Furthermore, since the stimulus is spatially structured the effect of various spatial frequencies of different patterns on the ERG wavelets could be examined.

METHOD

For both types of experiment to be described below the stimulus pattern was presented in Maxwellian view. The intensity of a 75 Watt Xenon high-pressure arc lamp (Osram) was controlled by means of neutral density filters (Schott). The pattern alternated at a rate of two displacements per second. The responses to both right and left movements were added together using a digital computer (PDP 11/40). 512 sweeps were averaged for each intensity setting using a sweep length of 70 ms. The records (512 points) were digitally smoothed by repeating the algorithm of a three-point Hanning filter 1000 times (attenuation of 40 dB at 100 Hz). By subtraction of the smoothed function, thus obtained, from the unfiltered waveform the fast components were isolated. The ERG was recorded (Tektronix 122 and 502, frequency response 0.2 Hz–10 kHz) from the right eye against the right ear lobe, the left ear was grounded. The amplitude of both the b-wave and of the high-pass filtered wavelets was measured from the peak of a wave to the bottom of the preceding trough.

For the spectral sensitivity study, a circular field (diameter 46.5°) was used as stimulus filled with a coloured (grating monochromator, Schoeffel GM 250) checkerboard pattern (checksize 2°44′). With the pattern removed the maximum retinal illuminance at 670 nm was 3 photop. log Td (4.7×10^6 light quanta/sec/deg^2). A dark adaptation period of 30 min preceded the recording. Two adult colour-normal subjects (M.K. and I.R.) were tested.

For studying spatial effects of the stimulus on the ERG wavelets, vertically oriented square wave stripe and checkerboard patterns of varying spatial frequency were used covering a range of about 5 octaves. In contrast to the spectral sensitivity study, a small visual field (diameter 24°) was used in order to obtain patterns of sufficiently high spatial frequencies. The retinal illuminance with the pattern removed was 4.65 photop. log. Td. Three subjects (M.K., V.R., and R.R.) were tested.

RESULTS

Figure 1 shows superimposed unfiltered and digitally smoothed (a) as well as high-pass filtered (b) ERGs obtained with an alternating colourless checkerboard pattern under increasing photopic luminance levels. Wavelets were observed more clearly when they were superimposed on the ascending slope of the b-wave. With increasing intensity, the peak latency of the smoothed b-wave decreased at a higher rate than that of the wavelets. As a consequence, the amplitude of those wavelets occurring later in time than the peak of the b-wave were attenuated. Wavelets occurring earlier than the peak of the b-wave increased in amplitude.

Spectral Sensitivity

Figure 2 shows luminance curves of wavelets 1–4 for different wavelengths based on peak latency and amplitude values. As was noted in Fig. 1, the peak latency of the b-wave (dashed curve in Fig. 2) decreased at a higher rate than

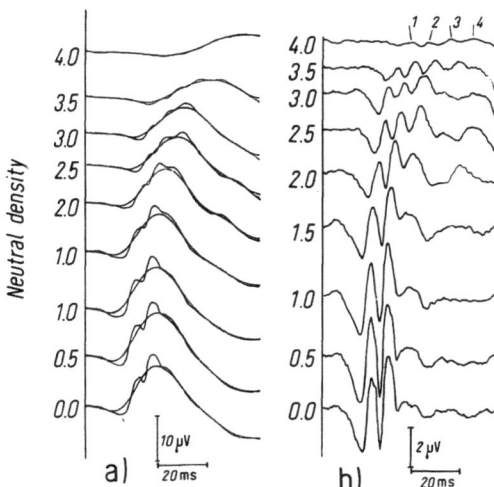

Fig. 1. ERGs obtained under increasing levels of photopic stimulation. (a) superimposed original and digitally smoothed ERGs. (b) High-pass filtered records obtained from a) by subtracting the smoothed from the unfiltered traces. The wavelets are labeled with consecutive numbers. All records are averages of six trials with a total of 3072 sweeps. Maximum retinal illuminance with the pattern removed 5.9 photop. log Td. White light. Subject M.K.

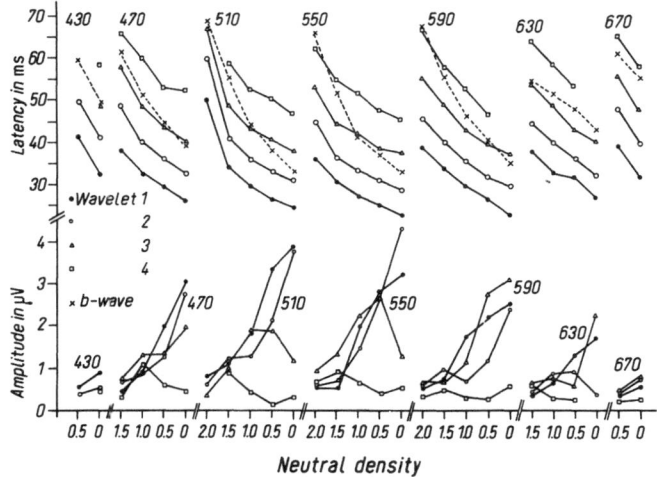

Fig. 2. Luminance curves of the ERG wavelets 1–4 based on latency (top) and amplitude (bottom) measurements. The numbers next to each curve (set of curves) refer to the stimulus wavelength in nm. All curves are averages of two trials. Subject I.R.

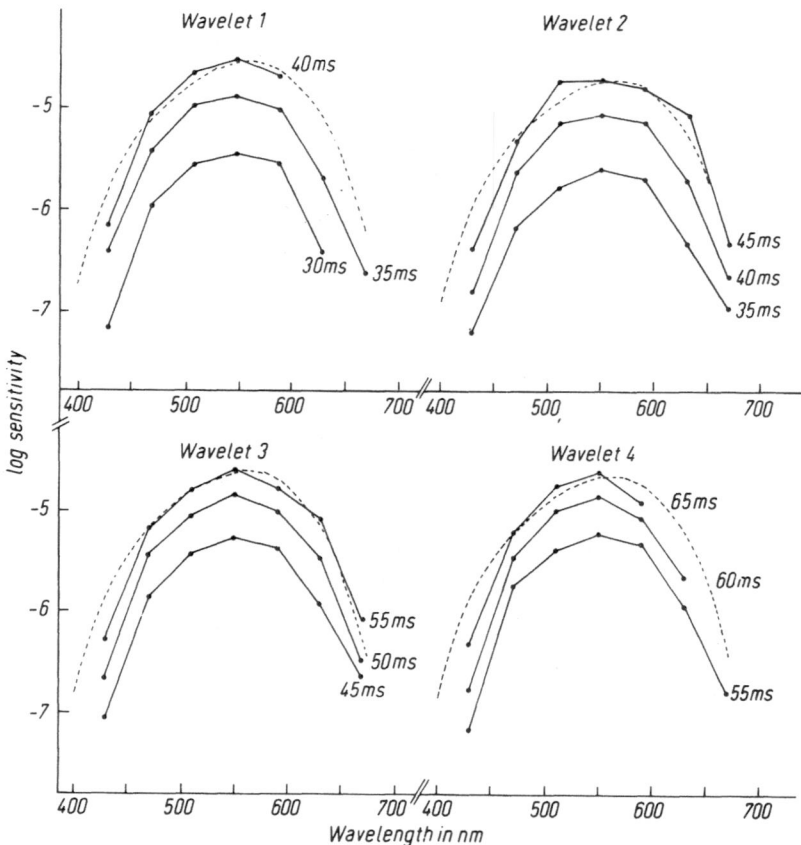

Fig. 3. Spectral sensitivity curves of wavelets 1–4 for different criterion latencies. The dashed curves are Wald's (1945) curve for the peripheral cones. Equal quantum intensity spectra. Subject I.R.

that of the wavelets. The decrease in amplitude of wavelet 3 at certain stimulus levels and the missing increase in amplitude of wavelet 4 can be explained from the observation that these wavelets occurred later in time than the peak of the b-wave. Since the peak latency curves of the wavelets show a monotonic decrease with increasing stimulus intensity spectral sensitivity was derived from smooth curves fitted "by eye" to the latency data points. The method of constant criterion response was used. At all adaptation levels studied, the spectral sensitivity of the wavelets (Fig. 3) could be described best by Wald's (1945) curve for the peripheral cones. Even at the lower intensities at which the wavelets became first noticeable they were of photopic nature and the shape of the spectral curves did not change significantly with decreasing criterion latencies (*i.e.,* increasing light adaptation).

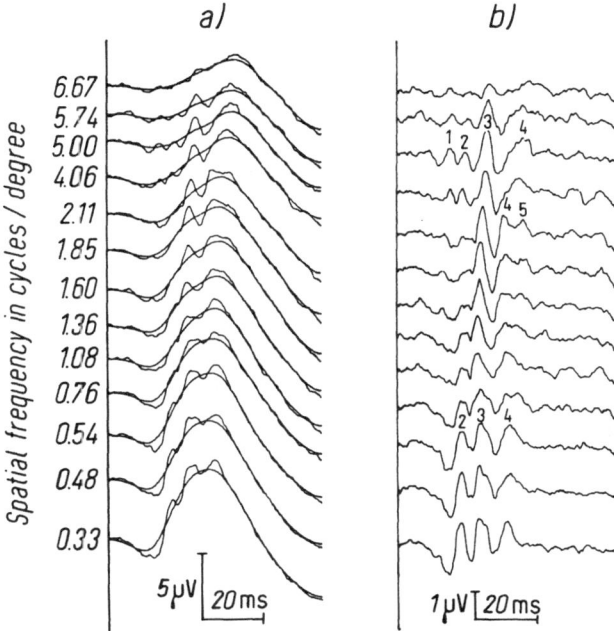

Fig. 4. ERGs obtained with square wave stripe patterns of different spatial frequencies. (a) Superimposed unfiltered and digitally smoothed ERGs (b) High-pass filtered records obtained from (a) by subtracting the smoothed from the unfiltered traces. The wavelets are labeled by consecutive numbers All records are averages of four trials with a total of 2048 sweeps. Subject M.K.

Spatial Selectivity

Superimposed original and digitally smoothed ERGs as well as high-pass filtered records obtained with alternating square wave stripe patterns of varying spatial frequency are shown in Fig 4a and b. Wavelets 1–5 showed typical changes in their number, waveform, amplitude, and temporal spacing as the spatial frequency was changed. At spatial frequencies higher than about 1 c/deg, up to five wavelets could be observed dominated by the amplitude of wavelet 3. Below 1 c/deg, only three wavelets were noticed.

The behaviour of the amplitude of wavelets 1–5 as a function of the spatial frequency of the stripe pattern is shown in Fig. 5a. Wavelet 2 showed a more or less monotonic decrease in amplitude with increasing spatial frequency. Wavelets 3 and 4 were of increased amplitudes between 2 and 5 c/deg and wavelets 1 and 5 were tuned to two different values of high spatial frequency. With decreasing spatial frequency below 1 c/deg the amplitudes of wavelets 2, 3, and 4 showed a steady increase. Over the entire spatial frequency range tested the behaviour of wavelets 2, 3, and 4 was similar for the three subjects tested. Wavelets 1 and 5, however, were observed only in subject M.K.

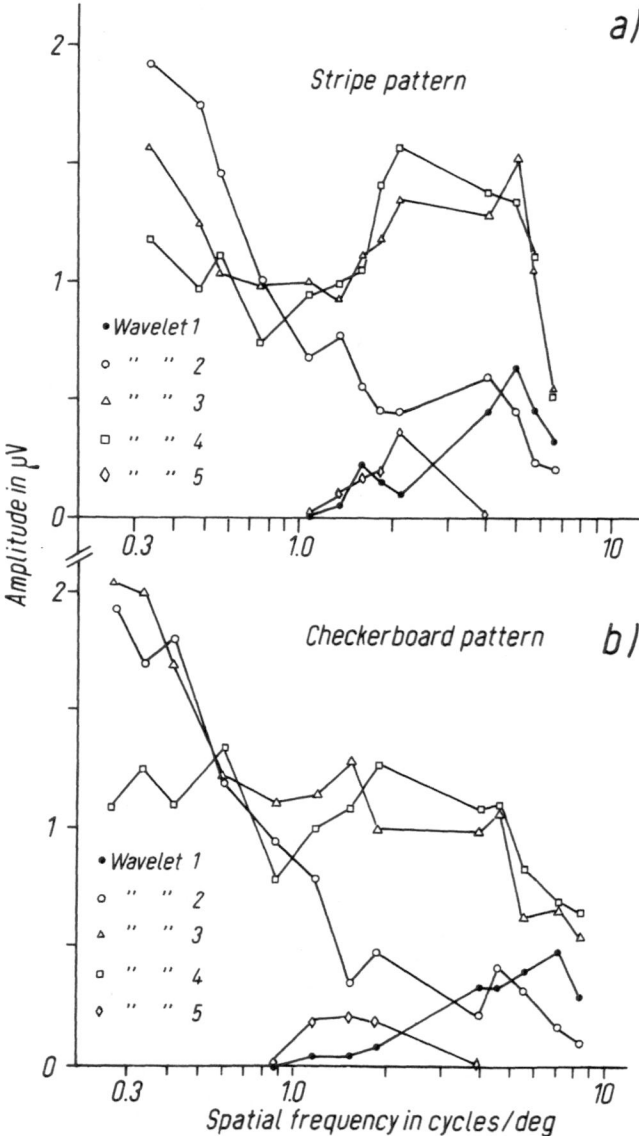

Fig. 5. Amplitudes of wavelets 1–5 as a function of the spatial frequency of the fundamental Fourier component of a square wave stripe (a) and of a checkerboard (b) pattern. Averages of four trials. Subject M.K.

The wavelets obtained with checkerboard patterns were similar in appearance to those shown in Fig. 4. The behavior of the wavelets' amplitudes as a function of the spatial frequency of the checkerboard's fundamental Fourier component is shown in Fig. 5b. The orientation of the fundamental component is on the 45° diagonals of the checkerboard pattern (Kelly, 1976). Wavelet 4 showed a weak tuning and wavelet 3 showed a plateau both occurring at spatial frequencies that were associated with the tuning peaks of wavelets 3 and 4 in Fig. 5a.

DISCUSSION

Figure 3 demonstrated that the wavelets 1–4 were of purely photopic nature. Thus, they offer the possibility of studying photopic retinal function unaffected by contributions of the scotopic system.

The different rates of decrease in peak latency of the b-wave and of the wavelets (Fig. 2) indicates that both ERG components represent two different mechanisms. However, they are not independent of each other since the wavelets were observed more clearly when superimposed on the ascending slope of the b-wave.

The contradictory results obtained with the spectral sensitivity studies mentioned in the introduction might be due to the different experimental procedures using different intensities of the adapting light as well as different durations of the flash and of the interflash interval. Since in the present study test and adaptation light were identical these variables were under control. Furthermore, luminosity functions of the wavelets that have been published so far were based on amplitude measurements carried out in different ways. Figure 2, however, indicated that peak latency measurements of the wavelets might provide a better means for determining spectral sensitivity than amplitude measurements.

The finding that the wavelets are of photopic origin is supported by the experiments studying the effects of different spatial frequencies on the wavelets. Only the cones can be expected to perform the high-spatial frequency resolution observed in Fig. 4. The wavelets showed a spatial tuning around a spatial frequency of 3 c/deg (Fig. 5). This observation might be related to Campbell and Robson's (1968) finding that the psychophysical contrast sensitivity function of the human visual system for square wave gratings peaks at a spatial frequency of 3 c/deg. Spatial selectivity at the retinal level has been demonstrated also for the "sustained"-type retinal ganglion cells of the cat (Enroth-Cugell and Robson, 1966; Maffei and Fiorentini, 1972).

The reduced spatial tuning behaviour of wavelets 3 and 4 observed with the checkerboard pattern (Fig. 5b) occurred in a spatial frequency range (of the checkerboard's fundamental Fourier component) comparable to that at which the corresponding tuning behaviour was noticed with the stripe pattern (Fig. 5a). This would indicate that the spatial selectivity of wavelets 3 and 4 can be predicted by two-dimensional Fourier analysis better than by feature analysis of a checkerboard pattern (Green et al., 1976; May and Matteson, 1976; De Valois et al., 1978).

The high-spatial frequency cut-off of the wavelets' amplitudes is determined by the modulation transfer functions of both the stimulating apparatus and of the subject's eye. The decrease in amplitude of the wavelets upon decreasing the spatial frequency from 2 to 1 c/deg (Fig. 5) can be attributed to the effects of lateral inhibition. With further decrease in spatial frequency, lateral inhibition seems to be ineffective and the amplitude of the wavelets increases again. Below 1 c/deg (Fig. 1 and 4), the wavelets resembled the "oscillatory" potentials commonly obtained with spatially unstructured single flashes of light.

REFERENCES

Adams, C.K. & W.W. Dawson. Fast retinal potential luminosity functions. *Vision Res.* 11: *1135–1146*, (1971).

Algvere, P. & S. Westbeck. Human ERG in response to double flashes of light during the course of dark adaptation: A Fourier analysis of the oscillatory potentials. *Vision Res.* 12: *195–214*, (1972).

Auerbach, E. The effect of slow intermittent light stimulation on the human ERG. *Docum. Ophthal.* 18: *376–391*, (1964).

Campbell, F.W. & J.G. Robson. Application of Fourier analysis to the visibility of gratings. *J. Physiol.* 197: *551–566*, (1968).

De Molfetta, V., D. Spinelli & F. Polenghi. Behaviour of electroretinographic oscillatory potentials during adaptation to darkness. *A.M.A. Arch. Ophthal.* 79: *531–535*, (1968).

De Valois, R.L., K.K. De Valois & E.W. Yund. Responses of striate cells to gratings and checkerboards. *Invest. Ophthalmol.* (Suppl.) 17: *174–175*, (1978).

Enroth-Cugell, Ch. & J.G. Robson. The contrast sensitivity of retinal ganglion cells of the cat. *J. Physiol.* 187: *517–552*, (1966).

Fujimura, K., Y. Tsuchida & J.H. Jacobson. Oscillatory potential of the human electroretinogram evoked by monochromatic light. *Invest. Ophthalmol.* 11: *683–690*, (1972).

Green, M., Th.R Corwin & V. Zemon. A comparison of Fourier analysis and feature analysis in pattern-specific color after-effects. *Science.* 192: *147–148*, (1976).

Jacobson, J.H., T. Hirose & A.B. Popkin. Oscillatory potential of the electroretinogram: Relationship to the photopic b-wave in humans. *A.M.A. Arch. Ophthal.* 78: *58–67*, (1967).

Johnson, E.P., L.A. Riggs & A.M.L. Schick. Photopic retinal potentials evoked by phase alternation of a barred pattern. In: Burian, H.M. & J.H. Jacobson (eds.) *Clinical electroretinography* (Suppl. 1 to Vision Res.): *57–91*, (1966).

Kelly, D.H. Pattern detection and the two-dimensional Fourier transform: Flickering checkerboards and chromatic mechanisms. *Vision Res.* 16: *277–287*, (1976).

Kojima, M. & E. Zrenner. Off-components in response to brief light flashes in the oscillatory potential of the human electroretinogram. *Albrecht v. Graefes Arch. klin. exp. Ophthal.* 206: *107–120*, (1978).

Maffei, L. & A. Fiorentini. The visual cortex as a spatial frequency analyzer. *Vision Res.* 13: *1255–1267*, (1973).

May, J.G. & H.H. Matteson. Spatial frequency-contingent color aftereffects. *Science* 192: *145–147*, (1976).

Stodtmeister, R. Purkinjeverschiebung oscillatorischer Potentiale im menschlichen Elektroretinogramm. *Deut. Ophth. Ges.* 71: *388–391*, (1972).

Stodtmeister, R. Human scotopic fast retinal potentials. Xth ISCERG-Symp. Docum. Opthal. Proc. Series Vol. 2: *199–203*, (1973a).

Stodtmeister, R. The spectral sensitivity functions of human ERG wavelets. *Ophthal. Res.* 5: *21–30*, (1973b).

Wachtmeister, L. On the oscillatory potentials of the human electroretinogram in light and dark adaptation. IV. Effect of adaptation to short flashes of light. Time interval and intensity of conditioning flash. A Fourier analysis. *Acta Ophthal.* 50: *250–269*, (1972).

Wachtmeister, L. On the oscillatory potentials of the human electroretinogram in light and dark adaptation. III. Thresholds and relation to stimulus intensity on adaptation to background light. *Acta Ophthal.* 51: *95–113*, (1973).

Wachtmeister, L. Luminosity functions of the oscillatory potentials of the human electroretinogram. *Acta Ophthal.* 52: *353–366*, (1974).

Wald, G. Human vision and the spectrum. *Science* 101: *653–658*, (1945).

Author's address:
Dr. Matthias Korth
Institut für Physiologie und Biokybernetik
Universität Erlangen-Nürnberg
Universitätsstr. 17
F.R.G.

Docum. Ophthal. Proc. Series, Vol. 23

STIMULUS FIELD, ELEMENT SIZE AND HUMAN VISUALLY EVOKED CORTICAL POTENTIALS

EMIKO ADACHI-USAMI

(*Hamamatsu-shi, Japan*)

ABSTRACT

The paper was concerned with spatial frequency (element size) characteristics at the central retina by use of a TV technique. Steady state VECP amplitudes as a function of spatial frequency were studied in a number of experiments in which orientation of a pattern, field size, retinal position, defocusing grade were altered. Also binocular and monocular stimulation were performed. It was shown that evaluation of VECP results concerning the above parameters is not seriously affected by the known disadvantages of our TV system.

INTRODUCTION

Using oscilloscope display methods Campbell and Maffei (1970) proved that the amplitudes of VECPs recorded from a human scalp reflect the psychophysical thresholds for various spatial frequencies. They used a stimulus of a repetitive sine-wave grating alternating in phase while keeping the space-average luminance constant. To produce spatial stimuli TV pattern generators have recently been used in clinical work because of its versatility. On the other hand certain limitations in using a TV system have been described (Arden *et al.*, 1977, Van Lith *et al.*, 1979, Adachi-Usami and Morita, 1979).

In this paper certain stimulus parameters which might affect spatial properties of human vision were studied by means of steady state VECPs making use of TV techniques.

METHODS

A multipurpose television pattern generator specially developed for VECP studies (Adachi and Morita, 1978, Adachi-Usami, 1979) was used. The stimulus consisted of either checkerboards or square wave gratings at constant average luminance and modulated sinusoidally at a reversal frequency of 12 Hz. The mean luminance of the TV screen was kept at 2.14 log ft-L (473 cd/m²). The contrast of the pattern was defined as

$$\frac{L_{max} - L_{min}}{L_{max} + L_{min}} \times 100\%.$$

Most of the experiment were performed with a constant contrast of 40%. The visual angle of the patterned field and the constituting elements of bars and checks were varied as required. The pattern was viewed monocularly with central fixation from a distance of 3 m; and occasionally from 0.6 and 1.2 m.

The VECPs were recorded by a scalp electrode placed 10% above the inion with a reference at the right earlobe. After passing through a preamplifier and a selective filter of 12 Hz (Q = 3.5), 100 responses were averaged and written out by an X-Y recorder. The pupil was dilated with 1% cyclopentrate to control the effects of pupil size and those of accommodation. An artificial pupil of 4 mm and ophthalmic lens correction for the proper viewing distance were always used. VECPs were measured for various bar or check sizes in a number of conditions where also other stimulus parameters were altered. In the case of bar stimulation the conventional term spatial frequency was used; for checks we preferred to indicate the size of the elements. The height between the peak and the trough of the sinusoidal output VECP was measured as the amplitude in all experiments.

Normal observers served as subjects.

RESULTS AND DISCUSSION

VECP amplitude vs. spatial frequency (element size) was studied by varying stimulus conditions in five ways.

1. *Orientation of the pattern*

It has been known from psychophysics that the human visual resolution is better by a factor of approx. 50% in the vertical and horizontal orientation than in the oblique orientation. In spite of a number of investigations in animals (Hubel and Wiesel, 1959, Pettigrew et al., 1968 and Mansfield, 1974), no definite explanation has been presented. In humans Maffei and Campbell (1970) found less sensitivity to the oblique orientations by measuring the amplitude of steady state VECPs, but such inequality was not found by recording the ERG. They suggested, thus, that orientational effects must arise between the site of origin of the ERG and the VECP. To see the effect of spatial frequency on such orientation effects, the following experiments were performed.

In a circular field of 4°, corresponding to a 3 m viewing distance, VECPs to square wave gratings presented vertically, horizontally and obliquely (45° and 135° by rotating the television set) were measured at spatial frequencies of 0.54, 1.1, 2.2, 4.4, and 8.7 cycles/degree. VECPs to checkerboards in corresponding element size of 56', 28', 14', 7' and 3.5' were also measured and comparison was made among the five kinds of pattern presented.

A representative set of VECP records is shown in Fig. 1. VECP amplitude vs. element size curves derived from three subjects are demonstrated in Fig. 2. Resulting data showed the following characteristics. (1) The maximum response for gratings (4.4 c/d) was found as smaller element size than for the checkerboards (14'). In general the response showed lower amplitudes for the gratings than for the checkerboard. (2) Orientation of the gratings affects only slightly the curves at spatial frequencies less than 4.4 c/d, but a marked decrease of the VECP amplitude to the oblique grating as compared to the vertical and horizontal ones was found with stimulation at higher spatial frequencies such

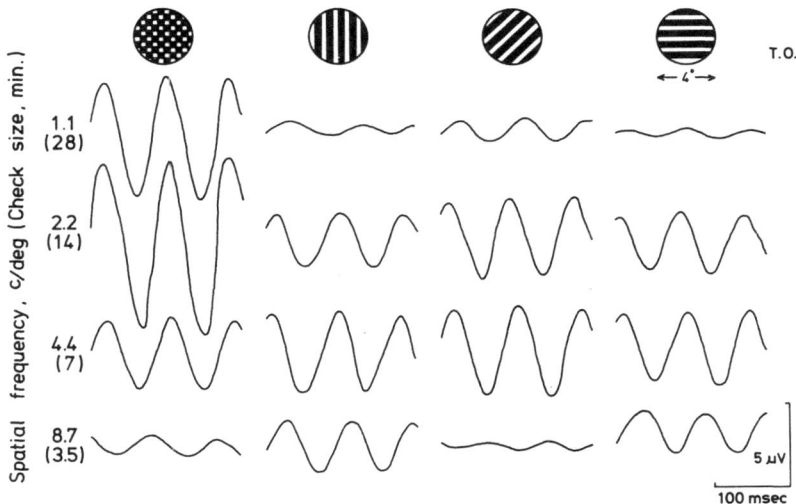

Fig. 1. VECP records in response to checkerboard, vertical, oblique, and horizontal grating pattern stimuli for four different element sizes (spatial frequencies). Reversal frequency 12 Hz, mean luminance 2.14 log ft-L, contrast 40%, 4° circular field viewed moncularly from a distance of 3 m with central fixation. Oz – right earlobe monopolar recording.

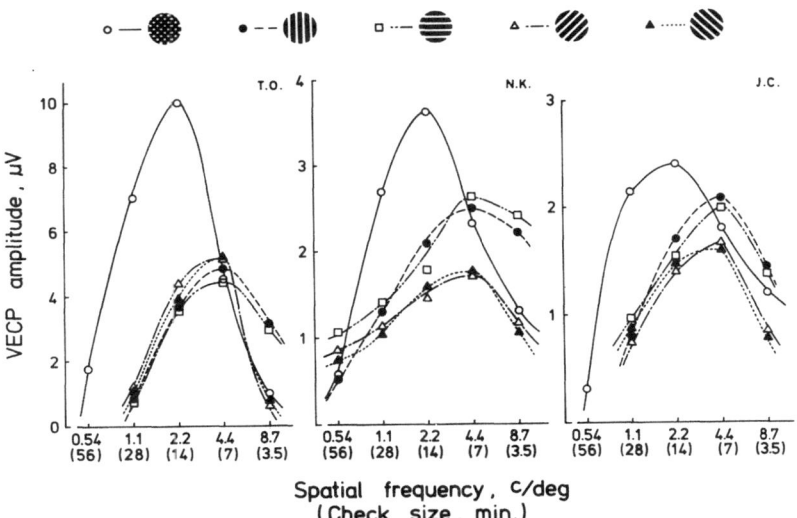

Fig. 2. VECP amplitude as a function of spatial frequencies (element sizes) for five different patterns in three subjects. Stimulus conditions were described in the legend of Fig. 1.

229

as 8.7 c/d. The higher the spatial frequency, the greater the decrease of sensitivity to the oblique orientation.

2. *Size of patterned field*

Spekreijse (1966) has reported that the amplitude of a steady state VECP for 10' check size saturated at a field size of 3.4° and concluded that only this central region of the retina corresponding to it contributed to the VECP. Only a few studies (Campbell and Maffei, 1970, Behrman *et al.*, 1972) have been reported on the relationship between field size and element size. In the following we report on the effect of field size on the VECP amplitude vs. spatial frequency curve using circular field of 1° to 24° both for checkerboard and vertical grating patterns.

In Fig. 3 the VECP amplitude as a function of stimulus field size for four element sizes are demonstrated.

Increasing the stimulus field, it appeared that the VECP amplitude to checkerboard stimulation increased up to a field size of approx. 6°, while in the case of gratings the point where the response no longer increases varies depending on the spatial frequency. The size of the stimulus field where saturation occurs depends on whether checkerboards or gratings are used. It is not dependent on the check size in checkerboard data. With grating stimulation, saturation occurs at larger field size and the amplitude remains very low

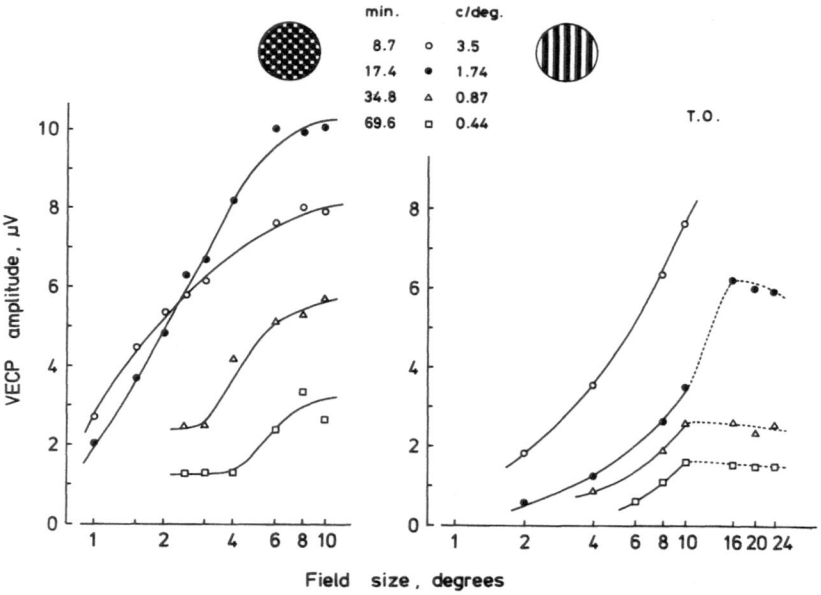

Fig. 3. VECP amplitude as a function of field size on a log scale for four different element sizes (of checkerboard, shown in the left half of the figure) spatial frequencies (of grating, in the right). Reversing frequency 12 Hz, mean luminance 2.14 log ft-L, contrast 40%, monopolar viewing, distance 1.2 m (0.6 m for data indicated with dotted lines in the right half of the figure).

230

when a pattern of lower spatial frequency is used. These data suggest that even a relatively low frequency grating hardly evokes a response from the peripheral retina. In Fig. 4, the effect of field size is demonstrated. On increasing the field size the peak of the amplitude vs. element size curve shifts towards larger element sizes and greater amplitudes. The VECPs to a grating did not show a maximum in the range of the element sizes used. Figure 2 as well as our previous study (Adachi and Chiba, 1979) with still higher spatial frequencies proved that there is indeed a peak at 4.4 c/d. Therefore beyond the range of Fig. 4.

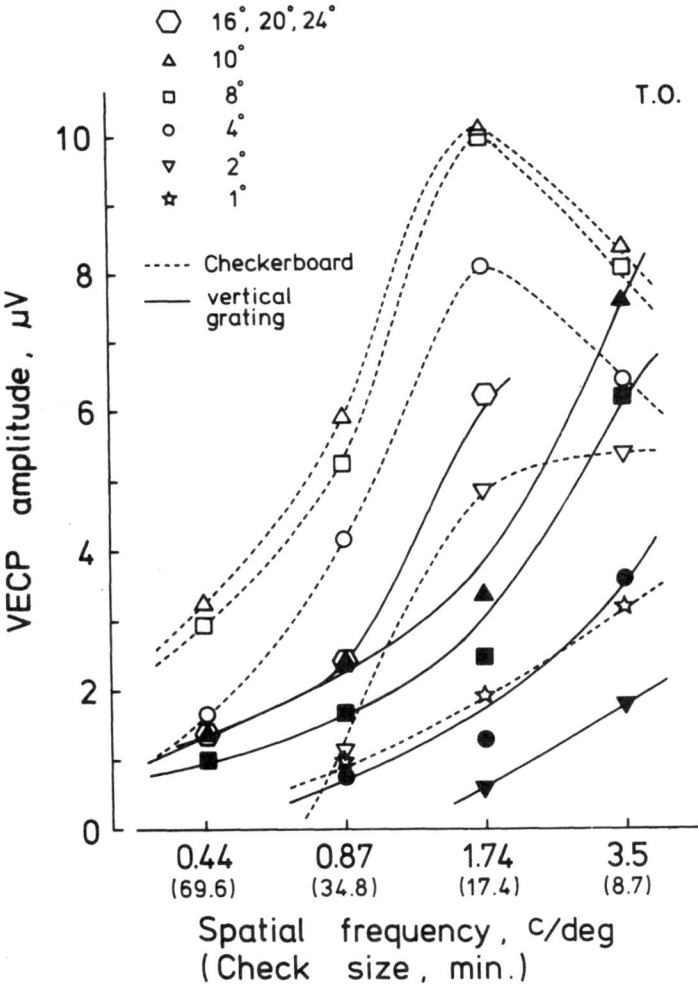

Fig. 4. VECP amplitude as a function of spatial frequencies (element sizes) for various sizes of stimulus field. Diameter of a circular stimulus field employed is shown in the figure. Dotted lines indicate data obtained from checkerboard stimulation and continuous lines for the grating.

The shift of the peak to smaller check sizes for smaller stimulus fields confirmed the large foveal contribution to the VECP as reported by Campbell and Maffei (1970). The fact that a 1° field yielded only 1/2 the VECP amplitude of a 2° field is somewhat surprising considering the expected domination of retino-centric projections. Possibly a minimum number of elements is important for the response.

3. Equal areal stimulation at different retinal sites

In view of the dependency in field size it was considered interesting to study the response from equal areas concentric to the macula.

A circular checkerboard pattern having a diameter of 8° and four annular patterns whose areas were equal to that of the 8° disc were used to elicit VECPs to different retinal positions at central fixation.

It is clear from Fig. 5 that the amplitude decreases as the retinal site stimulated, shifts towards periphery and this is definitely related to the check

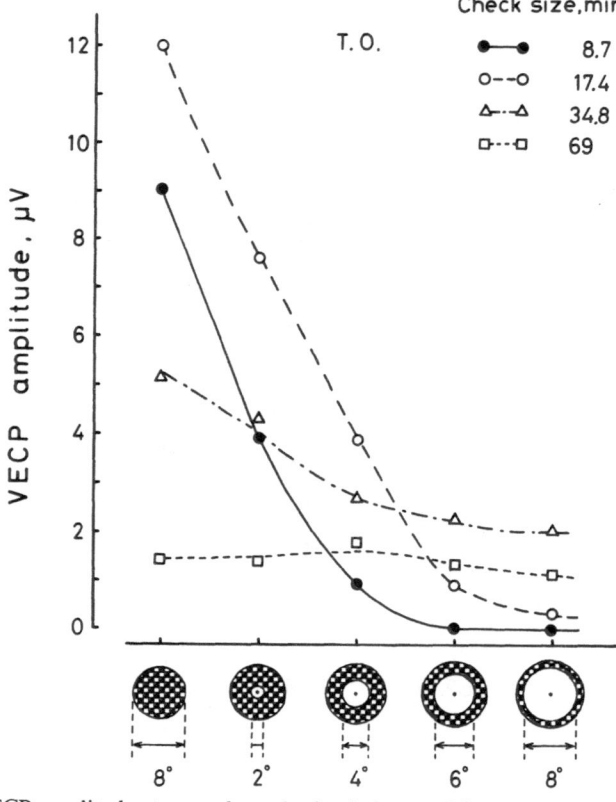

Fig. 5. VECP amplitudes to equal areal stimulation at different retinal sites centered around the fovea. Each annular field was areally equal to the circular area of 8° diameter. Central fixation. Reversal frequency 12 Hz. Mean luminance 2.14 log ft-L, contrast 40%, monocular viewing, distance 1.2 m.

size used. With relatively smaller check sizes such as 8.7′ and 17.4′, the decrease of amplitude caused by occluding the centre and displacing the stimulated site peripherally is much more evident than with larger checks. In other words, VECPs were remarkably greater when the central region of the retina was stimulated than when the paracentral area was stimulated. With greater check sizes of 34.8′ and 69′, the decrease of amplitude was not as evident possibly because of the much reduced amplitudes.

In Fig. 6 the amplitude is plotted against element size for four different retinal configurations. The peak of the curve does not alter by changing element size within an inner diameter of 4° at the fixation point. However, the

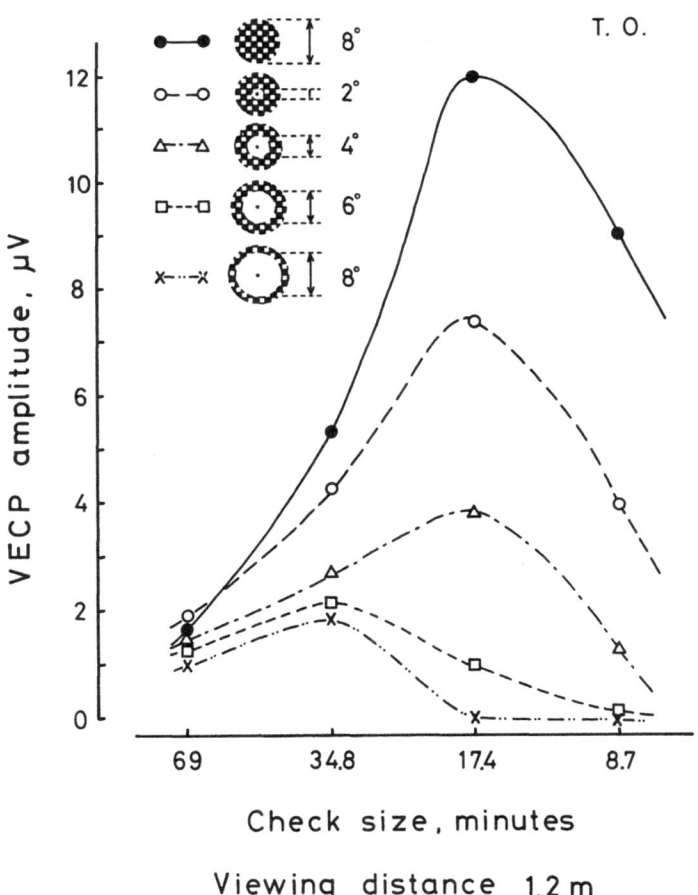

Fig. 6. Effects of equal areal stimulation at different retinal sites on VECP amplitude vs. check size curve. Stimulus conditions were described in the legend of Fig. 5.

233

peak shifts towards larger check sizes as the stimulated retinal area moves towards the periphery beyond 3° from the fovea. It should be noted that with such peripheral stimulation amplitudes were so small that reliable studies could not be made. This is in contradiction to results reported by others for instance Harter (1971), Michael and Halliday (1971), and Behrman *et al.* (1972) who reported easily measurable peripheral VECPs with large check size stimulation.

4. *Defocusing*

This was reported in detail elsewhere (Adachi-Usami, 1979). It may suffice to describe here that increasing the degree of defocusing, shifts the maximum sensitivity toward larger checks or bars, but sensitivity as a whole drops. This occurred more abruptly for smaller sizes. The VECP sensitivity decreased more than the psychophysical one especially for smaller sizes. No important difference was found between the results with bar and checkerboard patterns in this respect.

5. *Binocular and monocular stimulation*

With gratings it was found in a previous study (Adachi *et al.*, 1979) that the entire amplitude vs. spatial frequency curve was approx. 30% depressed with monocular compared to binocular stimulation. In both situations the peak of the curve lies at identical spatial frequency.

CONCLUSIONS

Spatial properties of bars and checks of relatively large dimensions produced by a TV system were studied in a number of stimulus conditions. In general spatial frequency characteristics were in good agreement with other authors (Regan and Richards, 1971, Freeman and Thibos, 1975, Marg *et al.*, 1976 and Sokol and Dobson, 1976) who used other devices. So far as the stimulus parameters studied in the present paper were concerned, the fine structure of the TV system and the presence of flicker did not seem to disturb VECP studies. Nevertheless, we should hold in mind certain disadvantages and limitations of the TV systems generally in use for carrying out experiments. Particularly at high spatial frequencies and low contrasts level.

REFERENCES

Adachi-Usami, E. & Y. Mortia. A new multipurpose television pattern generator and spatial frequency characteristics in man obtained by VECPs. *Folia Ophthalmol. Jpn.* 29: 787–789 (1978).

Adachi-Usami, E. A multipurpose television pattern generator (1979) pp. 161–165. in: Doc. Ophthal. Proc. Series XVIth ISCEV Symp. Morioka, 1978.

Adachi-Usami, E. & Y. Morita. Temporal contrast sensitivity characteristics of human vision as obtained by VECPs to checkerboard stimuli (1979) pp. 213–221. in: Doc. Ophthal. Proc. Series XVIth ISCEV Symp. Morioka, 1978.

Adachi, E. Binocular effects on the VECP amplitude vs. spatial frequency curve. *Acta Soc. Ophthal. Jap.* 83: *32–35* (1979).

Adachi-Usami, E. Comparison of contrast thresholds of bars and checks of large dimensions measured by VECPs and psychophysically at different accommodation. *Albrecht v. Graefes Arch. klin. exp. Ophthal.* 212: *1–9* (1979).

Adachi, E. & J. Chiba. Orientation effects on spatial frequency characteristics in human VECPs. *Acta Soc. Ophthal. Jap.* (1979).

Arden, G.B., D.J. Faulkner & C. Mair. A versatile television pattern stimulator for visual evoked potentials (1977), pp. 90–109. in: J.E. Desmedt, (ed.), Visual evoked potentials in man. Clarendon press, Oxford.

Behrman, J., S. Nissim & G.B. Arden. A clinical method for obtaining pattern visual evoked responses, (1972), pp. 199–206. in: G.B. Arden, (ed.), Advances in Experimental Medicine and Biology. Vol. 24. Plenum press, N.Y.

Campbell, F.W. & L. Maffei. Electrophysiological evidence for the existence of orientation and size detectors in the human visual system. *J. Physiol.* 207: *635–652* (1970).

Freeman, R.D. & L.D. Thibos. Contrast sensitivity in humans with abnormal visual experience. *J. Physiol.* 247: *689–710* (1975).

Harter, M.R. Visually evoked cortical responses to checkerboard pattern: effect of check size as a function of retinal eccentricity. *Electroenceph. Clin. Neurophysiol.* 28: *48–54* (1971).

Hubel, D.H. & T.N. Wiesel. Receptive fields of single neurons in the cat's striate cortex. *J. Physiol.* 147: *226–238* (1959).

Mansfield, R.J.W. Neural basis of orientation perception in primate vision. *Science*, N.Y. 186: *1133–1135* (1974).

Marg, E., D.N. Freeman, P. Pelzman & P.J. Goldstein. Visual acuity development in human infants. *Invest. Ophthalmol.* 15: *150–153* (1976).

Michael, W.F. & A.M. Halliday. Differences between the occipital distribution of upper and lower field pattern evoked response in man. *Brain Res.* 32: *311–324* (1971).

Pettigrew, J.D., T. Nikara & P.O. Biship. Responses to moving slits by single units in cat striate cortex. *Exp. Brain Res.* 6: *373–390* (1968).

Regan, D. & W. Richards. Independence of evoked potentials and apparent size. *Vision Res.* 11: *679–684* (1971).

Sokol, S. & V. Dobson. Pattern reversal visually evoked potentials in infants. *Invest. Ohpthalmol.* 15: *58–62* (1976).

Spekreijse, H. Analysis of e.e.g. responses in man evoked by sine wave modulated light. Thesis. Junk pub., The Hague. (1966).

Van Lith, G.H.M., H.E. Henkes & G.W. Van. Marle. Projector or TV as pattern stimulator? *Doc. Ophthal. Proc.* Series XVIth ISCEV Symp., Morioka 1978.

Author's address:
First Department of Physiology
Hamamatsu University School of Medicine
Handa-cho 3600
431–31 Hamamatsu-shi
Japan

VISUALLY EVOKED SCALP POTENTIAL FIELDS IN HEMIRETINAL STIMULATION[1]

D. LEHMANN AND W. SKRANDIES[2]

(Zürich, Switzerland)

ABSTRACT

Evoked potential data to hemiretinal checkerboard stimulation were recorded simultaneously in 47 channels from normal volunteers, and were used for the construction of scalp field distribution maps. Maximal electrical power of the evoked scalp fields defined response latency. Upper hemiretinal stimuli yielded shorter latencies than lower hemiretinal stimuli, and the presentation mode of the checkerboard pattern showed systematically increasing latencies from "on" to "reversal" to "off". Scalp locations of the responses also differed significantly between the modes of presentation.

The responses evoked by lateralized reversal stimuli were located over the hemisphere contralateral to the hemiretina stimulated for large targets, but tended towards the ipsilateral hemisphere for small targets.

We note that for practical clinical applications, not only the variance of latency and location across subjects, but also the effect of retinal location and presentation mode of the stimulus are crucial.

Visually evoked brain activity might be displayed as sequences of distributions of the electrical scalp fields, instead of conventional waveforms of potential differences between two points on the scalp, as a function of time. Sample results of the mapping procedure are shown in Figs. 1 and 2. All four map series of Figs. 1 and 2 were obtained with the same stimulus, a 2/sec checkerboard pattern reversal; the stimulus was presented to different retinal halves, and obviously, different scalp map series were the result. The EEG data for the scalp field maps were sampled simultaneously in 45 channels, using special A/D and formatting hardware, and then were further treated with a PDP-11 computer. The equipotential line plots were linearly interpolated between electrode positions (see Lehmann 1977).

When one examines the series of equipotential line maps in Figs. 1 and 2, it is quite obvious that there are times when the maps show maximal relief, *i.e.*, extreme peak and trough values. It is reasonable to assume that these times reflect maximal brain response activity. The times of maximal field relief (Lehmann 1977) may be determined by running computations of the amount of field power over time. Field power is calculated as the mean of the squared potential differences between all possible electrode pairs within the field, where the electrodes are about equally spaced over a large scalp area. If we

[1] Supported in part by Swiss National Science Foundation, EMDO, and Hartmann-Müller-Foundation.
[2] Supported by Roche Study Foundation, Basel.

right hemiretina

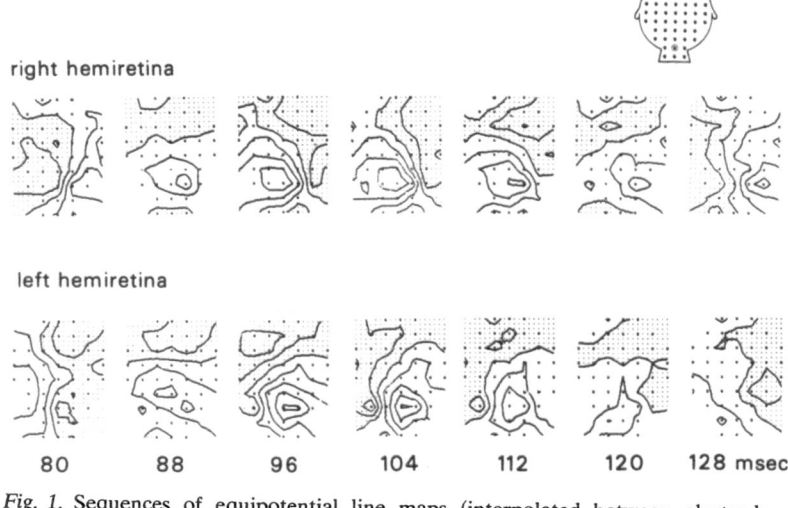

left hemiretina

80   88   96   104   112   120   128 msec

Fig. 1. Sequences of equipotential line maps (interpolated between electrode sites) of average scalp fields, evoked by checkerboard reversals to upper or lower hemiretina. Field lines in steps of 2.5 μV. Time in msec after reversal. Head seen from above, nose up; white areas indicate relative positivity, dotted areas relative negativity of the fields; electrodes are indicated by heavy dots; electrode array (45 channels) see inset, circled electrode at inion.

upper hemiretina

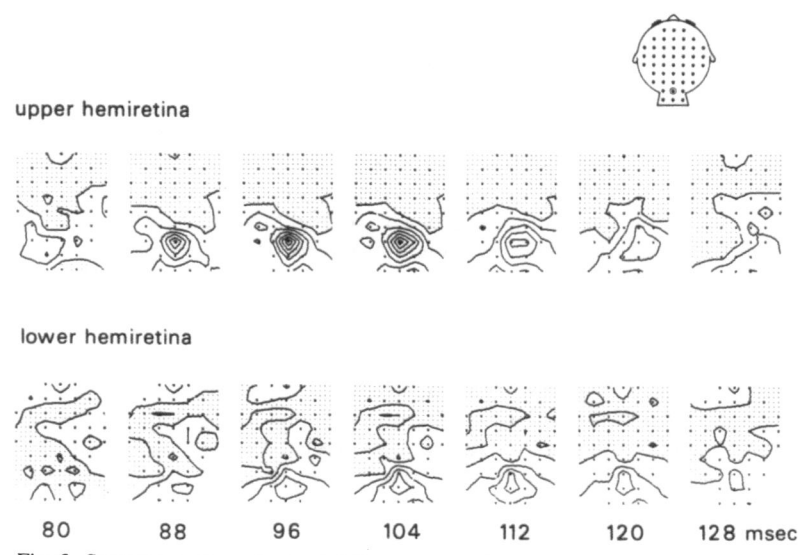

lower hemiretina

80   88   96   104   112   120   128 msec

Fig. 2. Sequences of equipotential line maps of average scalp fields, evoked by checkerboard reversals of 26 deg arc target to the right or left hemiretina. Field lines in steps of 1 μV. For other explanations, see Fig. 1.

238

examine the field power which was obtained with different retinal stimulus locations for times of maximal values (maximal field relief), it turns out that upper hemiretina stimuli cause an earlier response than lower hemiretina stimuli. On the other hand, the location of the occipital positive field peak at times of maximal field power is different for the four different locations of the stimuli, *i.e.*, it is located more anterior for upper than for lower hemiretina stimuli; and it is located on the left side for right hemiretina, and on the right side for left hemiretina stimuli. Thus, evoked potential scalp mapping of localized retinal stimuli appears feasible. However, there is a large literature which shows that stimuli of different physical parameters (size, contrast, color, presentation rate, etc.) evoke very different potentials (*e.g.*, Spekreijse *et al.*, 1977, White and Hintze, 1979). In addition, the mode of presentation (onset, offset, or reversal of a checkerboard pattern) has fundamental effects on the evoked potentials, as will be shown in the next paragraph. These observations necessitate a careful establishment of baseline values and their variance, before routine diagnostic use may be made of the method.

Upper vs. lower hemiretina

In fourteen subjects the right eye's upper or lower hemiretina was stimulated at random stimulus intervals (420–740 msec) with a checkerboard pattern (17×23 deg arc rectangular field, 1 deg arc checks white checks 0.9 log ft. Lambert, contrast 77.5%). The target was displayed on a TV screen with vertical scanning to ensure minimal (<0.1 msec) display time difference between upper and lower half. Responses for 3 conditions (onset, offset, and reversal) were averaged, using four midline electrodes between 3 cm below to 7 cm above the inion, referred to an anterior reference (at 30% of the distance nasion-inion). Since fields evoked by upper or lower hemiretina stimuli are concentric around the midline, the longitudinal electrode row sufficed for the assessment of latency and location. The maximal positive amplitude (indicative of maximal response power, as was demonstrated in scalp field distribution studies; see Lehmann and Skrandies 1979, and in prep.) between 80 and 140 msec after the stimulus was determined, and its latency and location was noted. The mean results over fourteen unselected, healthy subjects are given in Table I, which also indicates the significant differences between the conditions. Obviously, the mode of stimulus presentation (onset, offset, or reversal) has a striking effect on the response latency and location, and this must be kept in mind for practical applications.

Further, the response latencies and locations were significantly different (see Table I) for upper and lower hemiretina stimuli: there were significantly shorter latencies for upper than for lower hemiretinal stimuli; response location for onset was anterior, for offset significantly more posterior with upper hemiretina stimuli, but vice versa for lower hemiretinal stimuli.

We note that the smallest standard deviations were obtained with reversal stimuli presented to the upper hemiretina. Since lower hemiretina stimuli yield significantly longer latencies, a full-field stimulus is not recommended for latency testing. Rather, upper hemiretina stimuli which generally produce

Table 1. Mean latency (A) and location (B) and their SD's, over subjects (n), of the occipitally positive peak of maximal amplitude between 80 and 140 msec. Latency (A) in msec after the stimulus, location (B) in cm above the inion. Significances of differences are given for paired t-tests. In 4 of the 84 cases of 14 subjects, peaks did not occur during the analysis period $(n < 14)$.

A.		Onset msec	p	Revers. msec	p	Offset msec
Upper	x̄	98	<.001	103	<.001	120
	SD	10		4		8
	(n)	(13)		(14)		(14)
	p	<.025		<.001		<.16
Lower	x̄	109	<.15	111	<.001	123
	SD	12		7		6
	(n)	(11)		(14)		(14)
B.		cm		cm		cm
Upper	x̄	5.1	<.012	3.0	<.025	1.7
	SD	2.7		2.9		3.2
	(n)	(13)		(14)		(14)
	p	<.001		<.025		<.05
Lower	x̄	0.2	<.03	0.5	<.01	3.4
	SD	3.3		3.1		3.2
	(n)	(11)		(14)		(14)

larger amplitudes than lower hemiretina stimuli should be employed for routine tests (Lehmann and Mir 1976).

Right vs left hemiretina

Scalp topography of potentials evoked by right vs. left hemiretina stimuli was studied by several authors, using different parameters (including target sizes), a limited number of recording points, and examining conventional waveshapes (*e.g.*, Cobb and Morton, 1970, Shagass *et al.*, 1976, Blumhardt *et al.*, 1978), or scalp fields (Biersdorf and Nakamura, 1971, Lehmann *et al.*, 1969, Lehmann *et al.*, 1976). The reports disagree as to the ipsi- or contralateral scalp location of the response.

With 45-channel scalp field mapping, we studied in six healthy subjects average $(n = 125)$ potentials evoked by lateralized hemiretinal checkerboard reversal to circular, large and small (26 and 13 deg arc diameter) targets with 1 deg arc checks (white checks 1.45 log ft. Lambert, 93% contrast, tungsten bulb as source), using mirror reversal presentation with less than 1 msec reversal time.

Computation of evoked field power over time revealed no latency differences between left and right hemiretinal responses (105 ± 2.9 msec over the subjects). The electrode locations of maximal response amplitude (peak values of the fields) were determined for each subject within the 45 electrode array at the time of maximal field power. Figure 3 shows that for the small targets, the field peaks tended to the side ipsilateral to the stimulated hemiretina whereas for the large targets, the peaks tended to the side contralateral to the stimulated hemiretina. We note that the locations show some variance over subjects not only in the lateral, but also in anterior-posterior direction (our intra-electrode distance was on the average 3.5 cm). For routine applications it appears important to consider that, using one or few recording channels, one might easily miss the peak field values, and then a reliable interpretation of the results might become difficult.

In a next step, we examined the detailed configurations of the evoked fields. In order to study common features of field shapes in the subject population, we computed mean field distributions over subjects at maximal response time, after scaling of the individual fields so that all fields had equal amplitude; this ensured that idiosyncracies of individual subjects will have equal weight in the mean fields. Figure 4 shows that for small and large targets, the occipital

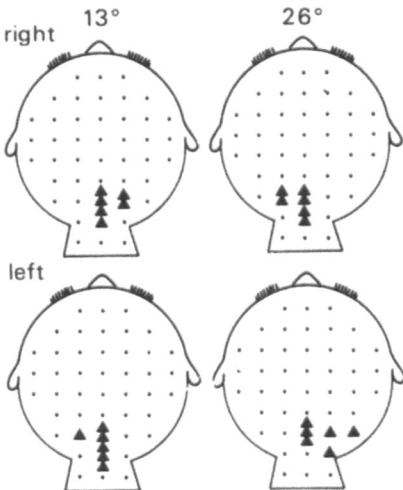

Fig. 3. Scalp locations of maximal, positive values of evoked, average scalp fields of six subjects (triangles), at latencies of maximal response power around 100 msec, for right (top) or left (bottom) hemiretinal checkerboard reversals of 13 or 26 deg arc target size. Display as in Fig. 1.

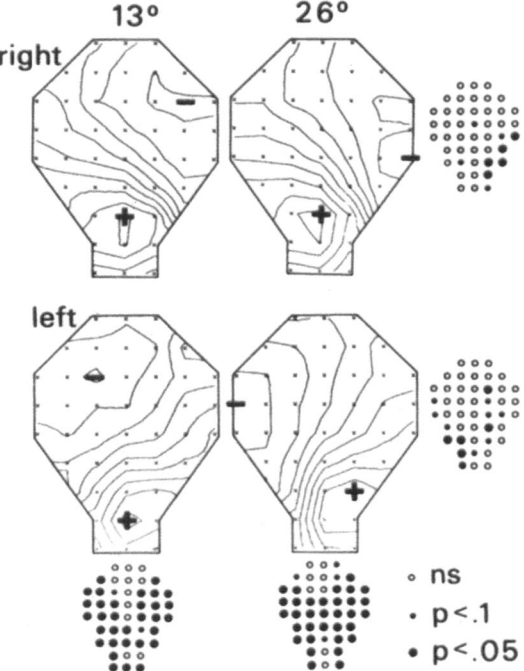

Fig. 4. Mean equipotential line scalp fields over six subjects, evoked by right (top) or left (bottom) hemiretinal checkerboard reversal stimuli of 13 or 26 deg arc target size. Individual average fields at latencies of maximal power of response around 100 msec were scaled for unity amplitude between subjects before mean computation. Head seen from above as in other figures; + indicates maximal, − minimal field value. Dot arrays indicate significances of differences at each electrode site (p values of paired t tests) between mean field values evoked by small and large target, and by right and left hemiretinal targets. Same data base as in Fig. 3.

right-left field gradients were steep over the hemisphere ipsilateral to the stimulated hemiretina, whereas the contralateral hemisphere tended to a flat plateau. These characteristics were most pronounced for large targets. Anterior areas showed gentle gradients. The t-test plots in Fig. 4 indicate that the differences between small and large target-evoked fields are largest over the side ipsilateral to the stimulated hemiretina. This means that large targets show a more pronounced lateralization (to the contralateral side). Since we know that absolute location of field peaks even tends to the ipsilateral hemisphere for small targets, it appears advisable to use large targets for more stable results.

According to these results of our field studies, conventional evoked waveshape recordings will show largest amplitudes over the hemisphere ipsilateral to the stimulated hemiretina in a bipolar left-right electrode chain, and contralateral from a unipolar left-right row of electrodes referred against a distant point (e.g., the mean of the two ears, or an anterior electrode).

The reported results which were obtained with hemifield stimulation indicate the principal problems for visual field mapping using evoked potentials. Our results demonstrate the data variance across subjects in terms of scalp locations, which may become quite problematic when only one or few channels are used. In addition, the results show that not only the retinal location of the stimulus, but also the mode of stimulus presentation (onset, offset, reversal) play a decisive role for latency and location of the evoked response.

REFERENCES

Biersdorf, W. R. & Z. Nakamura. Electroencephalogram potentials evoked by hemi-retinal stimulation. *Experientia* 27, 402–403 (1971).

Blumhardt, L. D., Barrett, G., Halliday, A. M. & A. Kriss. The effect of experimental "scotomata" on the ipsilateral and contralateral responses to pattern-reversal in one half-field. *Electroenceph. clin. Neurophysiol.* 45, 376–392 (1978).

Cobb, W. A. & H. B. Morton. Evoked potentials from the human scalp to visual half-field stimulation. *J. Physiol.* 208, 39–40 (1970).

Lehmann, D., Kavanagh, R. N., & D. H. Fender. Field studies of averaged visually evoked EEG potentials in a patient with a split chiasm. *Electroenceph. clin. Neurophysiol.* 26, 193–199 (1969).

Lehmann, D., Meles, H. P., & Z. Mir. Scalp field maps of averaged EEG potentials evoked by checkerboard inversion. *Biomed. Technik* (Stuttgart) 21, Suppl., 117–118 (1976).

Lehmann, D. & Z. Mir. Methodik und Auswertung visuell evozierter EEG-Potentiale bei Verdacht auf Multiple Sklerose. *J. Neurol.* 213, 97–103 (1976).

Lehmann, D. The EEG as scalp field distribution. p. 365–384 in: A. Rémond (ed.): EEG Informatics. Elsevier, Amsterdam (1977).

Lehmann, D., & W. Skrandies. Multichannel evoked potential fields show different properties of human upper and lower hemiretina systems. *Exp. Brain Res.* 35, 151–159 (1979).

Shagass, Ch., Amadeo, M. & A. Roemer. Spatial distribution of potentials evoked by half-field pattern-reversal and pattern-onset stimuli. *Electroenceph. clin. Neurophysiol.* 41, 609–622 (1976).

Spekreijse, H., Estevez, O. & D. Reits. Visual evoked potentials and the physiological analysis of visual processes in man. pp. 16–89 in: J. E. Desmedt (ed.): Visual Evoked Potentials in Man. Clarendon, Oxford 1977.

White, C. T. & R. W. Hintze. Color evoked potentials: Cortical and subcortical elements. pp. 431–442 in: D. Lehmann and E. Callaway (eds.): Human Evoked Potentials/Applications and Problems. Plenum, London, 1979.

Author's address:
Department of Neurology
University Hospitals
8091 Zürich
Switzerland

Docum. Ophthal. Proc. Series, Vol. 23

AMPLITUDE FLUCTUATIONS OF THE MONOCULAR CHECKERBOARD VER CAUSED BY BINOCULAR RIVALRY

J. PETERSEN

(*Göttingen, F.R.G.*)

ABSTRACT

The running average VER elicited by steady checkerboard reversal stimulation of one eye shows spontaneous periodic amplitude fluctuations. The modulation frequency is about 0.1 s^{-1}. Simultaneously the subjects see visual disturbances which are described as growing or shrinking and drifting clouds in the otherwise clear visual field. The fluctuation of the VER amplitude and the periodicity of the visual blurring are shown to correspond perfectly to each other. The observed effect is a rivalry phenomenon. The localisation within the visual pathway is not yet clear.

Pattern evoked potentials can be used for an objective method of refracting the eye (Millodet & Riggs 1970, Regan 1973). In such studies large short time variations of the VER amplitude are seen (Bostrom *et al.* 1978, Peterson 1979), which considerably confuse the refracting procedure. While refracting 18 persons we investigated these voltage fluctuations and found a psychophysical equivalent. The effect was studied in detail on two subjects.

Our experimental setup allows us to record the VER amplitude continuously with time using two channel lock-in detection. The reference inputs of the demodulators are separated $\pi/2$ in phase thus locking to the in-phase and quadrature component of the signal. From the demodulator outputs an analogue $\text{sqt}(a^2 + b^2)$ circuitry computes the magnitude of the voltage vector. In this way the influence of phase is eliminated. Filters are set to pass 1 to 30 Hz, the integrating time constant is 3s. The input to the visual system is supplied by means of a TV-screen presenting an alternating checkerboard pattern. Details of the stimulus are: field $10° \times 14°$, checksize 17 arc min, pattern reversal 13/s, contrast nearly 100%, mean luminance 0.8 log foot Lambert. The local luminance on the TV-screen is a square wave function of time.

In spite of the stimulation conditions remaining constant the recorded VER amplitude changes with time. In Fig. 1 three examples of the oscillations are depicted. All three curves show records of the VER amplitude versus time with: (a) the reversal frequency changing, (b) the correcting spectacle lens changing and (c) with stationary experimental conditions and 13 Hz stimulation. The amplitude fluctuates about 20 to 30% in a 0.05 to 0.1 Hz rhythm. Although the quantitative aspects are variable, the greater part of the subjects produce such voltage oscillations.

When looking monocularly at the TV screen subjective changes of the visual impression are noticed. Grey clouds appear on the checkerboard pattern which enlarge, shrink and drift through the stimulated field. Sometimes the visual impression breaks down over the whole field, resulting in a second of effective blindness. The disturbances alternate with clear periods in a rhythm of a few seconds.

To establish a correlation between subjective impression and VER amplitude, the subjects were requested to specify the moments when the clouds appeared and disappeared. These periods are marked in Fig. 1 by bulky plotting. The correlation between subjective pattern fading and decrease of the VER amplitude is convincing.

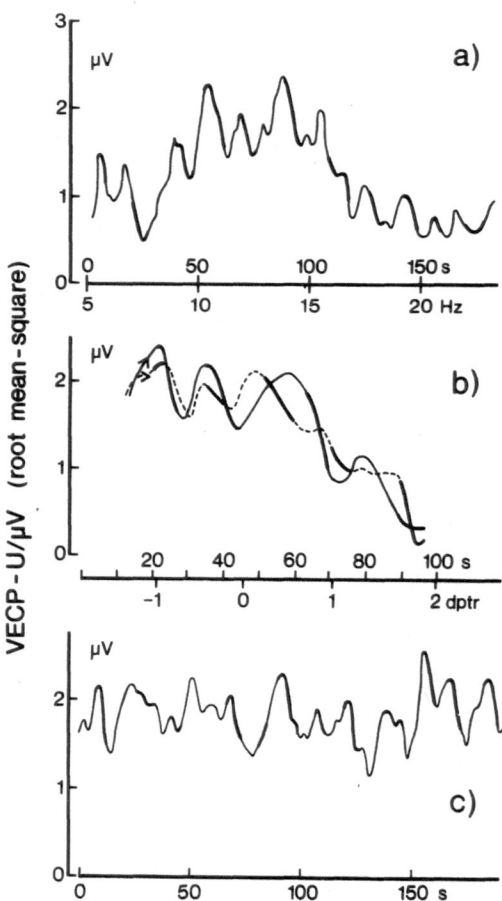

Fig. 1. Amplitude of VER as a function of time: (a) Frequency of checkerboard reversal is changing (b) Correcting lens power is changing (c) Constant stimulation at 13/s. The periods, when the subject reported visual disturbances, are marked by bulky plotting.

246

Principally the voltages of the lock-in outputs can vary due to variations of amplitude, phase or frequency of the input signal. So one has to look at the EEG signal itself. On a CRT screen no characteristic changes of the EEG (α-activity for instance) could be detected while the subjects saw clouds. Thus we summed up the responses during clear and disturbed visual impression into two separated channels of a computer averager. As a result we found both signals equal in frequency and phase but differing in amplitude by 20 to 30%.

One well known parameter modulating the VER amplitude is the refractive state of the eye, which can be changed by accommodation. The following arguments show that accommodation does not explain the observed effects. Defocussing always blurs the whole picture, while the disturbances seen by the subjects only pertain to parts of the visual field, the rest remaining sharp. Furthermore there is experimental evidence against accommodation. Bostron et al. (1978) compared VER recordings with and without a 1 mm pinhole before the eye. Effects due to refraction should be reduced drastically by the pinhole. The VER fluctuations were not. Correspondingly amplitude fluctuations can be seen in cycloplegic subjects too.

In order to find out the origin of the effect described above, we studied the influence of frequency, contrast and checksize. No dependence on these parameters could be detected. The visual impairment happens even if one avoids fixing one's eyes on a special checkerboard point. On the other hand, blinking reestablishes clear vision reliably for a moment. The leading eye is less subject to the disturbances. No clouds emerge when looking binocularly.

These findings show that the observed effect belongs to rivalry phenomena. The restriction to varying parts of the visual field and rhythmic appearance are well known (Levelt 1968, Bishop 1973). Binocular rivalry in VER has been demonstrated in an experimental situation, where both eyes were stimulated by differing patters (Cobb et al. 1967). The authors found agreement between subjective pattern perception and VER (phase being the measured quantity). Our experimental situation is an extreme case of differing patterns to both eyes: checkerboard reversal to the one and no stimulus by occlusion to the other eye. So binocular rivalry is expected to occur.

Levelt (1968) distinguishes rivalry during monocular stimulation, which he calls spurious rivalry, from true binocular rivalry, when both eyes are stimulated. He suggests spurious rivalry to be a retinal mechanism. In contrast true binocular rivalry must happen at higher levels of the visual system, where the information from both eyes converges. In principle the localisation of our rivalry effect within the visual pathway can be determined by electrophysiological means, too. The VER fluctuations have to be compared with the variations of the simultaneously recorded checkerboard ERG. Unfortunately experimental obstacles prevent such a measurement. The pattern evoked ERG is nearly an order of magnitude smaller than the VER. So more averaging must be done to get a reliable response. In our case of lock-in detection it turns out that the integrating time constant must be chosen longer than 10 s. But this necessarily smooths out the eventual 0.1 Hz variations. Alternatively one can sum up the ERG and VER voltages during clear and disturbed vision into four separated channels of a computer averager. So far we have not done this. Thus the localisation of the observed effect is subject to further investigation.

The local pattern fading is only found in monocular vision. It does not occur when looking binocularly. But the VER does show variations in amplitude under binocular conditions as well. The magnitude of these fluctuations is nearly the same as in the monocular case, while the amplitude of the VER itself is increased by about 50%. So one is led to the idea that the rivalry process is present in binocular vision too. Subjective disturbances are not to be expected. The fading areas in the field of the one eye can be complemented by nearly identical information coming from the other eye. Only time dependent losses in stereoscopic vision would result. On the other hand the existence of mechanisms modulating the VER amplitude other than rivalry can not be excluded.

REFERENCES

Bishop P.O. Neurophysiology of binocular single vision and stereopsis: in Handbook of Sensory Physiology, Vol. VII/3, Springer Berlin-Heidelberg-New York, 1973.

Bostrom C., Keller E.L. & E. Marg. A reconsideration of visual evoked potentials for fast automated ophthalmic refraction. *Invest. Ophth.* 17, *182* (1978).

Cobb W.A., Morten H.B. & G. Ettlinger. Cerebral potentials evoked by pattern reversal and their suppression in visual rivalry. *Nature* 216, *1123* (1967).

Levelt W.J.M. On binocular rivalry. Mouton, The Hague-Paris, 1968.

Millodot M. & L.A. Riggs. Refraction determined electrophysiologically. *Vis. Res.* 10, *1365* (1970).

Petersen J. Schnelle Refraktometrie und Binokularabgleich mit VECP. *Ber. Dtsch. Ophthal. Ges.* 76, pp 000 (1979).

Regan D. Rapid objective refraction using evoked brain potentials. *Invest. Ophthalm.* 12, *669* (1973).

Author's address:
Dr. Jörgen Petersen
Augenklinik der Universität Göttingen
Gosslerstrasse 12
D-34 Göttingen
F.R.G.

248

Docum. Ophthal. Proc. Series, Vol. 23

ASYMMETRIC PATTERN EVOKED RESPONSES AND STIMULUS PARAMETERS

G.H.M. VAN LITH, H.E. HENKES AND S.M. VIJFVINKEL-BRUINENGA

(*Rotterdam, The Netherlands*)

ABSTRACT

By vertical half field stimulation with a pattern reversal movement and a pattern flash, both Halliday's results of an ipsilateral occipital response and those of Jeffreys of a contralateral occipital response could be confirmed. These discrepancies can be explained by assuming two occipital dipoles, in one of which is the origin of the C_I of Jeffreys, while in the other the origin of Halliday's main positive peak as well as C_{III} of Jeffreys can be located.

INTRODUCTION

Several papers have been published concerning the significance of asymmetric electric responses recorded over the hemispheres in case of hemianopic field defects (Vaughan, Katzman and Taylor, 1963; Kooi, Guvener and Bagchi, 1965; Oosterhuis et al., 1969; Wildberger et al., 1976). Though objective confirmation of the field defects could often be established, the results were in general not consistent enough to make electrophysiological examination in hemianopia a reliable procedure. Various reasons for this inconsistency may be brought up. On the one hand, asymmetries occur in normal individuals, likely due to asymmetries between the two hemispheres and/or the skull. On the other hand, asymmetric responses frequently are not found in circumstances, in which they are to be expected. This may be caused by stray light from the stimulated retinal half to the other one and/or by a less proper fixation at the edge of the stimulus field. Stray light problems have greatly been solved now that pattern stimulation instead of light flash stimulation is applied; fixation problems, however, still exist.

A third reason for not finding asymmetric responses, where they ought to be, has been brought forward by Halliday (Halliday and Michael, 1970). By placing an array of electrodes over the hemispheres, Halliday found that the electrode positions, often used, are not that appropriate to detect hemispheric asymmetries. The best results were obtained with a reference electrode placed in the midline, 12 cm above the nasion. Paradoxical in the results of Halliday's group was that the highest responses were found at the electrode over the non stimulated hemisphere, *i.e.* from the ipsilateral electrode (Blumhardt, Barrett and Halliday, 1977; Blumhardt et al., 1978). Their explanation is that this ipsilateral response is generated by a dipole located in the contralateral hemisphere, but directed to the electrode on the other side (see Fig. 4). The electrode at the same side, referential to the midline electrode above the nasion, measures more or less perpendicularly to this dipole, consequently will register a much smaller potential.

The results of Halliday are just the opposite of those described by Jeffreys (Jeffreys and Axford, 1972a, 1972b). Jeffreys found the largest responses over the contralateral hemisphere which may be explained by the fact that he measured referentially to the ear lobes. Furthermore, he used pattern flashes instead of the pattern reversal stimulation, applied by Halliday.

In order to know which method gives the most reliable results for clinical purposes we compared both stimulus techniques, a pattern reversal and a pattern flash, registering the potentials according to Halliday, referentially to a midline electrode placed 12 cm above the nasion.

METHOD

Figure 1 shows our recordings of a pattern reversal (1A) and a pattern flash (1B) response, using in both types of stimulation a symmetrical field stimulus. In the response to a pattern reversal stimulation, the main positive peak (P) has been measured. In the pattern flash response, we see the positive C_I of Jeffreys, the negative C_{II} and the positive C_{III}. This latter peak was very small in Jeffreys' recording conditions and was not evaluated by him. Since in our recordings both C_I and C_{III} were well developed, C_{III} generally even being the largest, we paid attention both to C_I and C_{III}. As was already found by Jeffreys, C_{II} did not produce large differences between the hemispheres. Of 30 normal subjects, one eye was examined using half field pattern stimulation, both at the right side and at the left side; 60 examinations could thus be evaluated.

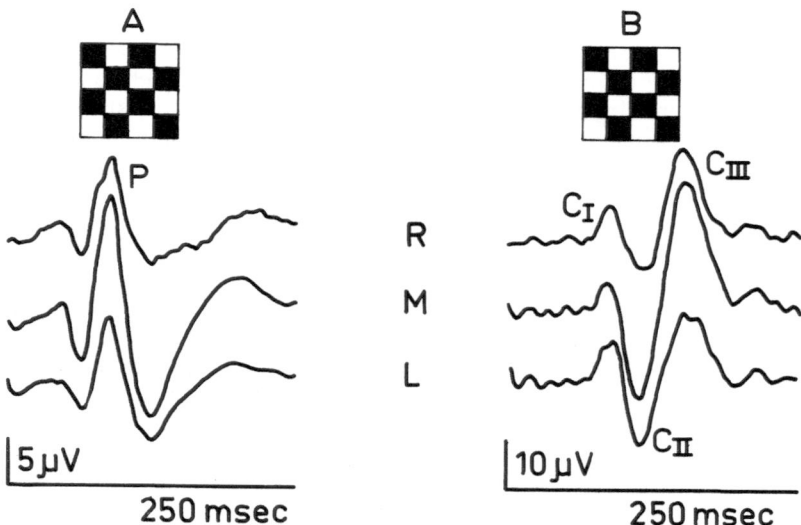

Fig. 1. VEPs to a pattern reversal stimulus (A) and to a pattern flash stimulus (B). Recordings of electrodes over the right occipital lobe (R), in the midline (M) and over the left occipital lobe (L). P: main positive peak of the pattern reversal response; C_I, C_{II}, C_{III}: positive, negative and positive peak according to Jeffreys.

Stimulus frequency was two per second, check size being 1° for the pattern reversal stimulus with 90% contrast and 40′ for the pattern flash of 40 msec, with 40% contrast.

The percentage difference between the potentials of the two occipital electrodes has been calculated as follows:

$$\frac{A_r - A_L}{\frac{1}{2}(A_r + A_L)} \times 100\%$$

in which A_r stands for the amplitudes of the potentials obtained from the right occipital electrode and A_L for those of the left occipital electrode. After symmetrical stimulation also differences between the right and left electrode have been found. Standard deviation of these differences was approximately 25%. Therefore, only differences of more than 50% have been assessed by us as statistically significant. Differences smaller than 25% have no meaning at all.

RESULTS

Halliday's finding of an ipsilateral response after half sided pattern reversal stimulation could be confirmed (Fig. 2); of the 60 examinations, however, only half of them produced differences between the hemispheres of more than 50%, while more than 10 showed only differences of less than 25%.

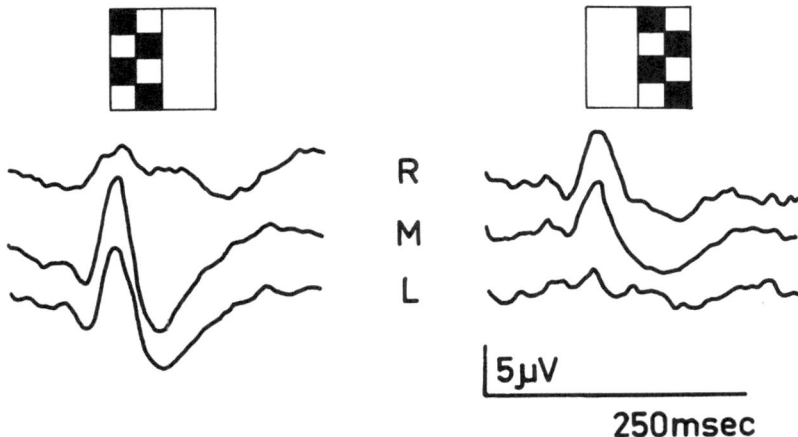

Fig. 2. VEPs to half field pattern reversal stimulation. See further Fig. 1.

The fact that only in half of the examinations a significant asymmetry was obtained, implies to the clinician that an asymmetry of more than 50% points to an abnormality, but which is much more important that the absence of such an asymmetry does not exclude pathology.

By applying pattern flashes we could also confirm Jeffreys' results for C_I, being largest at the contralateral side (Fig. 3). Most interesting however, is the fact that C_{III} behaves opposite to C_I, being highest at the ipsilateral side, *i.e.* according to Halliday's results. This gives evidence that the differences be-

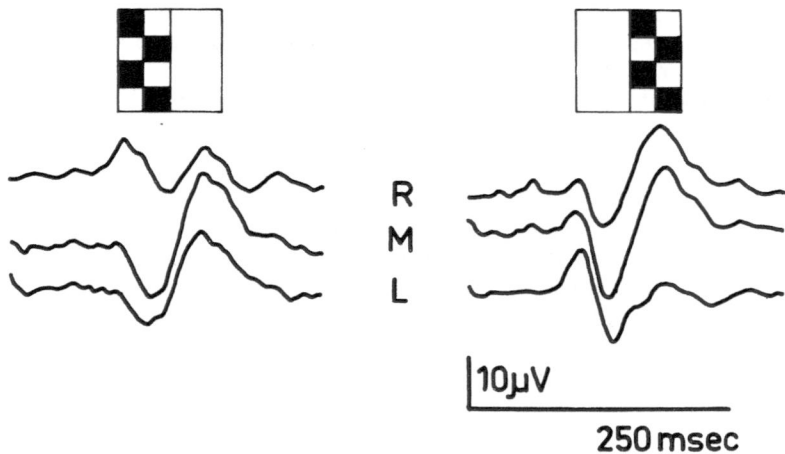

Fig. 3. VEPs to half field pattern flash stimulation. See further Fig. 1.

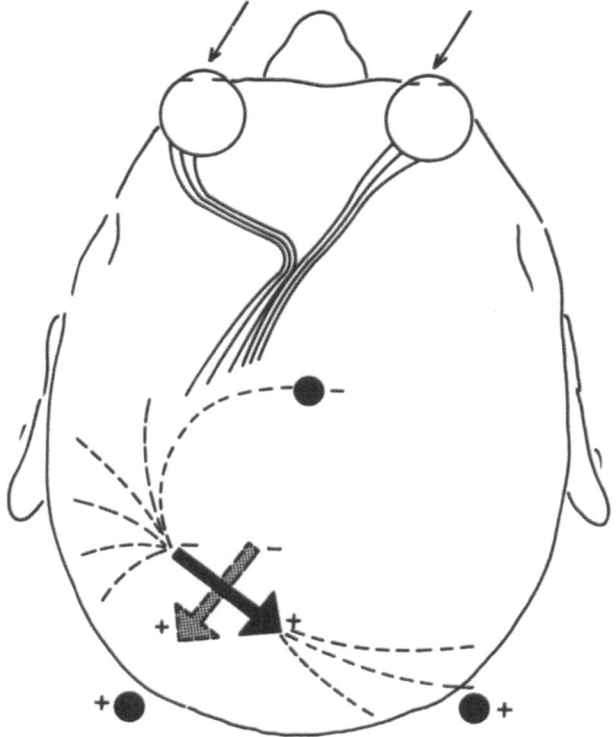

Fig. 4. Dipoles in the left occipital lobes after right half field pattern stimulation. Black arrow: dipole of Halliday, probably also the origin of C_{III} of Jeffreys. Grey arrow: dipole, which may cause C_I of Jeffreys.

tween Halliday and Jeffreys have nothing to do with the electrode position! We suppose that C_{III} has its origin in the same dipole as Halliday's main positive peak of the pattern reversal response, but that C_I is caused by another dipole, situated perpendicular to the first one (see Fig. 4).

As to the reliability of finding an asymmetrical response, pattern flash stimulation gave somewhat better results than pattern reversal stimulation. For C_{III} a difference of more than 50% was seen in 40 out of the 60 examinations, for C_I this was 44 times. C_I, however, was too small to be evaluated in 9 examinations.

REFERENCES

Blumhardt, L.D., Barrett, G. & A.M. Halliday: The asymmetrical visual evoked potential to pattern reversal in one half field and its significance for the analysis of visual field defects. *Brit. J. Ophthal.* 61: *454–461* (1977).

Blumhardt, L.D., Barrett, G., Halliday, A.M. & A. Kriss: The effect of experimental 'scotomata' on the ipsilateral and contralateral responses to pattern-reversal in one half-field. *Electroenceph. Clin. Neurophysiol.* 45: *376–392* (1978).

Halliday, A.M. & W.F. Michael: Changes in pattern-evoked responses in man associated with the vertical and horizontal meridians of the visual field. *J. Physiol.* 208: *499–513* (1970).

Jeffreys, D.A. & J.G. Axford: Source locations of pattern-specific components of human visual evoked potentials. I. Component of striate cortical origin. *Exp. Brain Res.* 16: *1–21* (1972a).

Jeffreys, D.A. & J.G. Axford: Source locations of pattern-specific components of human visual evoked potentials. II. Components of extrastriate cortical origin. *Exp. Brain Res.* 16: *22–40* (1972b).

Kooi, K.A., Guvener, A.M. & B.K. Bagchi: Visually evoked responses in lesions of the higher optic pathways. *Neurology* 15: *841–854* (1965).

Oosterhuis, H.J.G.H., Ponsen, L., Jonkman, E.J. & O. Magnus: The average visual response in patients with cerebrovascular disease. *Electroenceph. Clin. Neurophysiol.* 27: *23–34* (1969).

Vaughan, H. G., Katzman, R. & J. Taylor: Alterations of visual evoked response in the presence of homonymous visual defects. *Electroenceph. Clin. Neurophysiol.* 15: *737–746* (1963).

Wildberger, H.G.H., Lith, G.H.M. van., Wijngaarde, R. & G.T.M. Mak: Visually evoked cortical potentials in the evaluation of homonymous and bitemporal visual field defects. *Brit. J. Ophthal.* 60: *273–278* (1976).

Authors' address:
Department of Ophthalmology
Erasmus University
Eye Hospital
Schiedamse Vest 180
3011 BH Rotterdam
The Netherlands

Docum. Ophthal. Proc. Series, Vol. 23

SIMULTANEOUSLY RECORDED RETINAL AND CORTICAL POTENTIALS ELICITED BY CHECKERBOARD STIMULI

A. GRONEBERG

(*Frankfurt/M. and Bad Nauheim, F.R.G.*)

ABSTRACT

Human electroretinograms and visually evoked cortical potentials to centrally viewed checkerboard patterns were recorded simultaneously.

With increasing testfields, small checks (4.6′) produce little or no amplitude increase in both the ERG and VECP while with large checks (46′) an amplitude increase is seen. With increasing check sizes an amplitude increase is seen in the ERG only for larger testfields (12° to 16°) while in the VECP there is an amplitude increase for check sizes of 4.6′ to 10′ for all testfields (5° to 16°). The curve relating VECP amplitude to check size shifts from a peak response at 10′ at smaller testfields (5° to 8°) to 46′ at bigger fields (12° to 16°).

Using annular testfields of 14° an increase of the blanked center from 7° to 13° diminishes preferably the responses to smaller check sizes both in the ERG and VECP.

INTRODUCTION

Alternating pattern visually evoked cortical potentials (VECP) have been extensively investigated as a function of various checksizes and retinal areas. All these studies agree that the VECP shows spatial tuning, *i.e.* peak responses with contrast stimuli of medium (10–20′) check size with stimulation of the central retinal area. Detailed studies of the pattern-ERG have been performed by Riggs *et al.* (1964), Johnson *et al.* (1966), Armington (1968, 1971), Sokol (1972, 1977), Lawwill (1974a, 1974b) and Lawwill *et al.* (1977). While the flash ERG represents more a summed retinal response, mainly because of scattered light, an ERG from circumscript areas can now be obtained by use of the phase reversal technique (Riggs *et al.*, 1964). Thus, photopic VECPs and ERGs can be recorded with this new method under appropriate stimulus conditions.

Armington (1968) reported that the pattern ERG shows a monotonic increase in amplitude with increasing checksize while the VECP indicates spatial tuning with a preference for checks of medium size. The spatial tuning of the VECP has been explained by postulating lateral inhibition between the center and the surround of the receptive fields (Armington, 1971). Hence, in the central retinal area we would expect small receptive fields and accordingly the largest VECP response to small checks while more peripheral areas should produce a large response to larger checks. These investigations were directed toward determining if a similar behaviour is also seen in the pattern ERG.

METHODS

Checkerboard pattern reversal contrast stimuli were produced by a pattern generator (Medelec-system) on a TV-monitor. Checks ranged from 4.6' to 68' of arc with a 7 Hz reversal rate. Total mean luminance was 0.85 log foot lamberts. The testfield size was varied from 5° to 16° by placing a black cover with a circular center in front of the TV-screen. While the subjects sat in a shielded room and looked monocularly, the ERG was recorded using a Henkes contact lens. The VECP was recorded with a standard gold disk electrode 3 cm above the inion on the midline and the reference electrode was placed on the earlobe. With the contact-lens in place all subjects were corrected to a visual acuity of 20/20. The output of the preamplifiers were led to a computer (Nicolet 1072). Low and high frequency cutoffs for the ERG and VECP were 1 to 30 Hz. After 256 responses were accumulated, each trial was plotted on a X-Y plotter. Amplitudes were measured by peak to trough method.

Seven subjects with normal acuity took part in the experiments. Their ages ranged between 15 and 32 years.

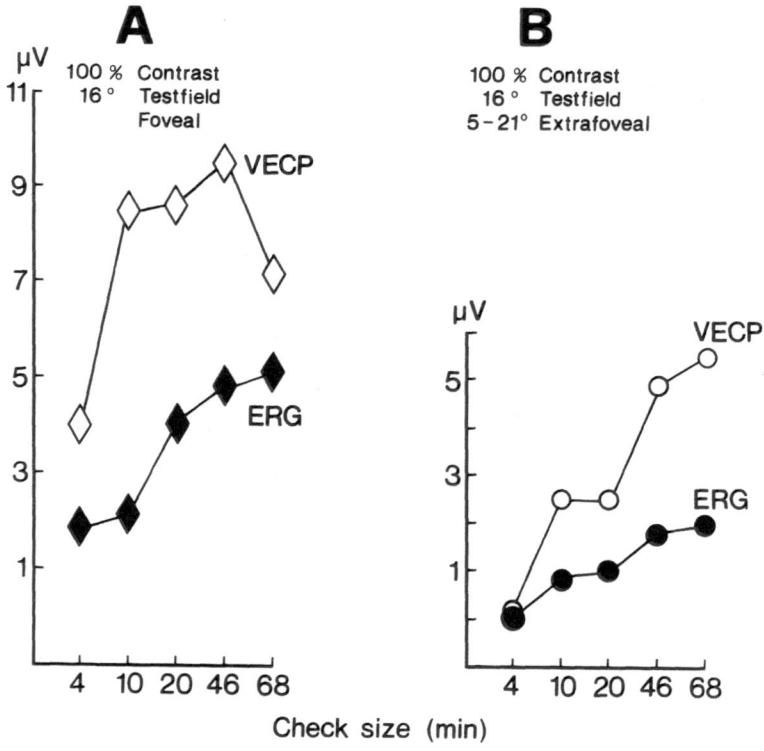

Fig. 1. Monocularly viewed averaged (N = 256) ERG and VECP potentials vs. different checksizes. A foveal, B extra-foveal stimulation.

RESULTS

In agreement with Armington *et al.* (1971) we found higher amplitudes with increasing checksize in the ERG while the VECP showed a peak at a checksize 46 min of arc when the control testfield was 16° degree (Fig. 1A). When the 16° testfield was centered 13° extrafoveally, all responses were smaller in amplitude and the maximum in the VECP was produced by the 68 min check (Fig. 1B). Checks below 10 min resulted in a unmeasurable response both for the ERG and the VECP.

We determined the relationship between ERG and VECP amplitude as a function of area by increasing the size of the testfield from 5° to 16°, centrally viewed. This resulted in almost no increases of amplitude of the ERG and VECP responses evoked by small checks. For the 46' check increasing test-fields produced an increase in amplitude both in the ERG and VECP (Fig. 2 A and B). On the other hand using a 10 min check the ERG showed a monotonic increase in amplitude as testfield size increased, while the VECP showed no amplitude increase as a function of testfield area (Fig. 2 C).

We made an attempt to determine the contribution of different parts of the peripheral retina to the ERG and VECP checkerboard pattern in response to different checksizes by blanking out parts of the central testfield. For this purpose parts of the central visual field were occluded, ranging from 7° to 13° in a testfield of 14°. When the smallest check (4.6 min) was presented in the annular region outside the 5° blanked center it produced a borderline response both in the VECP and in the ERG (Fig. 3 A and B). As the area of the annular region decreased, the VECP and ERG also decreased in amplitude, but the order was such that the response to the smallest check disappeared first, while the largest check was still able to evoke a response even with the smallest annular region. Figure 4 graphically summarizes the ERG and VECP data including the responses for a 14° testfield without occlusion of the central visual field.

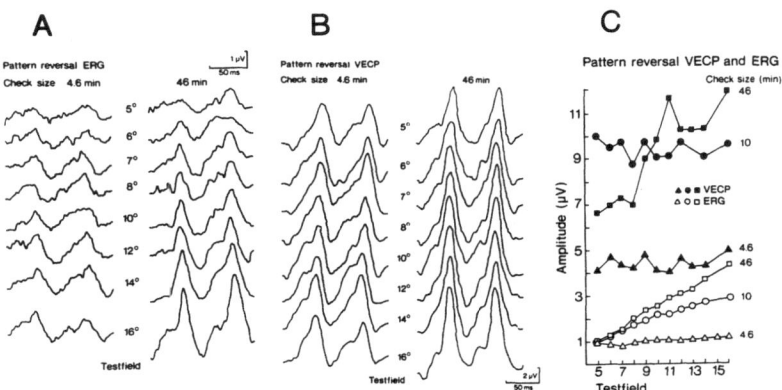

Fig. 2. ERG (A) and VECP (B) waveforms (N = 256) for small (4.6') and large (46') checksizes presented at increasingly larger testfields. Averaged ERG and VECP amplitudes (C) at increasingly larger testfields with checksizes of 4.6', 10' and 46' of arc.

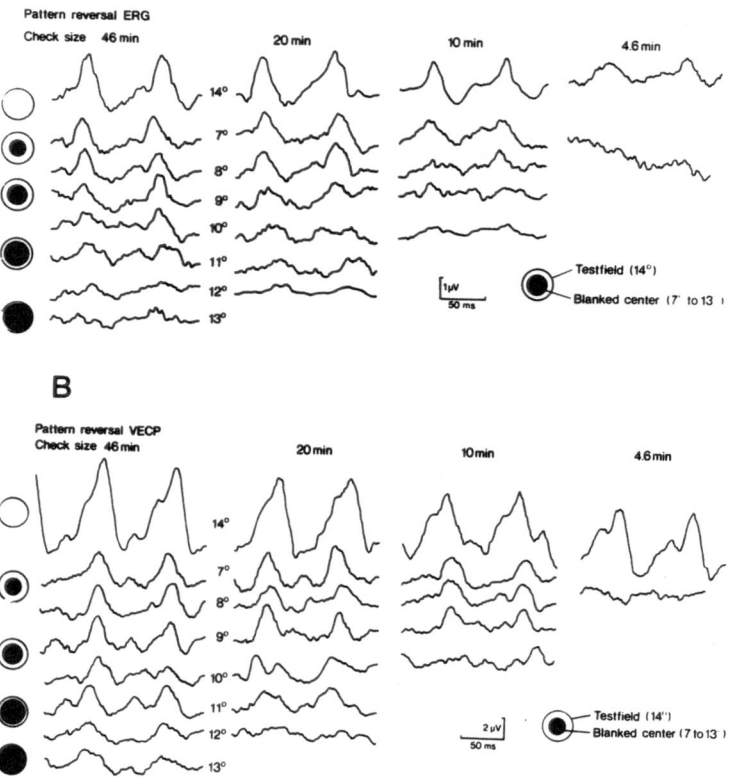

Fig. 3. ERG (A) and VECP (B) waveforms (N = 256) without (above) and with increasing blanked center (7° to 13°, below) in a 14° testfield.

When the checksize of the pattern reversal stimulus was increased from 4.6 to 68 min of arc, differences in the change of amplitude were noted for the ERG and the VECP. For small (5° and 8°) testfields, the VECP showed a maximum response for a 10 min and a 20 min checksize. With larger testfields (12° and 16°) it was found that now a 46 min checksize evoked the largest response in the VECP (Fig. 5 B).

By contrast, for the small testfields little or no increase was seen in the amplitude of the ERG as the function of checksize. It was only with larger testfields that the ERG showed a monotonic increase in amplitude as checksize increased (Fig. 5 A).

Figure 6 graphically summarizes the ERG and VECP data obtained for various checksizes and testfields.

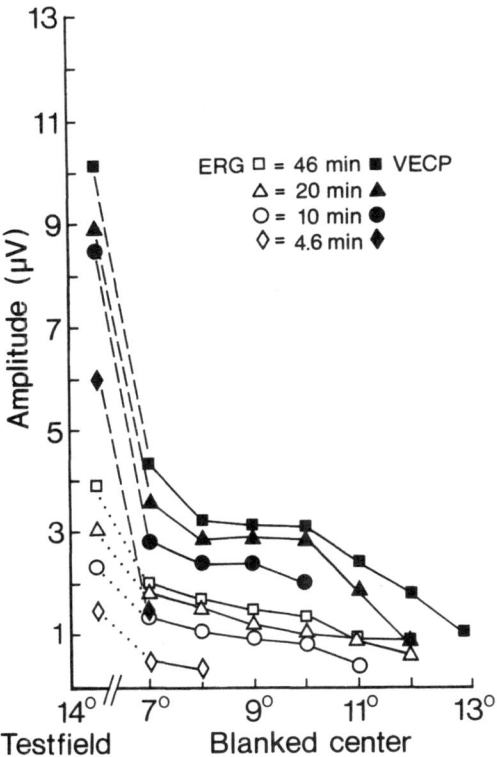

Pattern reversal VECP and ERG

Fig. 4. Averaged ERG and VECP amplitudes of 3 subjects without (left) and with increasing blanked center (7° to 13°) in a 14° testfield.

DISCUSSION

The results of these experiments indicate that under certain conditions a parallel behaviour of the pattern-ERG and -VECP can be demonstrated. Especially when various annular regions were stimulated with a number of checksizes it was found that a larger area-summation generates a larger response, both in the ERG and VECP in comparison with more central retinal areas, where smaller checks evoke the maximum response. A possible explanation of the larger spatial summation manifested by both the peripheral ERG and VECP, is that the receptive fields are bigger. The similarities found with large and small checks, when the annular testfield area grew, indicates that the neural organization of the peripheral retina may differ not very much at retinal

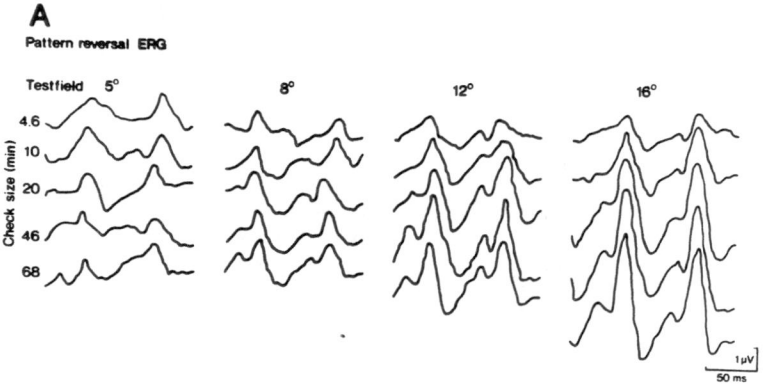

A

Pattern reversal ERG

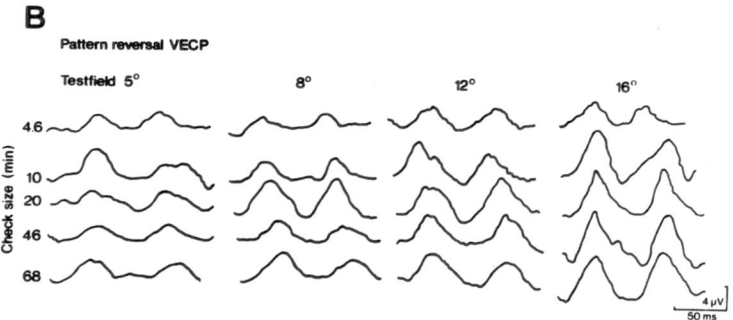

B

Pattern reversal VECP

Fig. 5. ERG (N = 256, A) and VECP (N = 64, B) waveforms for several test-fields at different checksizes.

and cortical level. Thus, these data are consistant with the belief that receptive field size increases with eccentricity.

It does not seem justified to take these results as the effects of the area alone. If the amplitudes of the checkerboard ERG were simply related to the number of receptors or retinal units stimulated in a given area then it should not matter what size of the pattern was used. However, the ERG amplitude does in fact depend on what checksize was employed.

Moreover the shift of the amplitude-peak of the VECP to larger checksizes in the larger testfield is consistent with the view that receptive field size increases with eccentricity. However, the VECP shows spatial tuning while the ERG does not. According to Armington et al. (1971) the antagonistic center-surround organization of the receptive field is responsible for the spatial tuning of the VECP. While it is true that the checksize and thus possibly the receptive field organization influences the ERG, it does not evidence spatial tuning. An explanation may be that at retinal level a fitting or larger checksize in comparison to receptive field size results in a maximum response while at

260

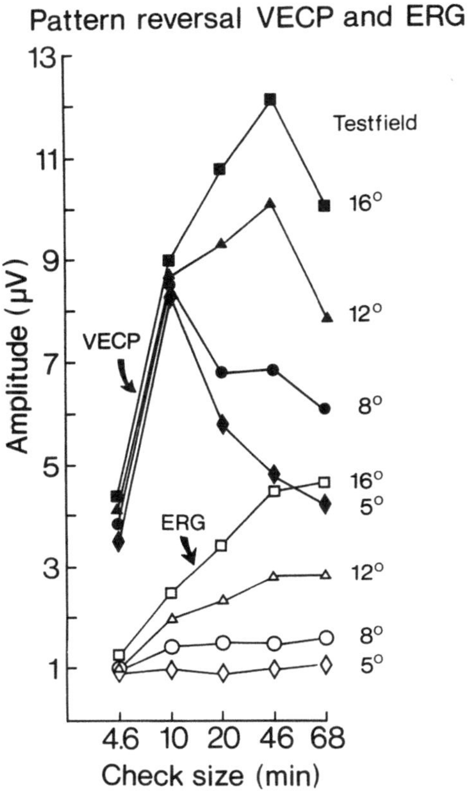

Pattern reversal VECP and ERG

Fig. 6. Averaged ERG and VECP amplitudes of 3 subjects for small (5° and 8°) and larger (12° and 16°) testfields vs. different checksizes.

cortical level more selective behaviour to ideal checksize is noted because of post retinal processing of visual information. Furthermore, a reorganization of the retinal receptive field structure has to be considered at the cortical level resulting in a sharpening of contrast.

REFERENCES

Armington, J.C. The electroretinogram, the visual evoked potential, and the area-luminance relation. *Vision Res.* 8: *263–276* (1968).

Armington, J.C., Corwin, T.R. & R. Marsetta. Simultaneously recorded retinal and cortical responses to patterned stimuli. *J. Opt. Soc. Amer.* 61: *1514–1521* (1971).

Johnson, E.P., Riggs, L.A. & Amy M.L. Schick. Photopic retinal potentials evoked by phase alteration of a barred pattern. In Burian, H.M. and Jacobson, J.H.: *3rd ISCERG Symposium, Illinois, 1964.* Suppl. to Vision Res. pp. 75–91, Pergamon Press, New York 1966.

Lawwill, T. Pattern stimuli for clinical ERG. In Dodt, E. and Pearlman, J.T. *11th*

ISCERG Symposium, Bad Nauheim 1973, Doc. Ophthal. Proc. Ser. 4: 353–362, Dr. W. Junk, The Hague 1974a.

Lawwill, T. The bar-pattern electroretinogram for clinical evaluation of the central retina. Am. J. Ophthal. 78: 121–126 (1974b)

Lawwill, T., Walther, C. & S. Crockett. The scotopic and photopic bar-pattern ERG— contributions of the central and peripheral retina. In Lawwill, T.: 14th ISCERG Symposium, Louisville 1976. Doc. Ophthal. Proc. Ser. 13: 287–291, Dr. W. Junk, The Hague 1977.

Riggs, L.A., Johnson, E.P. & Amy M.L. Schick. Electrical responses of the human eye to moving stimulus pattern. Science 144: 567 (1964).

Sokol, S. An electrodiagnostic index of macular degeneration. Arch. Ophthal. 88: 619–624 (1972).

Sokol, S. & B.H. Bloom. Macular ERG's elicited by checkerboard pattern stimuli. In Lawwill, T. 14th ISCERG Symposium, Louisville 1976, Doc. Ophthal. Proc. Ser. 13: 299–305, Dr. W. Junk, The Hague 1977.

Author's address:
Universitäts—Augenklinik
Frankfurt Main

Max Planck Institut für
Physiologische und Klinische Forschung
Bad Nauheim
F.R.G.

EXPERIENCE AND RESULTS OF PERIMETRIC INVESTIGATION BY MEANS OF VECP

WINIFRIED MÜLLER, E. HAASE, J. GAUSS AND G. HENNING

(*Erfurt, G.D.R.*)

ABSTRACT

The authors report the results obtained with electroperimetry in 106 patients, using the so-called Ilmenau-Erfurt perimeter 1. The instrument and method were introduced in earlier publications. In the course of the last few years the percentage of coincidence with the subjective visual fields has been improved to about 85 per cent due to a programme change.

INTRODUCTION

Starting out from the awareness that all that is seen must necessarily end in a change in the potential in the occipital centre of vision (area 17–19), we took and we still take the use of VECP as a signal for perimetric investigation just as a question concerning the technological and systematical efforts, which, however, is feasible and promising. In earlier studies we have published our considerations and the method we adopted (see the references). The first systematic structure we used for determining the electro-perimetric visual fields, the so-called Ilmenau–Erfurt perimeter I has been modified completely and newly designed in the meantime on a basis of comprehensive studies during recent years. Provision has been made for a new structure that will be disclosed at another passage. For a better understanding we present the illustration that shows the systematic structure (Figs. 1 and 2) and the block diagrams of the 1st and 2nd hardware intended for electroperimetry (Figs. 3 and 4).

In the course of this article we should like to report on the experience gained in applying electroperimetry within the scope of clinical diagnostics. P. Weber and G. Henning report on the accurate mathematical problems (see page 273). The computers applied are two optionally programmable process computers. Every kind of electroperimetry–whose result ought to be an objective visual field–aims at an automatic detection of signals and evaluation by the computer. We applied electroperimetry from the following clinical points of view:

1. To check up our method we searched for characteristic defects of the visual field in patients who can state safe and reproducible data in the application of the conventional method. In doing so we resorted to defects produced by retinal disorders and which depend on the affection of the visual pathway.
2. In patients showing great differences in conventional subjective perimetry we carried out the electroperimetric investigation in order to be able to dispose of an additional decision aid in the evaluation.

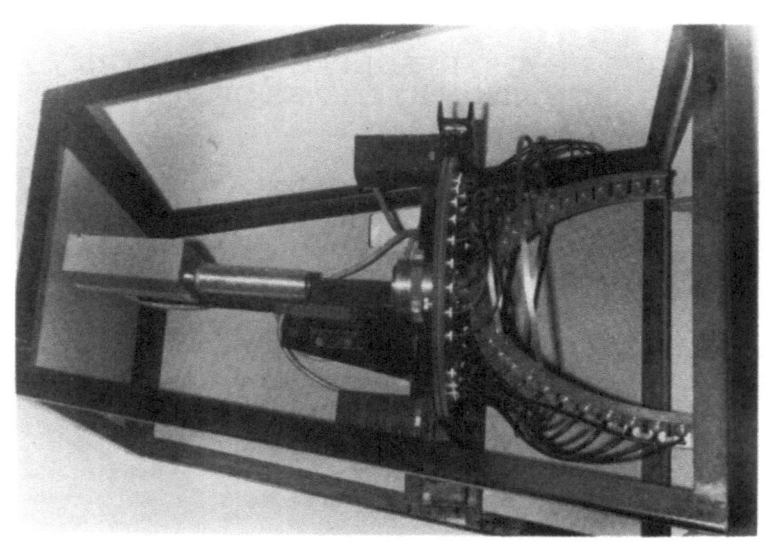

Fig. 2. Ilmenau-Erfurt perimeter II.

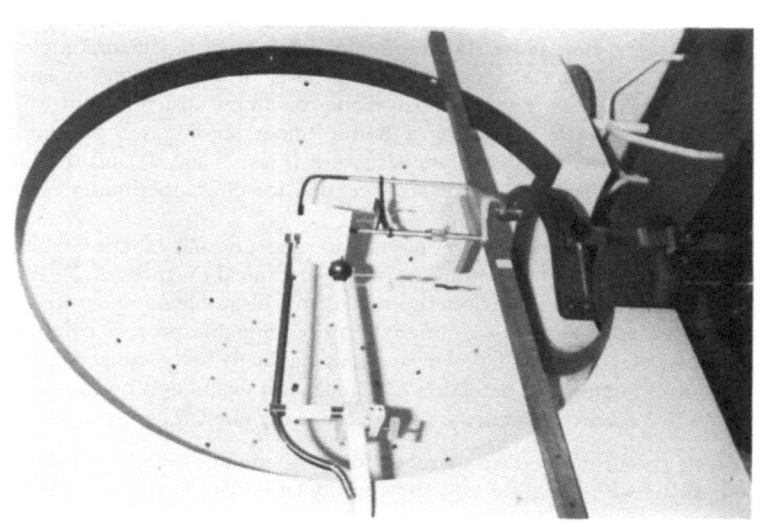

Fig. 1. Stimulation device of the Ilmenau-Erfurt perimeter I.

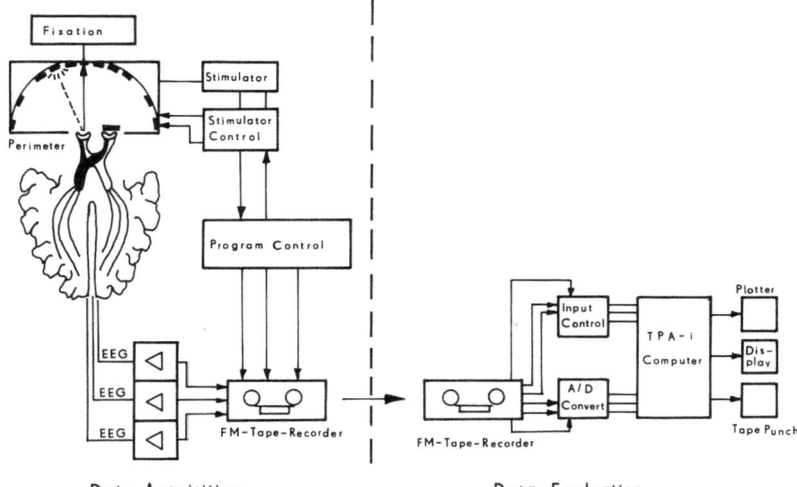

Fig. 3. Block diagram of the IEP I

electroperimeter (structure)

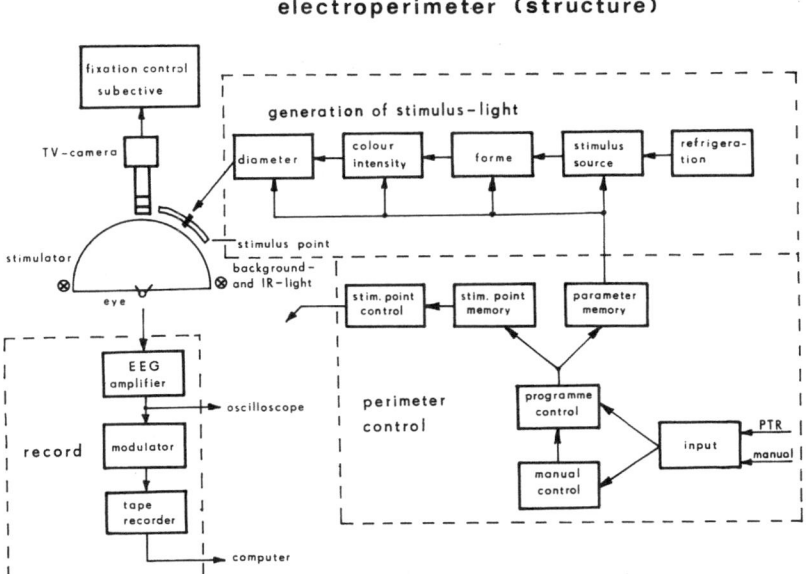

Fig. 4. Block diagram of the IEP II.

3. We examined persons who did not make any indication on the visual field, for they were not in a position to do so for the most various reasons.

4. We carried through electroperimetric checks of the visual field in persons in the case of whom the clinicians suspected the indications on the subjective visual field. These checkups were intended to assist the physician in charge in his assessment with the intention to obtain the actual result and to avoid any injustice to the patient. This group also includes those persons who are frequently made out as a sham patient without the necessary criticism.

It goes without saying that we evaluated the electroperimetric findings relative to the visual field and described in the complex of problems, itemized 2nd to 4th, by exercising much restraint and expressing criticism.

The VECP was evaluated by one single investigator who, at that time, was not aware of any result obtained with subjective conventional perimetry. The investigator made use of the following documents:

1. The analogue-averaging curve of two unipolar and one bipolar recordings.
2. The digital display of the minima and maxima.
3. Partially also computer-aided information on signal detection that is to say the computer has automatically detected whether there was a potential or there was not in the stimulation of a certain areal.

The following guideline was applied in the personal evaluation:

1. The centre answer formed the reference point of evaluation for all the curves. In the case of a failure of a centre answer, an answer, that was well defined and adjacent to the centre, was used as sample curve.
2. In the case of the analogue curve only the presence of N_2 was evaluated for the yes/no decision. The standard peak time relative to N_2 is approximately $110 \, ms \pm 20 \, ms$ in persons whose eyes and visual pathways are sound. The peak time was of no importance for the perimetric evaluation.
3. The answers were rated positive, provided the potential was detected in two recordings. The rating was negative in those cases in which there was no recording at all. If the decision were not to be made clearly the decisions in these cases were being coded as to be positive probable (+?) or negative probable (−?), or as no decision (?).
4. In case of artifacts during the recording the recording was rejected on the whole.
5. The minima and maxima values were compared with the result obtained in visual correlation. As far as the computer has processed automatic signal detection on the data obtained the latter were subjected to comparison.

We report on the results obtained with 106 patients (54 female and 52 male). The average age amounted to 38.5 years, 160 eyes were examined, 583 EEGs were recorded. Altogether, perimetric stimulation took place with 6831 stimuli points. Owing to technical faults in the recording process there was trouble with the computer in 7.5 per cent of all cases so that the curves had to be left out of consideration from the very beginning. In this connection we had to do without an accurate classification of the diagnoses. The visual field defects in 35 cases were due to retinal or optic nerve diseases, in 47 cases due to disorders of the visual pathway, in 6 cases aggravation was suspected, and in 18 cases the result obtained had to be considered as clinical obscure. We classified the results – as far as comparison with the subjective visual fields was feasible – into

(a) coincidence
(b) limited coincidence
(c) no coincidence
(d) cannot be evaluated

We indicate the results we obtained in Table 1.

Table 1. Evaluation of the electroperimetry visual fields in the time from 1973 to 1978.

71 % (123)	in coincidence and limited coincidence with conventional perimetry
11 % (19)	with no coincidence
18 % (31)	no evaluation feasible

These percentages should be taken as a basis indicating that perimetry is feasible with the methods applied by us. As it becomes obvious from other data we learned in the past to steadily improve the quota of results by changing the programme (Table 2). We are of the opinion that the new stimulation device and the comprehensive software will advance electroperimetry and make it more efficient. In conclusion it can be stated: while 6 years ago the feasibility of electroperimetry by means of VECP was doubted to a large extent, the steadily increasing number of publications on this problem recently has shown that electroperimetry from the most various points of view represents a present-day and future-oriented topic.

Table 2. Classification of the electroperimetric results obtained with visual fields in two-year groups.

1973 1974 } 55 %	in coincidence and limited coincidence with conventional perimetry
1975 1976 } 71 %	— " —
1977 1978 } 85 %.	— " —

REFERENCES

Forth, E., G. Henning, R. Berndt, E. Schmöger, W. Müller, E. Haase & W. Höhne. Beitrag zur Problematik der objektiven Perimetrie. Wiss. Z. TH Ilmenau 19; 3/4: *137–146*, (1973).

Henning, G., W. Müller, R. Berndt, E. Haase & G. Elsmann. Investigations on objective perimetry. Digest of the 10th Internat. Conference on Med. and Biological Engineering, Dresden 1973. S. 202 (1973).

Henning, G. Apparativer und methodischer Beitrag zur objektiven Perimetrie. Diss. TH Ilmenau (1974).

Müller, W., E. Haase, W. Höhne, E. Schmöger & G. Henning. Contribution to objective perimetry by means of the VER. Proc. XIth ISCERG-Symp., Bad Nauheim 1973; ed. by E. Dodt and J. T. Pearlman, p. 323–327, Den Haag, Junk (1974).

Müller, W., E. Haase, G. Henning & R. Berndt. Untersuchungen zur objektiven Perimetrie. *Albrecht v. Graefes Arch. klin. exp. Ophthalmol.* 190: *329–340* (1974).

Müller, W., E. Haase, & G. Henning. Vergleichende Untersuchungen von subjektiv und objektiv ermittelten Gesichtsfeldern. *Albrecht v. Graefes Arch. Klin. exp. Ophthalmol.* 194: *143–152* (1975).

Müller, W., E. Haase & J. Gauss. Gutachtliche und differentialdiagnostische Anwendungsbereiche des Verfahrens der objektiven Perimetrie. *Dt. Ges. Wesen* 31: *1886–1891* (1976).

Müller, W., E. Haase, J. Gauss, G. Henning & U. Pieper. Anwendung der objektiven Perimetrie in der klinischen Diagnostik. 21. *Internat. Wiss. Kolloquium TH Ilmenau*, 2: *241–243* (1976).

Müller, W. E. Haase & R. Niedlich. Zu einigen Problemen bei der elektroperimetrischen Untersuchung mittels VECP. *Albrecht v. Graefes Arch. klin. exp. Ophthalmol.* 207: *51–59* (1978).

Pieper, U. & G. Henning. Untersuchungen zur Effektivität der Averaging-Methode beim Nachweis evozierter Potentiale. 21. Internat. Wiss. Kolloqium TH Ilmenau 2: *241–243* (1976).

Schauer, M., G. Henning & W. Müller. Zur Problematik des Streulichteinflusses bei der lokalisierten Stimulation der Retina. *Albrecht v. Graefes Arch. klin. exp. Ophthalmol.* 197: *283–291* (1975).

Walther, A. Experimentell analytische Weiterentwicklung der Verfahrensgrundlagen und die Realisierung einer sich daraus ergebenden neuen Elektroperimetrie- Konzeption. Diss. TH Ilmenau (1977).

Author's address:

Prof. Dr. med. habil. W. Müller
Augenklinik der
Medizinischen Akademie Erfurt
Nordhäuser Str. 74
DDR-506 Erfurt
German Democratic Republic

Docum. Ophthal. Proc. Series, Vol. 23

A NEW PERIMETER FOR ELECTROPERIMETRY

A. WALTHER

(*Karl-Marx-Stadt, G.D.R.*)

ABSTRACT

The author represents a new perimeter based on the evaluation of the visual evoked cortical potentials (VECP). The equipment provides for stimulus diameter, duration, intensity, colour, and other parameters. The VECP signal is amplified, modulated, and is printed according to connected programs.

The co-operative team of the Technical College Ilmenau (section Biomedical engineering) and of the Medical Academy Erfurt (eye clinic–electrodiagnostic lab.) has already reported on its activities (Müller *et al.* (1974), Henning (1974)).

I should like to acquaint you with the advanced electroperimetry conception based on the objective perimetry method described (Beinhocher *et al.* (1966), Henkes (1966)). The conception is neither intended to develop automatic perimetry, think of the successful work by Frankhauser *et al.* (1972), nor is it to substitute conventional perimetry. Electroperimetry complements perimetry to a large extent. The choice of visual evoked cortical potential (VECP) results from the causalty between stimulus and VECP, and thus the methods can be applied on the whole.

The VECP dependencies on stimulus parameters as stimulus intensity, frequency, colour, as well as the dependence on the stimulus point on the retina are extensively described (Shipley *et al.* (1965); (1966), Henkes *et al.* (1966); (1974)). By these dependencies the conception (Walther (1977), (1978)) has to lay the foundation for the well defined diagnostics, and thus the following problems should be solved:

1. develop the stimulus parameters and hold those once selected at a constant level,
2. reduce the intraindividual and interindividual VECP variations under optimum conditions,
3. enable stimulus point control, at least in form of eye monitoring,
4. prevent physiological fatigue and possible habituation.

The team started out from the following biotechnical conditions:

1. Xenon flash light,
2. spherical stimulus area,
3. patient lying on an investigation table,
4. about 800 stimulus points in the stimulus area,
5. 65 stimulus points per visual field as a maximum within the investigation program in one session,
6. semi-automatic investigation course.

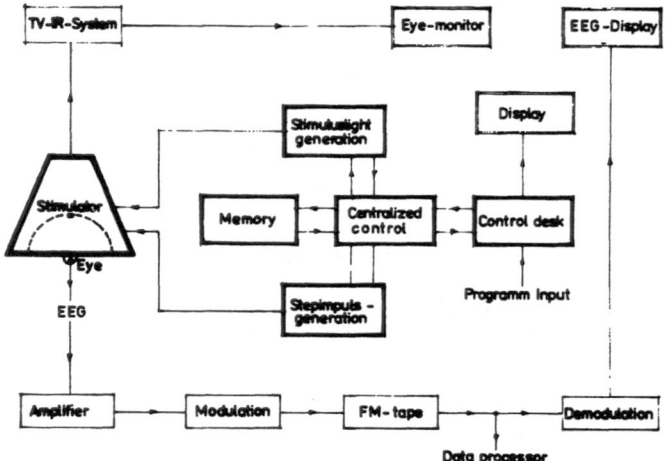

Fig. 1. Block diagram of the described electroperimeter.

Figure 1 shows the block diagram of the electroperimeter. By means of the input unit the investigation program can be read manually or entered on a perforated tape. The centralized control unit provides for stimulus coordinates, stimulus light parameters and patient parameters in several memory structures, and ensures the timing of all perimeter elements. Stimulus coordinates in the spherical stimulus area are produced by means of a step motor controlled by a rotating glass-fiber system. This transformation takes place at an accuracy, the stimulus field appearing statically. Stimulus point motion is invisible to the patient. Stimulus light parameters are supplied by an electronic flash tube control. The lighting equipment provides for stimulus duration, -intensity, -colour, -frequency as well as the stimulus diameter. The chromatic light is produced by a monochromatic filter system, mutually correcting the intensity. Stimulus point monitoring takes place by monitoring of some part of the eye by means of an infrared television system. The patient fixes a statistically pulsed fixation pattern. The VECP signal is amplified, modulated and is printed according to the programme, including the patient's number and parameters as code information on the FM tape recorder. The essential technical parameters of the electroperimeter are:

1. stimulus field diameter 720 mm,
2. stimulus points in the sphere 840,
3. stimulus distance in spherical coordinates 6°,
4. stimulus intensity max. 10^7 cd/m^2,
5. stimulus colour 461, 510, 589, and 650 nm,
6. stimulus diameter 3.5 and 5 mm,
7. background illumination 10 1x white.

CONCLUSION

The electroperimeter is capable of isolating the stimulus parameters accurately. Several memory structures allow the investigator to work up connected programs with 3 deviations from the main parameters in one session. Investigations are performed in Erfurt by means of this electroperimeter according to this conception.

The results are in conformity to the conception. Statistically determined results ought to be published in 1979 at the Congress of the Biomedical Society of the GDR in Berlin.

REFERENCES

Beinhocker, G.D., Brooks, E., Anfenger & R.M. Copenhaven, Electroperimetry, *IEEE Trans. bio.-med. Eng.* 13: *11–18* (1966).

Frankhauser, F., P. Koch. & A. Roulier. On Automation of Perimetry. *Albrecht v. Graefes Arch. Klin. Exp. Ophthal.* 184: *126–150* (1972).

Henkes, H.E. Die diagnostische Bedeutung der okzipitalen Antwort auf Lichtreize. *Klin. Wochenschr. Wien.* 23: *413–416* (1966).

Henkes, H.E., G.H.M. van Lith. Electroperimetry. *Ophthalmologica* 169: *151–159* (1974).

Henning, G. Methodischer und experimenteller Beitrag zur objektiven Perimetrie. Dissertation A, TH Ilmenau, (1974).

Müller, W., E. Haase, G. Henning & R. Berndt Untersuchungen zur objektiven Perimetrie. *Albrecht v. Graefes Arch. klin. exp. Ophthal.* 190: *239–340* (1974).

Shipley, T., R.W. Jones & A. Fry. Evoked Visual Potentials and Human Colour Vision. *Science* 150: *1162–1164* (1965).

Shipley, T, R.W. Jones & A. Fry. Intensity and Evoked Human Occipitogramm *Vis. Res.* 6: *657–667* (1966).

Walther, A. Experimentell analytische Weiterentwicklung der Verfahrensgrundlagen und die Realisierung einer sich daraus ergebenden neuen Elektroperimetrie-Konzeption. Dissertation A, TH Ilmenau, 1977.

Walther, A. Patentschrift WPA 61B/203690, 1978.

Author's address:
Bezirkskrankenhaus Karl-Marx-Stadt
DDR-9010 Karl-Marx-Stadt
German Democratic Republic

271

FIRST EXPERIENCE GATHERED IN COMPUTER-AIDED DETECTION OF ELECTROPERIMETRIC VECP

P. WEBER AND G. HENNING
(Ilmenau and Erfurt, G.D.R.)

ABSTRACT

For carrying out electroperimetry the authors have developed a computer-aided evaluation method processing analog data. A system of programs is represented, enabling evaluation of various detection criteria. As a result the computer provides for the following decisions: VECP detected, not detected or no detection possible.

For several years the Section of Biomedical Engineering and Bionics of the Ilmenau Institute of Technology has been working in the field of the computer-aided detection of visually evoked cortical potentials (VECP) for application in electroperimetry. The aim is to free the physician from routine work and to objectify the strategy of detection. The foremost point of this study is not the determination and quantitative evaluation of VECP parameters, but VECP detection.

The EEG is registered with a perimeter on three channels. Stimulation is done by means of flashes produced by Xenon lamps having a discharge power of 0.2 Ws and a stimulus mark diameter of 8 mm, the frequency of stimuli being 1 Hz. 45 single stimuli were set per stimulating point.

Treatment is done off-line by a PRS 4000 type process control computer. For analog conversion a system of programs has been established which has proved its usefulness in daily work for about three years. The usual averaging and the nexus of computer-aided detection of the evoked potentials had been combined in the evaluation program.

Figure 1 shows the print-out of the averaging results. The columns correspond to the three EEG channels; the rows represent the respective results obtained at one stimulating point. A gauge mark 5 μV (at the upper left) as well as the auxiliary lines at 80 and 160 ms are included. Furthermore, the patient's code number and the information about the angle leading to the stimulating point are recorded. The results obtained with an extremum analysis of the averaging curve are contained in an additional record.

Up to now these data have formed the basis for the decision on the presence of an evoked potential by the ophthalmologist. Since about two years an additional record concerning computer-aided detection of potentials has been made available. In order to put computer-aided detection of VECPs into practice we first searched for criteria reconstructing the evaluation algorithm practiced by the ophthalmologist (Fig. 2). Such criteria are:

- "external" correlation,
- maximum analysis, and
- the analysis of the "area" under the VECP.

273

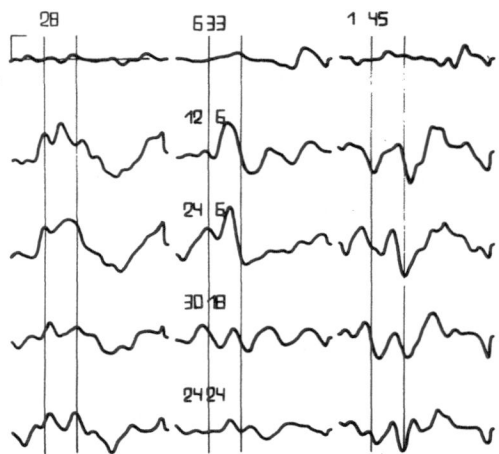

Fig. 1. Print-out of the averaging results.

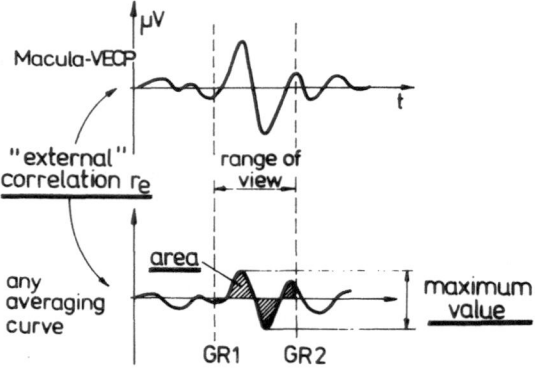

Fig. 2. Criteria of dedection of VECP.

In the "external" correlation process the averaging curves are compared correlatively to the averaging done with macula stimulation, and then the correlation factor is used for evaluation. The starting point is that there is some probability for the VECP to be present with macula stimulation, to serve as a model. We claim that the VECP is detected provided that the correlation factor exceeds a certain limit.

The two other criteria are due to the statement of the ophthalmologist according to which the evoked potentials must have a minimum amplitude. The "area" under the VECP is equivalent to the evoked potential energy.

Further criteria are due to signal analyses the evaluating physician cannot provide by means of the averaging curves. Such a criterion is:

– the "internal" correlation

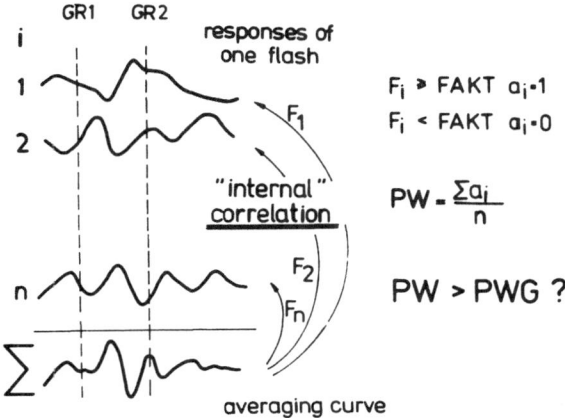

Fig. 3. Criteria of detection of VECP.

which has proved itself to be particularly efficient (Fig. 3). Here again, every averaging result is correlated to every single stimulus from which it is the average. The percentage PW of those single responses is determined, the correlation of which must be considered more extensive than a predetermined factor FAKT. This method is based on the fact that despite the signal attenuation of the VECP that to a large extent is compared to the EEG evidently stimulus-synchronous portions may be seized correlatively. An evoked potential is detected provided that PW exceeds a limit PWG.

The Fourier analysis, the double sum of cross products, an analysis of the temporal site of the extrema and of their amplitudes, as well as further criteria are under work, however, they do not yet yield satisfactory results.

All detection criteria refer to a temporarily defined VECP signal section (GR1–GR2).

The results have shown that a single criterion must be deemed very inaccurate for the detection of evoked potentials. Therefore, combinations of the criteria have been tried in a statistical experiment. With such tests 3 decisions of the computer can be performed:

1. VECP detected (YES) – X
2. no VECP present (NO) – ϕ
3. no statement possible – ?

To achieve this, two methods have been applied for the time being:
– search for a decision vector by means of discriminance analysis;
– search for decision parameters which will be applied to the data material according to a principle of priority.

The decision vectors and parameters found, they were experimented with a subject and patient material of 91 derivations by means of the perimeter. The material comprises 567 YES decisions and 314 NO decisions.

275

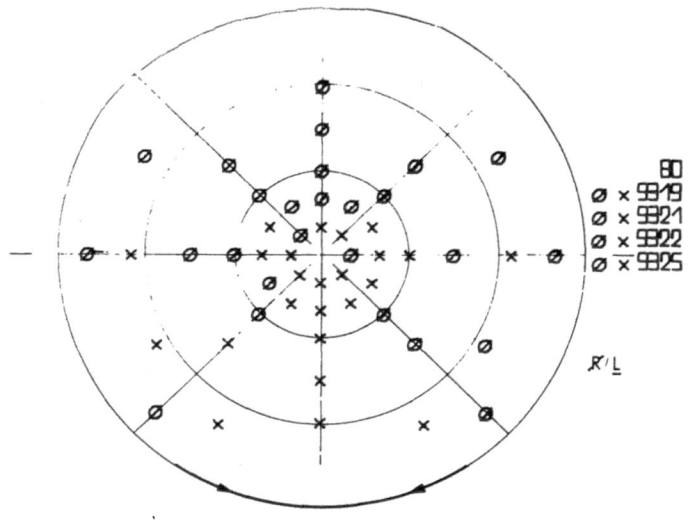

Fig. 4. Visual field with an 80 per cent decision certainty.

With the discriminance analysis the most favourable combination resulted using criteria:

"internal" correlation, "area", and "external" correlation. In 90 per cent of cases, agreement of computer results with the results obtained by the ophthalmologist could be achieved both in YES and NO decisions. Taking into consideration all the results the computer provide no decision (?) in 30 per cent of all cases. By combining parameters according to fixed parameters and priorities using criteria
– "internal" correlation and maximum analysis
an 80 per cent correspondence of the computer results with no decisions (?) made.

On the basis of this combination the ophthalmologist has provided the record mentioned above, containing the decisions of the computer. We distinguish between two variants having an 80 p.c. and a 90 p.c. decision certainty, respectively.

The 80 per cent variant realizes the condition of testing all averaging curves as regards a possible VECP and of deciding whether YES or NO. The 90 per cent variant supplies the certain decision and may contain "?" decisions.

Another program permits the summing up of the computer results of several derivations in one blank. In this case too, the visual fields are established separately according to the 80 and 90 per cent variants. Figure 4 shows a visual field with an 80 per cent decision certainty.

The method for computer-aided detection of VECP, which has been presented here, is continuously dealt with and completed. By testing further criteria it might be possible to further increase decision certainty and to objectify detection.

Summarizing we can state that computer-aided detection of VECP with reasonable errors occurring is also possible under the disadvantageous conditions of electroperimetry.

REFERENCES

G. Henning, U. Spittel, W. Müller & P. Weber. An attempt to computer-aided detection of VER for electroperimetry. (see pages 279–282, this volume).

Author's address:
Dipl. Ing. Peter Weber
Technische Hochschule Ilmenau, Fachbereich Biomedizinische
Technik und Bionik
DDR-63 Ilmenau
German Democratic Republic

Dr. Ing. Günther Henning
Medizinische Akademie Erfurt
Nordhäuser Strasse 74
DDR-50 Erfurt
German Democratic Republic

Docum. Ophthal. Proc. Series, Vol. 23

AN ATTEMPT TO COMPUTER-AIDED DETECTION OF VECP FOR ELECTROPERIMETRY

G. HENNING, U. SPITTEL, W. MÜLLER
AND   P. WEBER
(*Erfurt and Ilmenau, G.D.R.*)

ABSTRACT

The computer-aided evaluation of VECP depends on the signal-to-noise ratio of the VECP signal. The authors report on the rank correlation test and the results obtained with this method. Although the unfavourable conditions of electroperimetry cannot be considered optimum, computer-aided detection of VECP at a tolerable rate of error seems to be practicable.

The use of evoked potentials for objective clinical sensory function tests requires an adequate technique for signal evaluation. The determination of the presence or absence of potentials in a great many cases is the primary goal. In general, this decision is made by an experienced interpreter by estimation of the averaged potentials. This subjective analysis is one of the critical points of the objective test methods. For this reason it is our aim in this study to search for a possible technique for automatic computerized detection of VECP under the special conditions as they prevail in electroperimetry.

For realising an objective decision, signal – no signal, at least two different ways are imaginable:
– signal shape-dependent methods which are based on a computer simulation of the subjective decision process or on correlative techniques using a signal model,
– signal shape-independent methods which do not require any premise with regard to the similarity of signal and model.
The latter in some cases have the advantage that no signal template – neither an empirical nor a theoretical one – is necessary for signal detection. The detection efficiency of one possible realisation of this type — the rank correlation test – is the object of this paper.

MATERIALS AND METHODS

The rank correlation technique is based on the Friedman-test (Friedman (1937); it was first used for AEP-detection by Salomon (1974) and Maresch (1977). Rank correlation is a distribution-independent homogeneity test for dependent samples of measured data. The independence on the distribution of the data – which in practical cases is generally unknown for EP series – is obtained by conversion of the EP time series into rank values (Fig. 1). In the

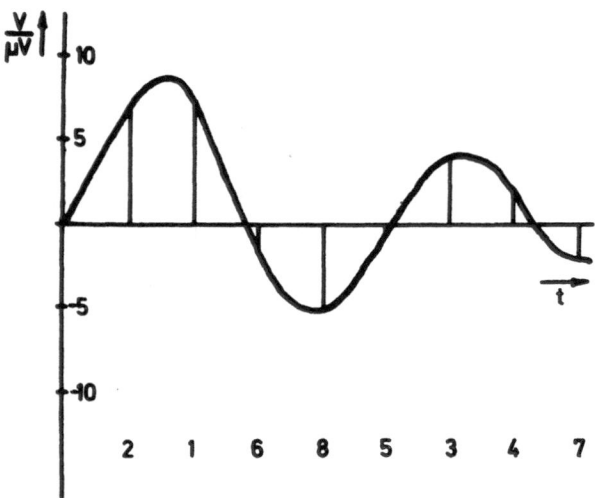

Fig. 1. Conversion of a sampled analog signal sweep (top) into a rank value series (bottom).

first approach these rank values will be randomly distributed for independent time series (e.g. stationary background EEG); yet there will appear significant differences between the rank values for dependent time series (e.g. EEG with EP-activity). The significance for this hypothesis may be computed by means of an algorithm described by Salomon (1974).

The efficiency of this method for the detection of VECP-activity was experimentally tested. We used VECP-data from 40 eye-healthy, cooperative subjects; the EEG was recorded occipitally in 3 channels by means of AgAgCl-electrodes. Six selected points from the central and peripheral visual field were tested ("positive" test points); at the beginning, in the middle and at the end of each data set, an EEG-record (without stimulation) was included ("negative" test points). Each of the positive test points was stimulated by 50 Xenon light flashes (luminance $5 \cdot 10^4$ cdm^{-2}, stimulation frequency about 1 Hz, visual angle 0.6°).

For our investigations we so had available 1080 records (720 positive, 360 negative) of electroperimetrical VECP-data. The evaluation of this material was accomplished off-line using a small computer TPA-i in a computer laboratory in the Medical Academy Erfurt. The whole primary data material was worked up several times with different operating parameters (different time windows; with/without digital low pass filtering); the rank correlation results were read out digitally, and analogously and additionally recorded on a digital magnetic tape for statistical evaluation.

RESULTS AND DISCUSSION

The VECP-rank correlation results obtained first of all show a clear increase in the test value Z_N – and with it for the likelihood of the presence of an EP – for

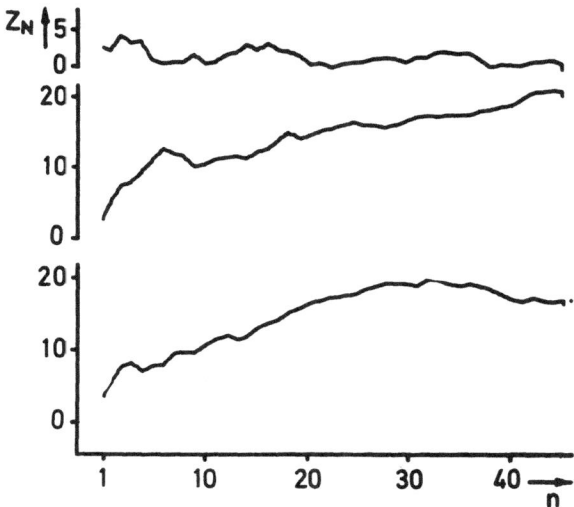

Fig. 2. Test value Z_N in dependence of number n of included single potentials (top: "negative" test point, middle and bottom: "positive" test points).

positive records compared with negative ones. With an increasing n (number of included single potentials) also Z_N increases for positive records, while it remains nearly constant at low values in negative records (Fig. 2). For $n > 30$ Z_n increases only unessentially. The statistical evaluation results emphasize this statement. Figure 3 shows as an example the distribution of Z_N for selected positive and negative records. For positive records there is to state a clear displacement of the distribution function to higher probability values; the mean value of Z_N is about four times higher than those in negative records. A

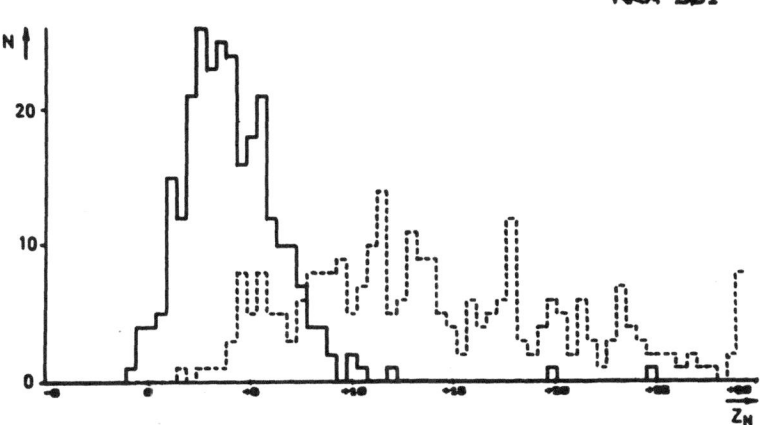

Fig. 3. Distribution of test value Z_N for negative test points (continuous line) and positive test points (broken line).

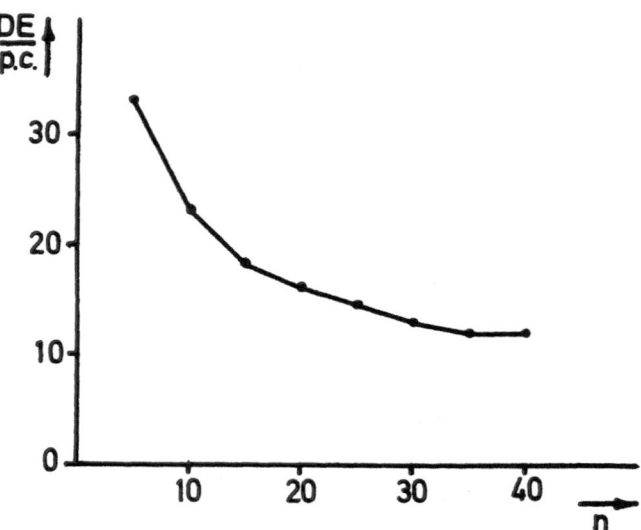

Fig. 4. Detection error DE for optimized decision value Z_N over n.

well defined separation of both groups, however, is not so easy because of the high variability of the signal parameters; the distribution functions have an overlapping range due to the presence of coherent signal components (*e.g.* α-activity) in negative records as well as by the unsatisfactory S/N-ratio in some positive records. For a possible application of the method for computer-assisted VECP-detection, therefore, it seems useful to compute an optimized decision value Z_N, for which the decision error DE – resulting from false positive and false negative decisions – becomes a minimum. Figure 4 represents the dependence of DE for optimized decision value Z_N from the number n of included single potentials. The decision reliability achieved by this method is at least in the same order as for subjective signal evaluation by an experienced ophthalmologist. This fact allows the conclusion that an objective computer-aided VECP-detection on the base of rank correlation test seems to be practicable at a tolerable error rate also under the unfavourable conditions of electroperimetry.

REFERENCES

Friedman, M. The use of ranks to avoid the assumption of normality implicit in the analysis of variance. *J. amer. statist. Ass.* 32: *675–701* (1937).

Maresch, H. Dissertation. Technische Universität Graz 1977.

Salomon, G. Electric response audiometry (ERA) based on rank correlation. *Audiology* 13; *181–194* (1974).

Author's address:
Dr. Ing. Günter Henning
Medizinische Akademie Erfurt
Nordhäuser Str. 74
DDR-50 Erfurt

SENSITIVITY OF SNELLEN, VER, AND ARDEN GRATING ACUITY ESTIMATIONS AS INDICATORS OF MACULAR AND OPTIC NERVE DISEASES*

HAROLD W. SKALKA

(*Birmingham, Alabama, U.S.A.*)

ABSTRACT

Patients with various macular and optic nerve abnormalities underwent Snellen, transient VER, and Arden grating "acuity" testing. Snellen acuity was the coarsest of the three evaluations, generally falling after Arden and VER acuity had already undergone significant degradation. The Arden gratings appeared to be the most sensitive of the three tests, essentially equalling VER performance in optic nerve diseases, and surpassing it in macular diseases. Variations in results between the different tests are generally understandable if one considers the functions tested by each and the anatomic derangements caused by the diseases in question. The Arden grating test appears to be an excellent and sensitive screening test for central visual disturbances.

For clinicians, visual function is usually described in terms of Snellen (or comparable target) acuity and visual field. These subjective tests of what may perhaps be termed the "quantity" of vision are easily standardized, do not require elaborate instrumentation, and are relatively economical of time. Their acceptance is such that the parameters they measure form the lingua franca of visual discourse and define our categories of vision and blindness.

When considering disorders of the optic nerve, visual field parameters may not always be, and acuity determinations often are not, the most useful terms in which to describe visual compromise. In macular disease, visual field tests usually are not, and high-contrast Snellen optotypes may not be, the most relevant of measures.

What may be referred to as the "quality" of vision is a somewhat elusive concept, not as easily compartmentalized and standardized. Modulation transfer functions provide a way of approaching this concept, but have generally required sophisticated laboratory resources. The recent development of the Arden grating test[1] has provided a means of looking at contrast sensitivity in a simple, rapid and reproducible manner.

We compared Snellen acuity, transient VER "acuity" to high-contrast alternating checks, and Arden grating "acuity" in patients with a variety of macular and optic nerve diseases, in order to evaluate the efficacy of each in detecting early deterioration of visual function (in a loose sense, the "quality" of the visual image). These are clearly not equivalent visual stimuli, differing in

---

* From the Combined Program in Ophthalmology, The University of Alabama in Birmingham-Eye Foundation Hospital, Birmingham, Alabama.

such parameters as contrast, field subtended, and dynamism of presentation. While congruence of results is to be expected in the absence of disease, it would be surprising indeed to find these test parameters equally affected by disease states.

MATERIAL AND METHODS

Patients with macular or optic nerve diseases were examined wearing their refractive corrections, including near adds where appropriate. Snellen acuity was recorded in the conventional manner, utilizing a projected image at a distance of 20 feet in a darkened room. Arden grating scores were obtained under standardized lighting conditions (7 ft. candles), all tests being performed by the same examiner to ensure uniformity of test administration.

VER "acuities" were obtained using monopolar leads 1 cm above the inion and recorded using the Nicolet CA-1000 system with television pattern generator. High-contrast black and white alternating check stimuli were presented at an alternation rate of 3.75 Hz, and 128 transient responses covering the 200 msec following each alternation were averaged. At our testing distance, the entire screen subtended 10° 42' horizontally and 8° 1' 30" vertically. End points were considered the smallest checks yielding recognizable responses (check sizes were reduced stepwise by half).

Our patient sample included a variety of macular and optic nerve diseases. Among these were senile macular degeneration, macular dystrophies, cystoid macular edema, pre-macular fibrosis, retrobulbar neuritis, ischemic optic neuropathy, traumatic neuropathies, tumors, etc.

RESULTS

Snellen acuity did not prove to be a good screening test for macular or optic nerve dysfunction. The high-contrast, familiar Snellen targets, read by the

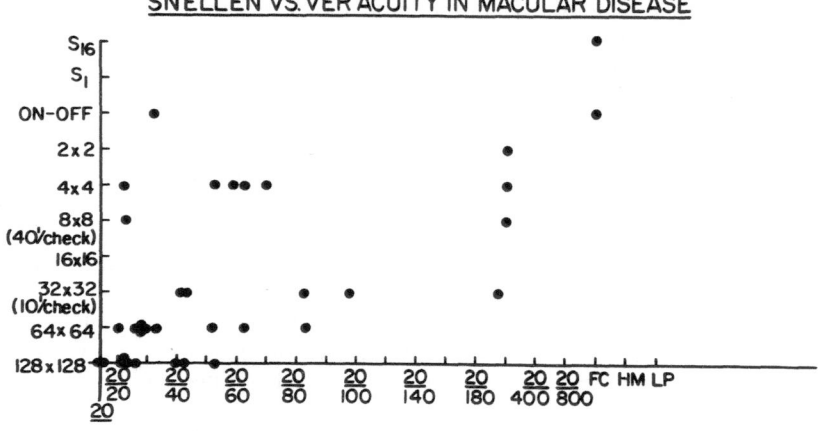

Fig. 1. Snellen acuity (abscissa), compared with VER "acuity" in a group of patients with various macular diseases. Ver acuities in this and succeeding figures are described in terms of numbers of checks on the stimulator screen (check size indicated twice for reference); S1 and S16 refer to Grass PS 22 photostimulator settings.

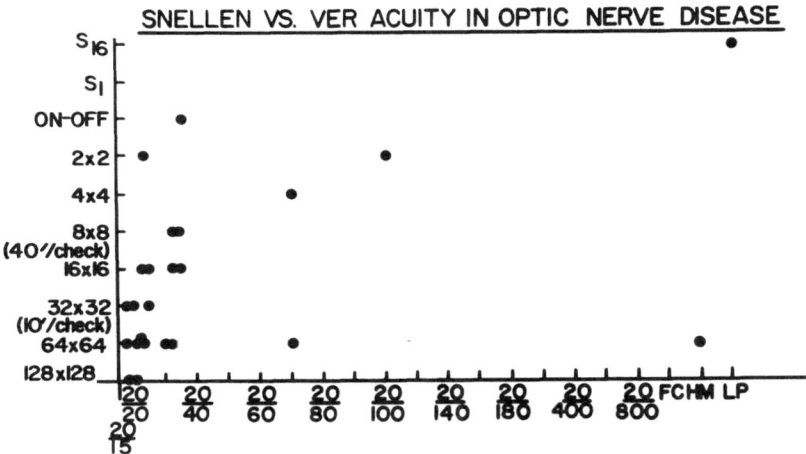

Fig. 2. Snellen acuity (abscissa) compared with VER "acuity" in a group of patients with various optic nerve diseases.

subjects at their own chosen speed, were relatively insensitive to subtle visual disturbances.

VER responses to alternating high-contrast black and white checks provided an objective test, and proved to be intermediate in sensitivity. While not clearly superior to Snellen determinations overall in macular diseases (Fig. 1), the VER was definitely more sensitive in reflecting optic nerve dysfunction (Fig. 2).

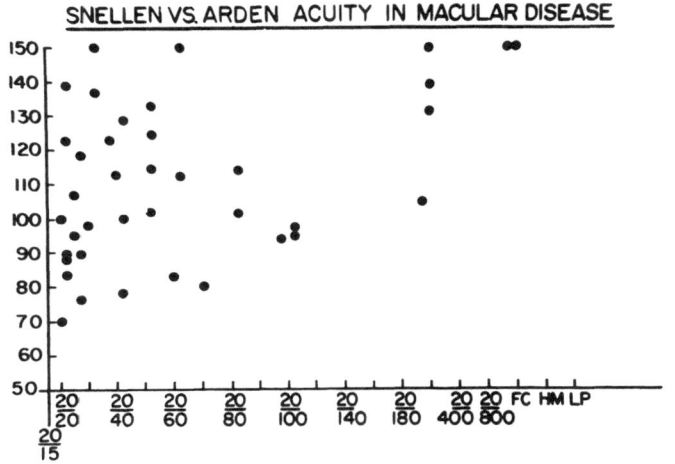

Fig. 3. Snellen acuity (abscissa) compared with Arden "acuity" in the macular disease patient group.

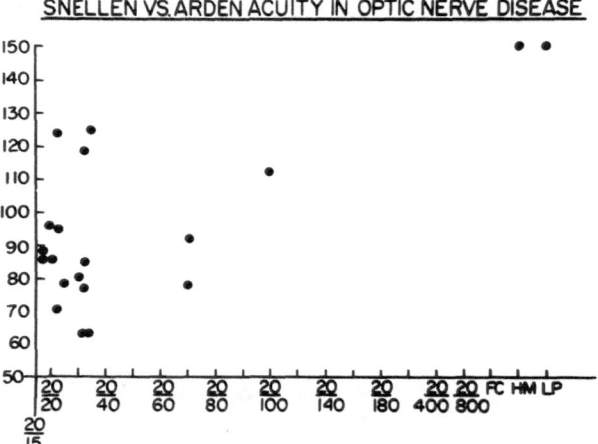

Fig. 4. Snellen acuity (abscissa) compared with Arden "acuity" in optic nerve disease patients.

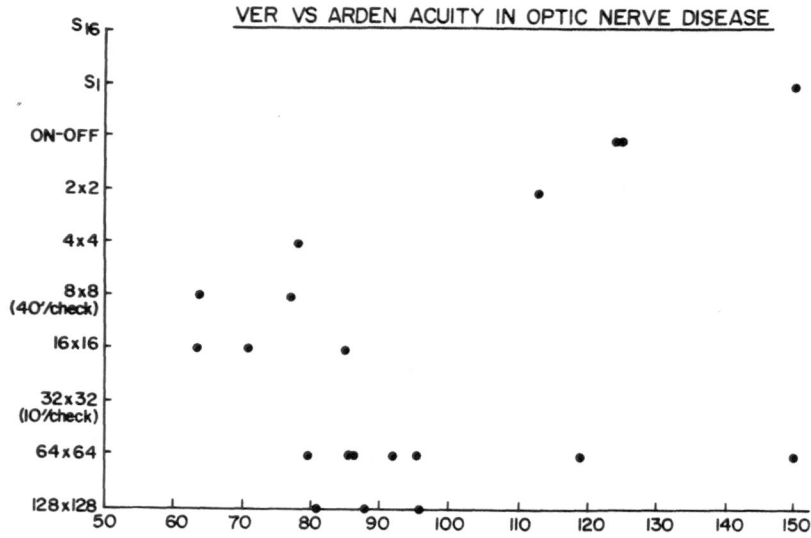

Fig. 5. Arden "acuity" (abscissa) compared to VER "acuity" in macular disease patients.

286

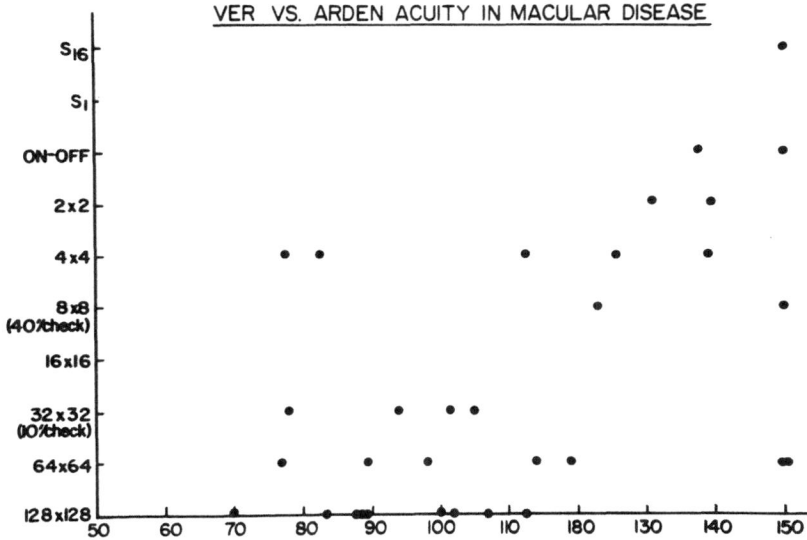

Fig. 6. Arden "acuity" (abscissa) compared to VER "acuity" in macular disease patients.

The Arden grating test presents the subject with unfamiliar targets of varying low contrast (and size), and requires a prompt response (on penalty of a poorer score). This test proved, in general, to be the most discriminating of the three in detecting abnormalities. In general, "quality" appeared to degrade before "quantity". The Arden gratings were clearly superior to Snellen testing in the detection of both macular and optic nerve dysfunction (Figs. 3 & 4). Arden grating scores fell, on average, about as early as VER performance in optic nerve diseases (Fig. 5), but were clearly more sensitive than VER responses as an early indicator of subtle macular disease (Fig. 6).

DISCUSSION

Not surprisingly, VER responses seemed most sensitive to optic nerve (transmission) problems. For example:

Case I – 22 y. o. female with pituitary adenoma. Small central scotoma and Marcus-Gunn pupil OD. Snellen acuity 20/30 –OD, 20/20 OS. Arden grating scores 63.5 OD, 62.5 OS (both normal). VER – low voltage OU, with detectable response to 20 min. checks OS, but not OD.

Case II – 39 y. o. male with resolving retrobulbar neuritis OS. Snellen acuity 20/20 OD, 20/40+ OS. Arden grating scores 66 OD, 125 OS. VER response good to 2.5 min. checks OD, non-recordable to 80 min. checks OS (and delayed to light flash stimuli).

287

In evaluating general macular (image detection) diseases, Arden gratings were easily the most sensitive indicator of dysfunction (neither Snellen nor VER estimations were, overall, superior to the other). Example:

Case III – 71 y. o. female with surface wrinkling retinopathy OU. Snellen acuity 20/30 −2 OD, 20/60 OS. VER responses to 5 min. checks either eye. Arden gratings totally non-discernible OU (score of 150 each eye).

Snellen acuity appeared to recover sooner than VER acuity in resolving macular problems, again underlining its relative coarseness as a determinant. Example:

Case IV – 54 y. o. male six weeks post cataract extraction OS. Resolving cystoid macular edema (fluorescein-proven). Snellen acuity 20/25 +3. VER responses barely recordable with 40 min. checks and non-recordable with 20 min. checks. (Arden score 123).

While Snellen and VER (as performed in this study) testing evaluate resolution of high-contrast macular targets, the Arden gratings present a sinusoidally-distributed series of contrast variations to the posterior pole. Accordingly, one would expect less interference with Arden acuity in focal foveal photoreceptor abnormalities, and this expectation was also borne out in practice. Example:

Case V – 8 y. o. male with central form of cone dystrophy. Discrete central scotomas OU, 483 errors on Farnsworth 100-hue test. Snellen acuity 20/80 − 20/200 OD, 20/70 − 20/100 OS. VER responses poor to 80 min. checks with each eye, non-recordable with 40 min. checks. Arden grating scores only slightly elevated, to 82.5 OD, 77.5 OS.

The objective, occipitally-recorded VER should not be affected by malingering or hysteria, and should likewise be unaffected by disorders of higher centers which could affect the subjective and interpretational aspects of the Snellen and Arden grating tests. This factor is illustrated by the following example:

Case VI – 13 y. o. female, bacterial meningitis several years previously. Slight nystagmus, right esotropia, temporal disc pallor with mildly amaurotic pupil OD. Snellen acuity hand movements at 4 ft. OD, 20/70 OS. Arden grating scores 150 OD (non-detectable), 92 OS. VER – good responses to 5 min. checks with each eye.

VER stimuli may be infinitely varied with the aid of appropriate electronics. Such instrumentation is expensive and elaborate, and such testing rather time-consuming. Furthermore, as responses decrease with more subtle stimuli, end-points must be extrapolated from levels of stimulation strong enough to yield responses clearly distinguishable from background "noise". The qualitative appreciation of various visual stimuli is a tapestry richer in variety than the mere determination of high-contrast minimum separable ("quantity"), and can be evaluated by VER techniques using stimuli of varying size and contrast. The Arden grating test provides such information in a standardized, simple, inexpensive and portable form. The only variables are ambient light, rate of stimulus presentation, and age of patient (the last factor not noted by Arden). Age-adjusted normal values have been developed[2]. This grating test offers a sensitive avenue for the assessment of visual "quality" in suspected macular and optic nerve disorders in clinical practice.

REFERENCES

Arden, G.B. The importance of measuring contrast sensitivity in cases of visual disturbances. *British Journal of Ophthalmology*, 62, 4, *198–208* (1978).

Skalka, H.W. The effect of age on Arden grating acuity. *British Journal of Ophthalmology*. 64, 1, *21–23* (1980).

Author's address:
Harold W. Skalda, M.D., F.A.C.S.
Combined Program in Ophthalmology
1720 Eighth Avenue, South
Birmingham, Alabama 35233
U.S.A.